T0362539

Lyme Disease and the Expanded Spectrum of Blacklegged Tick-Borne Infections

Editor

ROBERT P. SMITH

INFECTIOUS DISEASE CLINICS OF NORTH AMERICA

www.id.theclinics.com

Consulting Editor
HELEN W. BOUCHER

September 2022 • Volume 36 • Number 3

ELSEVIER

1600 John F. Kennedy Boulevard • Suite 1800 • Philadelphia, Pennsylvania, 19103-2899.

http://www.theclinics.com

INFECTIOUS DISEASE CLINICS OF NORTH AMERICA Volume 36, Number 3
September 2022 ISSN 0891–5520, ISBN-13: 978-0-323-97292-5

Editor: Kerry Holland
Developmental Editor: Hannah Almira Lopez

Infectious Disease Clinics of North America (ISSN 0891–5520) is published in March, June, September, and December by Elsevier Inc., 360 Park Avenue South, New York, NY 10010-1710. Periodicals postage paid at New York, NY and additional mailing offices. Subscription prices are $357.00 per year for US individuals, $950.00 per year for US institutions, $100.00 per year for US students, $408.00 per year for Canadian individuals, $979.00 per year for Canadian institutions, $445.00 per year for international individuals, $979.00 per year for international institutions, $100.00 per year for Canadian students, and $200.00 per year for international students. To receive student rate, orders must be accompanied by name of affiliated institution, date of term, and the *signature* of program/residency coordinator on institution letterhead. Orders will be billed at individual rate until proof of status is received. Foreign air speed delivery is included in all *Clinics* subscription prices. All prices are subject to change without notice. **POSTMASTER**: Send address changes to *Infectious Disease Clinics of North America*, Elsevier Health Sciences Division, Subcription Customer Service, 3251 Riverport Lane, Maryland Heights, MO 63043. **Customer Service: 1-800-654-2452 (US). From outside of the US and Canada, call 1-314-447-8871. Fax: 1-314-447-8029. E-mail: JournalsCustomerService-usa@elsevier.com (print support) or JournalsOnlineSupport-usa@elsevier.com (online support).**

Infectious Disease Clinics of North America is also published in Spanish by Editorial Inter-Médica, Junin 917, 1er A 1113, Buenos Aires, Argentina.

Reprints. For copies of 100 or more, of articles in this publication, please contact the Commercial Reprints Department, Elsevier Inc., 360 Park Avenue South, New York, New York 10010-1710. Tel. 212-633-3874, Fax: 212-633-3820, E-mail: reprints@elsevier.com.

Infectious Disease Clinics of North America is covered in *MEDLINE/PubMed (Index Medicus), Current Contents/ Clinical Medicine, Science Citation Alert, SCISEARCH,* and *Research Alert.*

Contributors

CONSULTING EDITOR

HELEN W. BOUCHER, MD, FIDSA, FACP
Director, Infectious Diseases Fellowship Program, Division of Geographic Medicine and Infectious Diseases, Tufts Medical Center, Associate Professor of Medicine, Tufts University School of Medicine, Boston, Massachusetts, USA

EDITOR

ROBERT P. SMITH, MD MPH
Director, Division of Infectious Diseases, Maine Medical Center, Professor of Medicine, Tufts University School of Medicine, South Portland, Maine, USA

AUTHORS

SHEILA L. ARVIKAR, MD
Instructor in Medicine, Center for Immunology and Inflammatory Diseases, Massachusetts General Hospital, Harvard Medical School, Charlestown, Massachusetts, USA

PAUL G. AUWAERTER, MD
Sherrilyn and Ken Fisher Professor of Medicine, Sherrilyn and Ken Fisher Center for Environmental Infectious Diseases, Johns Hopkins School of Medicine, Baltimore, Maryland, USA

KELLY BALDWIN, MD
Maine Medical Center, Portland, Maine, USA

FELIPE CENTELLAS, MD
Cayuga Medical Center, Ithaca, New York, USA

TYLER CRISSINGER, MD
Maine Medical Center, Portland, Maine, USA

BRIAN E. DAIKH, MD
Tufts University School of Medicine, Boston, Massachusetts, USA; Department of Medicine, Consulting Rheumatologist, Maine Medical Center, Rheumatology Associates, Portland, Maine, USA

JEAN DEJACE, MD
Assistant Professor of Medicine, University of Vermont, Division of Infectious Disease, Department of Medicine, The UVM Medical Center Campus, Burlington, Vermont, USA

JOHN J. HALPERIN, MD
Overlook Medical Center, Summit, New Jersey, USA; Professor of Neurology and Medicine, Sidney Kimmel Medical College, Thomas Jefferson University

JASON A. HELIS, MD
Tufts University School of Medicine, Boston, Massachusetts, USA; Department of Pediatrics, Division of Pediatric Neurology, Barbara Bush Children's Hospital at Maine Medical Center, Portland, Maine, USA; Maine Medical Partners Neurology, Scarborough, Maine, USA

TAKAAKI KOBAYASHI, MD
Fellow Physician, Division of Infectious Diseases, Department of Internal Medicine, University of Iowa Hospitals & Clinics, Iowa City, Iowa, USA

PETER J. KRAUSE, MD
Division of Epidemiology of Microbial Diseases, Yale School of Public Health, Yale School of Medicine, New Haven, Connecticut, USA

DOUGLAS MACQUEEN, MD, MS
Cayuga Medical Center, Ithaca, New York, USA; Assistant Professor of Clinical Medicine, Weill Cornell Medicine

CAROL A. McCARTHY, MD
Division of Pediatric Infectious Diseases, Maine Medical Center, Portland, Maine, USA

ADRIANA MARQUES, MD
Laboratory of Clinical Immunology and Microbiology, National Institute of Allergy and Infectious Diseases, National Institutes of Health, Bethesda, Maryland, USA

PAUL MEAD, MD, MPH
Bacterial Diseases Branch, Division of Vector-borne Diseases, National Center for Emerging and Zoonotic Infectious Diseases, Centers for Disease Control and Prevention (CDC), Ft Collins, Colorado, USA

ANNE PIANTADOSI, MD, PhD
Assistant Professor, Department of Pathology and Laboratory Medicine, Department of Medicine, Division of Infectious Diseases, Emory University School of Medicine, Atlanta, Georgia, USA

BOBBI S. PRITT, MD, MSc
Professor, Department of Laboratory Medicine and Pathology, Division of Clinical Microbiology, Mayo Clinic, Rochester, Minnesota, USA

KYLE G. RODINO, PhD
Assistant Professor, Department of Pathology and Laboratory Medicine, Perelman School of Medicine, University of Pennsylvania, Philadelphia, Pennsylvania, USA

RICHARD V. SHEN, MD
Infectious Diseases, Southcoast Physicians Group, Fall River, Massachusetts, USA

ISAAC H. SOLOMON, MD, PhD
Assistant Professor, Department of Pathology, Brigham and Women's Hospital, Harvard Medical School, Boston, Massachusetts, USA

ALLEN C. STEERE, MD
Professor of Medicine, Center for Immunology and Inflammatory Diseases, Massachusetts General Hospital, Harvard Medical School, Charlestown, Massachusetts, USA

FRANC STRLE, MD, PhD
University Medical Center Ljubljana, Ljubljana, Slovenia

RAMI WAKED, MD
Division of Infectious Diseases, Maine Medical Center, Portland, Maine, USA

GARY P. WORMSER, MD
New York Medical College, Valhalla, New York, USA

Contents

> Lyme disease is the most common vector-borne illness in North America
> and Europe. The etiologic agent, Borrelia burgdorferi sensu lato, is trans-
> mitted to humans by certain species of Ixodes ticks, which are found
> widely in temperate regions of the Northern hemisphere. Clinical features
> are diverse but death is rare. The risk of human infection is determined by
> the distribution and abundance of vector ticks, ecologic factors influencing
> tick infection rates, and human behaviors that promote tick bite. Rates of
> infection are highest among children aged 5 to 15 years and adults aged
> more than 50 years. In the northeastern United States where disease is
> most common, exposure occurs primarily in areas immediately around
> the home. Knowledge of disease epidemiology is important for patient
> management and proper diagnosis.

> Erythema migrans, an expanding erythematous skin lesion that develops
> days to weeks following an Ixodes species tick bite, is the most common
> clinical manifestation of Lyme disease. Presentations in the United States
> differ somewhat from that in Europe, presumably because of the different
> etiologic agents. Diagnosis is based on the appearance of the skin lesion,
> rather than on laboratory testing. After treatment with an appropriate oral
> antibiotic for 10 to 14 days, the prognosis is excellent. Two conditions that
> cause a similar skin lesion following a tick bite, but are of unknown cause,
> are Southern tick-associated rash illness in the United States and tick-
> associated rash illness in Japan.

> Early disseminated Lyme disease can involve the peripheral or central ner-
> vous system, but with early diagnosis and treatment, prognosis for full re-
> covery is excellent. The typical clinical presentations of neuroborreliosis
> are highlighted, and an approach to diagnosis and treatment is described.

> Lyme carditis is an uncommon manifestation of Lyme disease. Most cases present with heart block of varying degrees, but the spectrum of disease includes other transient arrhythmias and structural manifestations, such as myopericarditis or cardiomyopathy. Antibiotics hasten the resolution of Lyme carditis, and cardiac pacing can be an adjunctive therapy. Outcomes are generally good, but there are rare fatalities associated with Lyme carditis. The latter underscores the continued need for improved modes of prevention of Lyme disease and the importance of its early recognition and treatment.

> Arthritis is the most common late manifestation of Borrelia burgdorferi infection in the United States, usually beginning months after the tick bite. In most patients with Lyme arthritis (LA) today, arthritis is the presenting manifestation of the disease. Patients have swelling and pain in one or a few large joints, especially the knee. Serologic testing is the mainstay of diagnosis. Responses to antibiotic treatment are generally excellent, although a small percentage of patients have persistent, postinfectious synovitis after 2 to 3 months of oral and IV antibiotics, which respond to anti-inflammatory therapies. Herein we review the clinical presentation, diagnosis, and management of LA.

> The central or peripheral nervous systems may be involved in up to 15% of patients with untreated infection with B burgdorferi sensu lato, characteristic involvement including meningitis, cranial neuritis, and radiculoneuritis. Diagnosis, based on a logical combination of clinical context and antibody-based testing, is usually straightforward, as is treatment. Misconceptions about what does and does not constitute neurologic disease, and about laboratory testing in this infection, have resulted in widespread anxiety that a broad range of other disorders may be attributable to nervous system Lyme disease. This article will review the reasons for these misunderstandings and the arguments against them.

> Lyme disease is now the most frequently reported vector-borne disease in the United States. The highest incidence is in children aged 5 to 9 years with a male predominance. The most common manifestation, erythema migrans, is sometimes not recognized, leading to risk of complications. Testing for Lyme disease should only be done if there is a consistent clinical syndrome with exposure in a Lyme-endemic area. Most forms of Lyme disease are successfully treated with short courses of oral therapy. Prevention and management of tick bites is important.

Standard 2-tier testing (STTT), incorporating a screening enzyme immunoassay (EIA) or an immunofluorescence assay (IFA) that reflexes to IgM and IgG immunoblots, has been the primary diagnostic test for Lyme disease since 1995. In 2019, the Food and Drug Administration approved a modified 2-tier test strategy using 2 EIAs: offering a faster, less expensive, and more sensitive assay compared with STTT. New technologies examine early immune responses to Borrelia burgdorferi have the potential to diagnose Lyme disease in the first weeks of infection when existing serologic testing is not recommended due to low sensitivity.

Most patients with Lyme disease will fully recover with recommended antibiotic therapy. However, some patients report persisting nonspecific symptoms after treatment, referred to as posttreatment Lyme disease symptoms (PTLDs) or syndrome (PTLDS), depending on the degree to which the individual's symptoms impact their quality of life. PTLDs occur in a portion of patients diagnosed with chronic Lyme disease (CLD), a controversial term describing different patient populations, diagnosed based on unvalidated tests and criteria. Practitioners should review the evidence for the Lyme disease diagnosis and not overlook unrelated conditions. Current evidence shows that prolonged antibiotic therapy provides little benefit and carries significant risk. Further research to elucidate the mechanisms underlying persistent symptoms after Lyme disease and to understand CLD is needed.

Human granulocytic anaplasmosis (HGA) is a bacterial infection caused by Anaplasma phagocytophilum and transmitted by the bite of the black-legged (deer tick) in North America. Its incidence is increasing. HGA can be transmitted after 24 to 48 hours of tick attachment. The incubation period is 5 to 14 days after a tick bite. Symptoms include fever, chills, headache, and myalgia. Complications include shock, organ dysfunction, and death. Mortality is less than 1% with appropriate treatment. Doxycycline is first line treatment for all ages. Start it empirically if symptoms and risk factors suggest HGA. PCR is the confirmatory test of choice.

Babesiosis is caused by intraerythrocytic parasites that are transmitted primarily by ticks, infrequently through blood transfusion, and rarely through transplacental transmission or organ transplantation. Human babesiosis is found throughout the world, but the incidence is highest in the Northeast and upper Midwestern United States. Babesiosis has clinical features that resemble malaria and can be fatal in immunocompromised and older patients. Diagnosis is confirmed by identification of

Babesia parasites on blood smear or Babesia DNA with polymerase chain reaction. Standard treatment consists of atovaquone and azithromycin or clindamycin and quinine for 7 to 10 days.

Powassan virus is an increasingly recognized cause of severe encephalitis that is transmitted by Ixodes ticks. Given the nonspecific clinical, laboratory, and imaging features of Powassan virus disease, providers should consider it in patients with compatible exposures and request appropriate testing.

In North America, several hard tick-transmitted Borrelia species other than Borrelia burgdorferi cause human disease, including Borrelia miyamotoi, Borrelia mayonii, and possibly Borrelia bissettii. Due to overlapping clinical syndromes, nonspecific tickborne disease (TBD) testing strategies, and shared treatment approaches, infections with these lesser known Borrelia are likely under-reported. In this article, we describe the epidemiology, clinical manifestations, diagnosis, and treatment of these less common Borrelia pathogens.

A consultation regarding Lyme disease can be challenging for the infectious disease physician when the referral question centers on the use of prolonged or empirical antibiotic treatment of Lyme disease and associated tick-borne infections. Patients who have been infected with Borrelia burgdorferi, and many who have been misdiagnosed, are confronted with a seemingly endless array of misinformation that is not in keeping with the current understanding of the clinical spectrum of Lyme disease and its response to evidence-based treatment. Preparing for these conversations with a good grasp of the public beliefs regarding Lyme disease and its treatment can be beneficial.

INFECTIOUS DISEASE CLINICS OF NORTH AMERICA

INFECTIOUS DISEASE CLINICS OF NORTH AMERICA

FORTHCOMING ISSUES

December 2022
Complex Infectious Disease Issues in the Intensive Care Unit
Sameer Kadri and Naomi P. O'Grady, editors

March 2023
Infections in Older Adults
Puja Van Epps and David H. Canaday, Editors

June 2023
Sexually Transmitted Infections
Jeanne Marrazzo, Editor

RECENT ISSUES

June 2022
Covid-19 Infection
Rachel A. Bender Ignacio and Paul E. Sax, Editors

March 2022
Pediatric Infections
Rebecca G. Same and Jason G. Newland, editors

December 2021
Infection Prevention and Control in Healthcare, Part II: Clinical Management of Infections
Keith S. Kaye and Sorabh Dhar, Editors

Preface

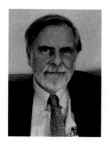

Robert P. Smith, MD, MPH
Editor

Tick-borne diseases are a growing public health concern across much of North America.[1] Black-legged ticks, in particular, continue their range of expansion in the northeast and upper midwestern United States, bringing with them an impressive list of human pathogens. Dr Mead puts the consequences of this phenomenon into context in our first article, entitled, "Epidemiology of Lyme disease." East of the Mississippi, the vector tick *Ixodes scapularis*, commonly called the deer tick, may transmit seven different pathogens. In the western United States and Canada, *Ixodes pacificus*, the western black-legged tick, transmits Lyme disease, *Borrelia miyamotoi* infection, and anaplasmosis, but with far fewer reported cases overall. In this issue of the *Infectious Disease Clinics of North America*, our authors provide expert reviews of the illnesses these ticks cause, with a particular emphasis on the most common, and, in some respects, most contentious, Lyme disease. Recognition of the seven diseases associated with black-legged tick infections is relatively recent, with the first clinical reports of babesiosis (1970) and Lyme disease (1977) followed in rapid succession by anaplasmosis (1994), deer tick virus (or Powassan virus lineage 2) encephalitis (2009), and infections due to *Ehrlichia muris eauclairensis* (2009), *B miyamotoi* (2013), and *Borrelia mayonii* (2016).

While the emphasis here is on pathogens transmitted by North American black-legged ticks, reference is also made to the differences in the epidemiology and clinical presentation of Lyme disease and other diseases transmitted by related *Ixodes* tick species (ie, *Ixodes ricinus* and *Ixodes persulcatus*) in Europe and Asia.

The next five articles provide current, evidence-based reviews of the clinical features of Lyme disease, such as erythema migrans, neurologic sequelae of early disseminated Lyme disease, Lyme carditis, and Lyme arthritis as well as rare neurologic complications of late disease. The article by McCarthy and colleagues highlights aspects of the presentation and clinical course of Lyme disease and other diseases transmitted by black-legged ticks in children. The article by Kobayashi and Auwaerter provides a review of sero-diagnostics for Lyme disease, including a discussion of the recent Food and Drug Administration endorsement of a modified two-tier diagnostic strategy.

Infect Dis Clin N Am 36 (2022) xiii–xvi
https://doi.org/10.1016/j.idc.2022.04.005
0891-5520/22/© 2022 Published by Elsevier Inc.

We also extend our discussion to less-well-understood aspects of *B burgdorferi* infection, including current research on possible causes for posttreatment Lyme disease symptoms (article by Marques). For clinicians and their patients, the medical and/ or social framing and public representation of Lyme disease are often contradictory and confusing, sometimes to the detriment of good patient care. We have included a discussion of the challenges the infectious disease specialist must meet when the consultation includes discussion of disparate views and public misperceptions of the scope and treatment of Lyme disease (article by Dejace).

Four subsequent articles provide overviews of major infections other than *B burgdorferi* transmitted by these ticks: anaplasmosis (MacQueen and Centellas); babesiosis (Waked and Krause); Powassan virus encephalitis (Piantadosi and Solomon); and infection by *Borrelia mayonii* or *Borrelia miyamotoi* (Rodino and Pritt). In a minority of cases, these pathogens may be transmitted as coinfections, presumably from a single tick bite. The commonest of these coinfections involves *B burgdorferi* and *Anaplasma phagocytophilum* or *Babesia microti*.

Molecular detection led to recent discoveries of human infection by *B mayonii* and *E muris eauclairensis*[2,3] in patient blood samples from the upper Midwest. Subsequent studies led to their detection in black-legged ticks in this region, the presumed vector for these infections.[4] Over a fourth of the 100 or more identified cases of *E muris eauclairensis* occurred in immune-compromised patients, but the clinical presentation and course have otherwise been similar to that of anaplasmosis and infection by the most common cause of erhlichiosis, *Erhlichia chaffeensis.*[2] Ehrlichiosis, which with the rare exception noted above, is transmitted by bites from the lone star tick, *Amblyomma americanum*, and is therefore not represented by a separate article in this issue.

Three species of ticks account for most transmission of human pathogens in the eastern and midwestern United States (**Figure 1**). The American dog tick (*Dermacentor variabilis*) is widely distributed, but its importance as a vector of disease (i.e., Rocky Mountain spotted fever, tularemia) varies regionally.Northward range expansion of the lone star tick (*A americanum*) in the northeast United States has led to a larger geographic overlap with the black-legged tick.[5] The growing regional complexity of exposure to tick-transmitted pathogens, coupled with human mobility, leads to a challenging panoply of tick-transmitted diseases for consideration in the acutely ill patient. If a patient presents with a combination of fever and leucopenia and/or thrombocytopenia, the initial differential diagnosis may include anaplasmosis, ehrlichiosis, *B miyamotoi* or *B mayonii*, babesiosis, and rickettsial diseases. Knowledge of regional epidemiology, and potential patient risk factors often helps to narrow the possibilities.[6,7]

Our understanding of the scope and public health burden of these diseases continues to evolve, and substantial gaps in our knowledge and ability to diagnose and treat them remain.

With the marked increase in incidence of anaplasmosis and babesiosis in the northeastern United States, it is notable that we have only one well-studied antibiotic available to treat severe anaplasmosis and just two combination therapies in use for babesiosis. Powassan encephalitis, caused by a lineage of Powassan virus or deer tick virus, is a severe and life-threatening infection for which no treatment is available.

Given increased attention to current gaps in diagnosis and treatment of infections transmitted by black-legged ticks, and rapid advances in the clinical science that underpins their diagnosis and treatment, we encourage our readers to use these state-of-the-art reviews as a framework for continuing assessment of new insights and strategies as they are published in the peer-reviewed literature.

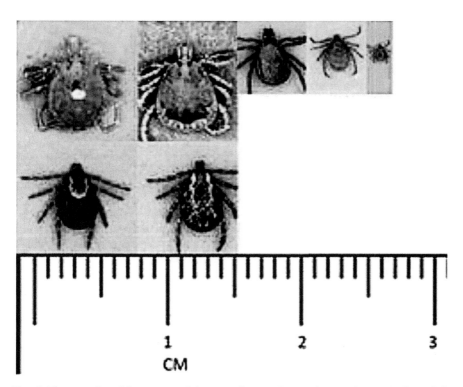

Fig. 1. Three major tick vectors of human diseases in North America. Top, from left, *Amblyomma americanum* female; A. americanum male, *Ixodes scapularis* female, I. scapularis male, I. scapularis nymph. Bottom, from left, *Dermacentor variabilis* female, D. variabilis male. (*Courtesy of* Smith LB, MaineHealth Institute for Research)

Prevention remains a challenge. Effective control strategies for the tick vectors often require a nuanced understanding of local ecologic and epidemiologic realities. Behaviors to prevent tick bites can be helpful, but difficult to sustain. To date, no preventive vaccines for these diseases are approved, although research efforts are underway on this front. Through a combination of informed medical care for those ill with tick-borne infections, and implementation of existing and novel strategies for their prevention, the rise in public health burden of these infections can be stemmed.

Robert P. Smith, MD, MPH
Division of Infectious Diseases
Maine Medical Center
Tufts University School of Medicine
41 Donald B Dean Drive, Suite B, South Portland
ME 04106, USA

E-mail address:
robert.smith@mainehealth.org

REFERENCES

1. Paules CI, Marston HD, Bloom ME, et al. Tickborne diseases—confronting a growing threat. N Engl J Med 2018;379:701–3.

2. Pritt BS, Sloan LM, Johnson DK, et al. Emergence of a new pathogenic Ehrlichia species, Wisconsin and Minnesota, 2009. N Engl J Med 2011;365:422–9.

3. Johnson DK, Schiffman EK, Davis JP, et al. Human infection with Erhlichia muris-like pathogen, United States, 2007-2013. Emerg Infect Dis 2015;21(10):1794–9.

4. Telford SR III, Goethert HK, Cunningham JA. Prevalence of Ehrlichia muris in Wisconsin deer ticks collected during the mid-1990s. Open Microbiol J 2011;5:18–20.

5. Molaei G, Little EAH, Williams SC, et al. Bracing for the worst–range expansion of the lone star tick in the northeastern United States. N Engl J Med 2019;381(23): 2189–92.

6. Centers for Disease Control and Prevention. Tickborne diseases of the US: a reference manual for health care providers. 5th edition. Centers for Disease Control and Prevention; National Center for Emerging and Zoonotic Infectious Diseases (NCE-ZID), Division of Vector-borne Diseases; 2018.

7. CDC: Diagnosis and management of tickborne rickettsial diseases: Rocky Mountain spotted fever and other spotted fever group rickettsioses, ehrlichioses, and anaplasmosis—United States. A practical guide for health care and public health professionals. MMWR Morb Mortal Wkly Rep 2016;65(2):1–43.

Epidemiology of Lyme Disease

Paul Mead, MD, MPH

KEYWORDS

- Lyme disease • Epidemiology • Incidence • *Borrelia burgdorferi*
- Tick-borne diseases • Human • Zoonosis • *Ixodes*

KEY POINTS

- An estimated ~465,000 Americans are treated for Lyme disease annually, although not all are necessarily infected.
- Cases are concentrated in 14 high incidence states, located in the northeast and north-central United States; discrete areas of risk exist in the Pacific coast states.
- Areas of risk have expanded substantially over the last two decades, leading to cases in previously non-endemic areas.
- Clinicians must consider epidemiologic factors when evaluating patients for possible Lyme disease.

INTRODUCTION

Lyme disease is a tick-borne zoonosis caused by certain genospecies of the spirochete *Borrelia burgdorferi* sensu lato.[1] The organism cycles naturally among small mammal and avian hosts, transmitted by ticks of the *Ixodes ricinus*-complex.[2] Human illness is characterized by diverse dermatologic, neurologic, rheumatologic, and cardiac abnormalities.[3,4] Also called Lyme borreliosis, Lyme disease is the most common vector-borne disease in both Europe and North America. More than 400,000 cases have been reported in the United States since 2004, accounting for 63% of all reportable tick, flea, or mosquito-borne illnesses nationwide.[5] Although the disease was named in the mid-1970s for a small Connecticut town, typical cases were described in Europe as early as 1883.[6,7]

As with other zoonoses, Lyme disease is first and foremost a disease of place. The intrinsic risk of a location depends on the local ecology, the virulence of circulating *Borrelia* spirochetes, and the feeding habits of specific tick vectors.[8] Human behavior

Disclosure: No interests or conflicts to disclose.
Bacterial Diseases Branch, Division of Vector-borne Diseases, National Center for Emerging and Zoonotic Infectious Diseases, Centers for Disease Control and Prevention (CDC), 3156 Rampart Road, Ft Collins, CO 80521, USA
E-mail address: pfm0@CDC.GOV

Infect Dis Clin N Am 36 (2022) 495–521
https://doi.org/10.1016/j.idc.2022.03.004
0891-5520/22/Published by Elsevier Inc.

id.theclinics.com

Table 1
Named genospecies of *Borrelia burgdorferi* sensu lato, as of January 2022, by geographic region

Detected in Humans	*Borrelia Genospecies*	Geographic Location			
		North America	South America	Europe	Asia
++++	*B. afzelii*			X	X
	B. americana	X			
	B. andersonii	X			
++	*B. bavariensis*			X	
+	*B. bissettiea*	X	?	X	X
++++	*B. burgdorferi*	X		X	
	B. californiensis	X			
	B. carolinensis	X			
	B. chilensis		X		
	B. finlandensis			X	
++++	*B. garinii*			X	X
	B. japonica				X
	B. kurtenbachii	X			
	B. lanei	X			
+	*B. lusitaniae*			X	
+	*B. mayonii*	X			
	B. sinica				X
+	*B. spielmanii*			X	
	B. tanukii				X
	B. turdi				X
+	*B. valaisiana*			X	X
+	*B. yangtzensis*				X

strongly influences the likelihood of exposure to infected ticks and the patterns of care-seeking required for diagnosis and treatment. These factors, along with medical and public health infrastructure, all shape the observed epidemiology of human Lyme disease.

Causitive Agent

Twenty-two named genospecies of *B. burgdorferi* sensu lato are currently recognized based on isolates obtained from ticks and reservoir hosts; 10 have been detected in humans (**Table 1**).[9,10] Additional genospecies have been proposed, and the list is likely to grow further. Worldwide, most human infections are caused by *B. afzelii*, *B. garinii*, and *B burgdorferi* sensu stricto (hereafter referred to simply as *B. burgdorferi*). *B. bavariensis*, a fourth genospecies that was previously considered a variant of *B. garinii*, is widely distributed in Europe and Asia. The other 6 genospecies, *B. bissetii*, *B. lusitaniae*, *B. mayonii*, *B. spielmanii*, *B. valaisiana*, and *B. yangtzensis* have been isolated from humans infrequently, and their public health importance is yet to be determined.

In North America, human infections are caused almost exclusively by *B. burgdorferi*, with occasional *B. mayonii* infections occurring in regions of the upper Midwest. Several other genospecies commonly present in North American ticks, such as

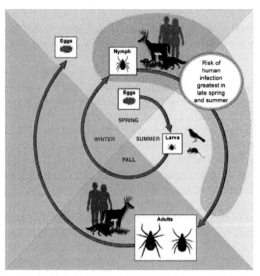

Fig. 1. Two-year life cycle of the black-legged tick, *Ixodes scapularis*, the principal vector of the Lyme disease spirochete.

B. andersoni, have not been detected in human samples.[11] A recent metagenomics-based analysis detected a dozen known pathogens in ~13,000 blood samples collected from patients with suspected tick-borne illness from throughout the United States. More than 100 *B. burgdorferi* sensu lato infections were identified; however, all were caused by either *B. burgdorferi* or *B. mayonii*.[12] The apparent absence of human infection with other genospecies may be due to differences in pathogenicity, transmission dynamics, or both.

Tick Vectors and Transmission

The principal known vectors of *B. burgdorferi* sensu lato are all members of *I. ricinus*-complex.[2] *Ixodes spp.* ticks have a 2 to 3-year life cycle, during which they take 3 blood meals, one each as a larvae, nymph, and adult (**Fig. 1**). Ticks are uninfected when they hatch from eggs and only acquire the spirochete if they feed on an infected reservoir host, typically a mouse, other small mammal, or bird. Infected ticks transmit the pathogen during subsequent feedings as a nymph or adult, thereby perpetuating the natural cycle. The spirochete has been detected in ticks of other genera feeding on infected hosts; however, laboratory studies suggest that these ticks are not competent vectors.[13] Humans are incidental or "dead-end" hosts that do not sustain large numbers of spirochetes in their tissues. Adult ticks feed preferentially on deer, which are generally immune to *B. burgdorferi* but play an important role in the ecology of disease by transporting ticks and supporting tick populations.[2]

Although multiple species of *Ixodes* ticks transmit *B. burgdorferi* sensu lato among animals, only 4 commonly bite humans. Two of these, *I. ricinus* and *I. persulcatus*, are the principal vectors in Europe and Asia, respectively. In the United States, the principal vector is the black-legged or "deer" tick, *I. scapularis*, which also transmits the bacteria *Anaplasma phagocytophilum* and *B. miyamotoi*, the parasite *Babesia microti*, and Powassan virus. These ticks are abundant in forested areas of the northeastern, mid-Atlantic, and northcentral states. In some areas, up to 60% of nymphal and adult ticks are infected with *B. burgdorferi*. A second *Ixodes* species, *I. pacificus*, transmits

B. burgdorferi in the western United States. Foci of *I. pacificus* ticks occur from the central California coast northward into southern British Columbia. Because of the hosts on which they feed, *I. pacificus* ticks are less often infected and therefore account for far fewer human infections.[2]

I. scapularis ticks also live in the southeastern United States but are less abundant there and very rarely infected with *B. burgdorferi*.[14] This situation seems to be driven by genetic, phenotypic, and local ecologic factors.[2,15] Whereas immature ticks in the Northeast feed primarily on small mammals, ticks in the southeast often feed on lizards, which are not competent reservoirs of the spirochete.[8] Questing habits also differ, and southern *I. scapularis* seem less prone to biting humans.[16] A few *B. burgdorferi* sensu stricto isolates have been identified in the Southeast collected from animals within a few miles of the Atlantic coast.[17] This distribution is notable in that the coastline is an important landmark for migratory birds, which may play a role in long-distance dispersal of infected ticks.[18]

Alternate modes of *B. burgdorferi* transmission have been investigated by several researchers. *B. burgdorferi* is able to survive when inoculated into blood and held under blood banking conditions; however, transfusion-associated transmission has never been documented. This contrasts with *Babesia* and *Anaplasma*, for which transfusion-associated transmission of has been demonstrated repeatedly, and may be due to the low levels of spirochetemia associated with human Lyme disease.[19,20] There is no credible evidence of transmission through sexual contact, semen, urine, or breast milk.[21,22] Rare instances of intrauterine infection associated with miscarriage and stillbirth have been reported among women infected during pregnancy; *B. burgdorferi* has also been identified in placentas of women with normal pregnancy outcomes.[23,24] A recent meta-analysis found that women with gestational Lyme disease who reported receiving antimicrobial treatment had fewer adverse birth outcomes than untreated women, providing indirect evidence of an association between infection and poor birth outcomes.[25] Nevertheless, large epidemiologic studies have identified no definable pattern of teratogenicity, and outcomes are generally good when pregnant women receive appropriate treatment.[26,27]

Reporting, Incidence, and Distribution Within the United States

Lyme disease has been a nationally notifiable condition in the United States since 1991. Health-care providers report cases to state or local health officials, who categorize these reports according to standardized surveillance case definitions developed by the Council of State and Territorial Epidemiologists.[28] Jurisdictions share their data with the Centers for Disease Control and Prevention (CDC) for annual publication; public release generally occurs the following year after all jurisdictions have certified their results. Case definitions are revised periodically, as in 1996 to clarify laboratory criteria, and again in 2008 to allow reporting of probable cases. Under the latest revision, effective January 2022, the national surveillance case definition captures cases from high incidence states, defined as those reporting greater than 10 cases per 100,000 population per year, based on laboratory testing alone.[28] This change was implemented to better standardize reporting across states, improve efficiency, and reduce surveillance costs. By convention, national surveillance data are reported by county of patient residence, and as a result, infections acquired during travel are occasionally reported from states where there is no evidence of local transmission. For example, among many suspected Lyme disease cases reported to Arkansas Department of Health during 2015 to 2016, only 2 could be confirmed, and when interview both patients reported recent out-of-state exposures in high incidence areas.[29]

Table 2
Reported vector-borne disease cases, United States, 2015 to 2019 (Ref 47)

Disease	2015	2016	2017	2018	2019	TOTAL
Lyme disease[a]	38,069	36,429	42,743	33,666	34,945	*185,852*
Anaplasmosis[a]	3656	4151	5762	4008	5655	*23,232*
Ehrlichiosis	1302	1399	1687	1832	3036	*9256*
Spotted fever rickettsiosis	4198	4269	6248	5544	5207	*25,466*
Babesiosis[a]	2100	1910	2368	2160	2420	*10,958*
Tularemia[b]	314	230	239	229	274	1286
Powassan virus infection[a]	7	22	34	21	43	*127*
Tick-borne diseases	49,825	48,410	59,081	47,460	51,580	*256,356*
Mosquito-borne diseases[c]	5819	47,461	6077	5410	4876	*69,643*

[a] Transmitted by *I. scapularis*.
[b] Includes fly-transmitted.
[c] Caused by Chikungunya virus, California serogroup arboviruses, Dengue viruses, Eastern equine encephalitis virus, *Plasmodium spp.*, St. louis encephalitis virus, West Nile virus, Yellow fever virus, and Zika virus.

Lyme disease accounts for most reportable vector-borne disease cases in the United States. During the 5 years from 2015 to 2019, more than 185,000 Lyme disease cases were reported, as compared with approximately 70,000 cases of other tick-borne infections, and a similar number of mosquito-borne disease cases (**Table 2**).[30] Case counts have increased substantially over time, from approximately 10,000 in 1992 to a peak of nearly 43,000 cases in 2017 (**Fig. 2**). Notably, cases of anaplasmosis, babesiosis, and Powassan virus infection have also increased in recent years (see **Table 2**). The growing cost of tallying Lyme disease cases has caused health departments in some high incidence states to curtail surveillance efforts, leading to sudden decreases in reported cases. The most extreme instance involves

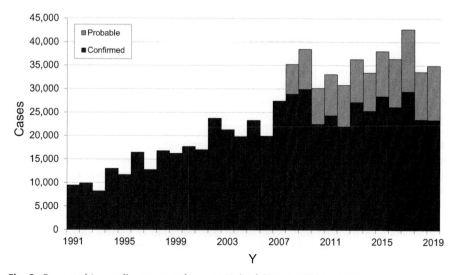

Fig. 2. Reported Lyme disease cases by year, United States, 1991 to 2019.

Massachusetts, where tallied cases decreased from 2933 in 2015 to only 7 in 2019. Other high incidence states have implemented similar measures, and recent trends in surveillance data should be interpreted with caution.

Even when functioning well, passive public health surveillance does not capture all cases occurring in the broader community. Underreporting may be particularly common for early forms of Lyme disease, which rely on clinician diagnosis and reporting, rather than more reliably captured laboratory data. Targeted studies conducted in the 1990s suggested that Lyme disease cases were underreported by 3-fold to 12-fold, depending on the state and method of estimation.[31] Although these values may seem large, they are on par with rates of underreporting for other nationally notifiable conditions.[32] In 2008, a nationwide evaluation using Lyme disease test results from commercial laboratories yielded an estimate of 288,000 infected source patients (range 240,000–444,000), approximately 8-fold greater than the number of cases reported that year.[33] A second analysis using insurance claims data for the overlapping period 2005 to 2010 yielded a roughly similar annual estimate of 296,000 to 376,000 clinician-diagnosed Lyme disease cases.[34] Finally, in the most recent national analysis of insurance claims data covering the 9-year period from 2010 to 2018, researchers estimated that ~476,000 patients were diagnosed and treated for Lyme disease annually in the United States (range 405,000–547,000).[35,36] Insurance claims data have limitations, and treatment of Lyme disease does not prove infection in all cases.

Within North America, Lyme disease occurs in 2 major foci. One encompasses the Northeast and mid-Atlantic regions, extending from Virginia north into Maine and west through Pennsylvania (Fig. 3A). The second focus involves the upper Midwest, principally the states of Minnesota and Wisconsin. Collectively, 14 states in these 2 foci account for more than 90% of reported US cases (Connecticut, Delaware, Maine, Maryland, Minnesota, New Hampshire, New Jersey, New York, Pennsylvania, Rhode Island, Vermont, Virginia, West Virginia, and Wisconsin).[37,38] Annual incidence rates in these states generally exceed 10 per 100,000 population, and in 6 exceeded 50 per 100,000 in 2019 (Table 3). Although accounting for a small percentage of total cases, focal areas of transmission also occur along the West Coast in California, Oregon, and Washington where *I. pacificus* is the vector.[2] In California, risk seems greatest in the coastal counties of Humboldt, Mendocino, and Santa Cruz.[39]

Although the geography of Lyme disease risk is focal, it is also dynamic.[40] During the last 20 years, both major foci of risk have expanded greatly in size, extending in all directions into neighboring states (Fig. 3B) and adjacent areas of Canada. States on the leading edge of this expansion 10 years ago (eg, Maine, Vermont, New Hampshire) have some of the highest reported incidence rates currently (see Table 2). More recently affected states include West Virginia, where annual incidence has climbed to 39 per 100,000 population, and Ohio, where incidence, although much lower, has increased 10-fold (see Table 3). Expansion into an area is often spotty at first. On the southern end of expansion, North Carolina continues to have an overall incidence of less than 1 case per 100,000 population. Nevertheless, a 2019 investigation identified 4 cases of Lyme disease among children attending a wilderness camp and an infection prevalence of nearly 20% among *I. scapularis* ticks collected in the area.[41]

As noted above, *I. scapularis* ticks are present in other areas of the southern United States where few or no human cases are reported. Nationwide data on the seroprevalence of *B. burgdorferi* antibodies in dogs supports the conclusion that this reflects a true absence of transmission.[42] Repeated assessments of canine seroprevalence reveal that in the 14 states where incidence of human illness is high, roughly 5% to 20% of dogs statewide are seropositive.[43] These values underscore the exquisite sensitivity of dogs as sentinels for the presence of *B. burgdorferi* in the environment.

A

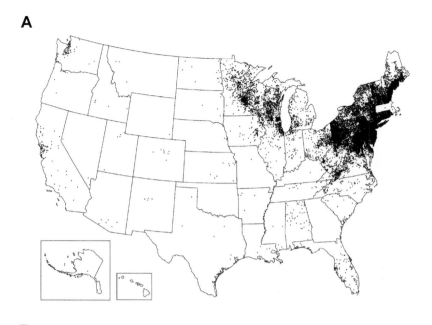

B

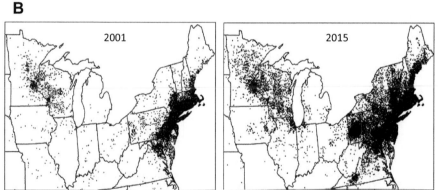

Fig. 3. (*A*) Geographic distribution of reported Lyme disease cases, United States, 2019. One dot per case placed randomly in county of patient residence. (*B*) Expanding distribution of reported Lyme disease cases, 2001 and 2015.

It is therefore notable that although millions of dogs in the southeastern and southcentral states have been tested, generally fewer than 0.5% are seropositive. This value is consistent with the false-positive rate for the assay,[44] and the occasional immigration of dogs from high-risk areas.[45] Occasionally higher percentages have been detected in nonendemic areas but in at least once instance, this seems to result from selective testing of dogs moved from high incidence areas.[46] Discordance between human infection and canine seroprevalence may also occur in areas where enzootic cycles involve ticks that feed readily on dogs but not on humans.[14]

Incidence and Distribution Outside the United States

In Canada, Lyme disease is a rapidly emerging public health problem, driven in part by climate change.[47] Infected *I. scapularis* ticks now are found in southern regions of

Table 3

Incidence of confirmed Lyme disease cases reported to Centers for Disease Control and Prevention by States and the District of Columbia, United States, 2010 to 2019

	2010	2011	2012	2013	2014	2015	2016	2017	2018	2019	3-y Average
Alabama	0.0	0.2	0.3	0.2	0.6	0.3	0.3	0.5	0.4	0.9	0.6
Alaska	1.0	1.2	0.5	1.9	0.7	0.1	0.8	1.1	1.1	0.1	0.8
Arizona	0.0	0.1	0.1	0.3	0.2	0.1	0.1	0.3	0.1	0.1	0.1
Arkansas	0.0	0.0	0.0	0.0	0.0	0.0	0.0	0.1	0.0	0.2	0.1
California	0.4	0.0	0.2	0.2	0.1	0.2	0.2	0.2	0.2	0.2	0.2
Colorado	0.0	0.0	0.0	0.0	0.0	0.0	0.0	0.1	0.1	0.1	0.1
Connecticut	55.0	56.0	46.0	58.7	47.8	52.2	34.6	38.5	35.5	22.3	32.1
Delaware	73.1	84.6	55.3	43.2	36.4	35.3	41.1	43.8	52.2	63.6	53.2
District of Columbia	5.7	N	N	5.1	5.3	11.6	9.7	8.9	8.1	8.1	8.4
Florida	0.3	0.4	0.3	0.4	0.4	0.6	0.6	0.6	0.5	0.4	0.5
Georgia	0.1	0.3	0.3	0.1	0.0	0.1	0.0	0.1	0.0	0.0	0.0
Hawaii	0.0	0.0	0.0	0.0	0.0	0.0	0.0	0.0	0.0	0.0	0.0
Idaho	0.4	0.2	0.0	0.9	0.5	0.2	0.5	0.9	0.3	0.3	0.5
Illinois	1.1	1.5	1.6	2.6	1.8	2.2	1.8	1.7	1.5	1.9	1.7
Indiana	1.0	1.2	1.0	1.5	1.5	1.5	1.9	1.4	1.1	1.5	1.3
Iowa	2.2	2.4	3.0	5.0	3.5	4.2	2.4	3.6	2.9	2.2	2.9
Kansas	0.2	0.4	0.3	0.6	0.4	0.4	0.6	0.4	0.3	0.4	0.4
Kentucky	0.1	0.1	0.2	0.4	0.2	0.3	0.4	0.1	0.1	0.3	0.2
Louisiana	0.0	0.0	0.1	0.0	0.0	0.0	0.1	0.2	0.0	0.2	0.1
Maine	42.1	60.3	66.6	84.8	87.9	74.7	86.4	106.6	83.0	121.2	103.6
Maryland	20.1	16.1	18.9	13.5	16.0	20.8	21.2	19.7	14.8	13.3	15.9
Massachusetts	36.3	27.3	51.1	57.0	54.1	43.0	2.1	4.7	0.2	0.1	1.7
Michigan	0.8	0.9	0.8	1.2	0.9	1.3	1.6	2.0	1.8	2.8	2.2

	24.4	22.2	16.9	26.4	16.4	21.4	23.6	25.2	16.9	16.2	19.5
Minnesota	0.0	0.1	0.0	0.0	0.1	0.1	0.0	0.0	0.0	0.1	0.1
Mississippi	0.1	0.1	0.0	0.0	0.1	0.0	0.0	0.0	0.0	0.0	0.0
Missouri	0.1	0.1	0.0	0.0	0.1	0.0	0.0	0.0	0.0	0.0	0.0
Montana	0.3	0.9	0.6	1.6	0.5	0.2	1.2	0.4	0.5	0.6	0.5
Nebraska	0.4	0.4	0.3	0.4	0.3	0.3	0.5	0.3	0.4	0.2	0.3
Nevada	0.1	0.1	0.4	0.4	0.1	0.2	0.1	0.2	0.2	0.1	0.2
New Hampshire	63.0	67.3	75.9	100.0	46.9	32.8	51.8	71.2	68.3	81.3	73.6
New Jersey	37.8	38.5	30.8	31.3	29.0	43.9	37.3	40.3	32.3	27.0	33.2
New Mexico	0.1	0.1	0.0	0.0	0.0	0.0	0.0	0.1	0.0	0.2	0.1
New York	12.3	16.0	10.4	17.9	14.4	16.4	13.3	17.6	12.5	14.6	14.9
North Carolina	0.2	0.2	0.3	0.4	0.3	0.4	0.3	0.7	0.5	0.9	0.7
North Dakota	3.1	3.2	1.4	1.7	0.3	2.0	1.2	1.6	1.8	1.8	1.8
Ohio	0.2	0.3	0.4	0.6	0.8	1.0	1.1	2.0	2.1	3.3	2.5
Oklahoma	0.0	0.1	0.0	0.0	0.0	0.0	0.0	0.0	0.0	0.0	0.0
Oregon	0.2	0.2	0.1	0.3	0.1	0.1	0.3	0.3	0.2	0.2	0.2
Pennsylvania	26.0	37.2	32.5	39.0	50.6	57.4	70.3	72.2	61.8	52.8	62.3
Rhode Island	10.9	10.6	12.7	42.2	54.0	53.4	50.6	56.2	62.5	49.7	56.1
South Carolina	0.4	0.5	0.7	0.7	0.4	0.3	0.5	0.3	0.2	0.3	0.3
South Dakota	0.1	0.2	0.5	0.4	0.2	0.6	0.9	0.5	0.5	0.8	0.6
Tennessee	0.1	0.1	0.0	0.2	0.1	0.1	0.1	0.2	0.2	0.3	0.2
Texas	0.2	0.1	0.1	0.2	0.1	0.1	0.1	0.1	0.1	0.1	0.1
Utah	0.1	0.2	0.1	0.3	0.2	0.1	0.4	0.3	0.3	0.2	0.3
Vermont	43.3	76.0	61.7	107.6	70.5	78.4	78.1	103.6	55.6	113.1	90.8
Virginia	11.4	9.3	9.8	11.2	11.7	13.1	11.6	12.3	8.7	9.2	10.1
Washington	0.2	0.2	0.2	0.2	0.1	0.2	0.2	0.4	0.1	0.2	0.2
West Virginia	6.9	5.8	4.4	6.3	6.1	13.2	16.2	27.7	30.7	39.2	32.5
Wisconsin	44.0	42.2	23.9	25.2	17.2	22.7	26.0	31.0	19.3	20.9	23.7
Wyoming	0.0	0.2	0.5	0.2	0.3	0.0	0.2	0.5	0.0	0.3	0.3
US Incidence	7.3	7.8	7.0	8.6	7.9	8.9	8.1	9.1	7.2	7.1	7.8

Values are confirmed cases per 100,000 population per year.
Abbreviation: N, not reportable this year.

Manitoba to Nova Scotia, and *I. pacificus* ticks are established in areas of southern British Columbia.[48] Human Lyme disease cases have increased nearly 20-fold during the last decade, from 144 in 2009 to 2634 on 2019.[49] Although Ontario accounts for the largest number of cases, Nova Scotia has the highest incidence (86 per 100,000 population), fully 12-fold greater than the national incidence (7 per 100,000 population). The high incidence among humans in Nova Scotia correlates with a high seroprevalence of anti-*Borrelia* antibodies among domestic dogs in the province.[50] Further changes in climatic conditions are expected to drive northward expansion of *Ixodes* populations, increasing areas of risk.[47]

Ixodes ticks are found in northeastern Mexico and in Baja; however, evidence for human Lyme borreliosis in Mexico is limited to a few case reports.[2,51,52] Serologic evidence of *Borrelia* infection was reported for 28% of ~600 adults and children with neurologic disease in one study; however, these results have been met with skepticism given the potential for nonspecific reactions.[53] Similarly, debate exists over the role of Lyme disease as a cause of carditis in Mexico.[54] More information is needed to sort out the validity of various claims. Further south, *B. burdorferi* sensu lato spirochetes have been detected by molecular methods in Ixodid ticks collected in Argentina,[55] Brazil,[56,57] and Uruguay.[58] In Chile, a recently described genospecies, *B. chilensis*, was cultured from *I. stilesi* ticks and long-tailed rice rats.[59] Whether these genospecies and their associated vectors pose a risk of human infection remains to be determined. A "Lyme-like" illness known locally as Baggio-Yoshinari syndrome has been described in Brazil; however, patients with this diagnosis lack serologic evidence of *Borrelia* infection.[60]

In Europe, risk for Lyme borreliosis is widespread but variable. *I. ricinus* is the principal vector and transmits all 3 major pathogenic genospecies. Populations of *I. ricinus* are found throughout western, central, and eastern Europe, generally at elevations less than 1300 meters (for current distribution see: https://www.ecdc.europa.eu/en/disease-vectors/surveillance-and-disease-data/tick-maps).[2,61] Rates of infection in adult ticks tend to be higher in eastern as compared with western Europe, and the relative frequency of infection with the different genospecies varies across regions. Ticks collected in northern and eastern regions of Europe (eg, Scandinavia, Baltic states, Czech Republic, Slovakia, Croatia, Bulgaria) are more likely to carry *B. afzelii*, whereas those from western Europe countries (eg, Austria, Switzerland, United Kingdom) are more likely to be infected with *B. garinii*.[62] The distribution of *I. ricinus* extends into the northern reaches of Morocco, Algeria and Tunisia, where infection with *B. lusitaniae* is more common.[2]

Reported rates of human infection are not easily compared among European countries due to differences in surveillance practices.[63–65] This should change with the implementation of standardized reporting for neuroborreliosis cases within the European Union.[66,67] In general, incidence seems higher in northeastern and central Europe and decreases moving west and south into Spain and Italy.[65,68–70] Annual rates of 100 cases per 100,000 population or more have been reported in areas of Sweden, Norway, Estonia, Lithuania, Poland, Germany, Austria, Slovenia, Switzerland, and the Netherlands.[68,71–76] Lower national rates of 20 to 90 cases per 100,000 population have been reported for Finland, Belgium, and France.[64,68,77,78] Rates in the British Isles average less than 10 cases per 100,000 population, except in the Scottish Highlands where peaks of 44 cases per 100,000 have been reported.[79–81] A mean annual rate of 7 has been reported for Bulgaria, and incidence in Italy, Spain, and Portugal is generally less than 1 per 100,000 population.[68,82,83] Iceland has seen growing incidence in recently years but all cases seem to be imported.[84]

Risk of Lyme borreliosis extends across Eurasia, from Eastern Europe through Turkey, Ukraine, southern Russia, portions of Mongolia, China, and into Japan.[85] The principal vector in this region is *I. persulcatus*, which overlaps with *I. ricinus* in Eastern Europe.[61] This tick species transmits *B. afzelii* and Asian and Eurasian variants of *B. garinii*; it is not known to transmit *B. burgdorferi* sensu stricto.[86,87] Reported incidence in endemic areas of Russia generally ranges from 5 to 10 cases per 100,000 population.[63] Older reports suggest higher rates in areas northeast of Moscow in Vologda oblast, in the Sverdlovsk (Urals) region, and western Siberia.[88] Infected ticks are found in Mongolia; however, information on human cases is scarce.[89] In China, at least 6 genospecies of *B. burgdorferi* sensu lato have been isolated from rodents and ticks.[90–92] Human infection seems widespread, with a few confirmed infections caused by *B. garinii*, *B. afzelii*, or *B valaisiana*.[93,94] A far larger proportion of cases are ascribed to an uncharacterized genospecies of *B. burgdorferi* sensu lato.[92] Both *B garinii* and *B. afzelii* have been isolated from patients in Japan; however, overall incidence is less than 0.1 case per 100,000 population. Most cases occur on Hokkaido Island in northern Japan, or less commonly, from exposures in subalpine-forested areas in central Japan.[95] A serosurvey of dogs in Sapporo found evidence of anti-*Borrelia* antibodies in 10%, suggesting a local enzootic transmission.[96] Enzootic cycles are established in Korea and Taiwan, and confirmed human infections with *B. yangtzensis* and *B. garinii* have been reported from Korea and Taiwan, respectively.[97,98]

Moving further south, an enzootic cycle involving *B. yangtzensis* and the tick *I. granulatus* has been reported recently from Sarawak, Borneo, and there is some serologic evidence of human *Borrelia* infection in Malaysia.[99–101] Seroreactivity has also been detected in North India, where *I. persulcatus* occurs.[102] Cases of Lyme-like illness have been reported in Australia; however, most assessments have concluded that evidence for local infection is lacking.[103] Similarly, reports of Lyme disease in South Africa and other African countries have been met with skepticism.[104] Interpretation of serologic evidence is complicated by the occurrence of relapsing fever *Borrelia* infections, especially in regions of Africa.

Seasonality

Lyme borreliosis occurs most often in the warmer months, influenced by the questing habits of ticks and the recreational tendencies of humans.[2,105] Nymphal ticks are thought to play a particularly important role in transmission due to their small size and relative abundance. Nymphal questing usually peaks in late spring or early summer, corresponding with a surge in human disease (**Fig. 4**).[38,106,107] Approximately 50% of US cases have onset in June and July. A slightly later peak in July and August has been reported in European countries.[69,70,72,77,108] Adult *I. scapularis* quest in the fall but are less abundant than nymphs, producing a smaller but discernible shoulder of cases that lasts into October (see **Fig. 4**). Due to longer and more variable incubation periods, seasonal fluctuations are slightly less pronounced for disseminated stages of infection, as compared with erythema migrans (EM).[38] Questing behavior is influenced by meteorologic factors,[109] and onset of human illness can vary from year to year based on climatic conditions.[110]

Occurrence by Age and Sex

Lyme disease occurrence is strongly influenced by patient age and sex. Incidence in most countries is bimodal, with higher rates among children and adolescents ages 5 to 15 years, lower rates among young adults, and higher rates among adults ages 50 years and over. In the United States, incidence has remained relatively stable

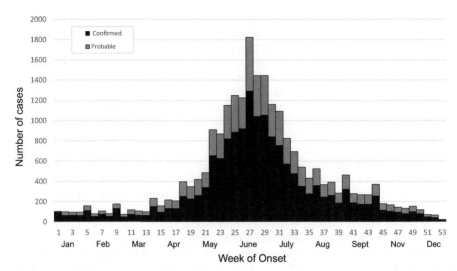

Fig. 4. Seasonal distribution of confirmed and probable Lyme disease cases, United States, 2019.

over the past decade among children, while increasing among older adults (**Fig. 5**). Incidence is higher among males in all age groups (**Fig. 6**), and males account for a growing percentage of US cases, increasing steadily from 51% in 1992 to 57% in 2019.[105,106] In contrast, females account for 51% to 60% of identified cases in many European series, and incidence can be far higher than for males in some age categories.[63,105,108,111] These varying patterns likely reflect behavior-related differences in exposure, although age and sex specific differences in susceptibility and care seeking behavior may also contribute. Differences in the age and sex distribution are observed within the United States when comparing high and low incidence areas,

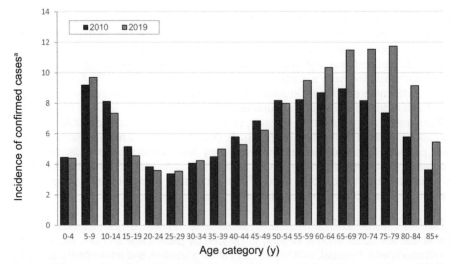

Fig. 5. Incidence of confirmed Lyme disease cases by age, United States, 2010 and 2019.
[a]Cases per 100,000 population per year.

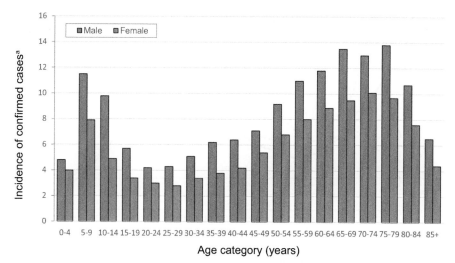

Fig. 6. Incidence of confirmed Lyme disease cases by age and sex, United States, 2019. [a]Cases per 100,000 population per year.

with adult women accounting for the majority of reported cases in low incidence areas.[38] Barring fundamental differences in risk factors for infection, this discrepancy suggests that a portion of cases reported from low incidence areas are actually due to other conditions, consistent with the lower positive predictive value of clinical and laboratory findings in low incidence setting.

Clinical Features

EM is universally the most common feature of Lyme borreliosis, occurring in 60% to 90% of cases in both North America and Eurasia.[4,38,112,113] EM reflects localized reproduction of spirochetes within the skin and typically begins 3 to 14 days after tick bite. EM is characterized by gradual expansion over days and often accompanied by symptoms of fatigue, fever, headache, mild stiff neck, arthralgia, or myalgia. Less common cutaneous manifestations include acute lymphocytoma and the chronic atrophy of acrodermatitis chronica atrophicans (ACA).[114] From the skin, spirochetes can disseminate to other parts of the body to cause neurologic defects (eg, facial palsy, meningitis, radiculopathy), cardiac abnormalities (eg, carditis with atrioventricular heart block), and monoarticular or oligoarticular arthritis. Clinical course is variable, and clinicians are referred to other sources for details of illness, diagnosis, and patient management *(see Chapters 2–8)*.[4,115]

Although the clinical features of Lyme borreliosis are broadly similar across populations, differences can be discerned related to geography and to patient age and sex. In the United States, where nearly all infections are caused by *B. burgdorferi*, arthritis is a commonly reported form of disseminated infection. Among cases with clinical information reported during 2008 to 2015, 27% were associated with arthritis, whereas only 12% had neurologic symptoms (usually facial palsy).[38] Arthritis was disproportionately common among children aged 5 to 15 years, whereas carditis, which accounted for ~1% of reported cases, was disproportionately common among men aged 20 to 40 years (**Fig. 7**).[38]

The most common infecting genospecies in Europe, *B. garinii* and *B. afzelii*, seem to have somewhat different tissue tropisms than *B. burgdorferi*, resulting in a shift in

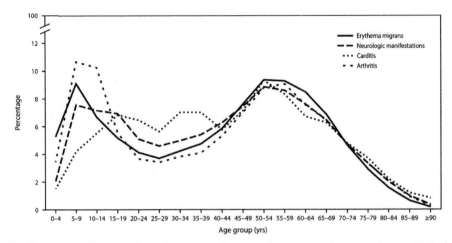

Fig. 7. Percent of reported, syndrome-specific Lyme disease cases by age category, United States, 2008 to 2015. (*From* Schwartz AM, Hinckley AF, Mead PS, Hook SA, Kugeler KJ. Surveillance for Lyme Disease — United States, 2008–2015. MMWR Surveill Summ 2017;66(No. SS-22):1–12. DOI: https://doi.org/10.15585/mmwr.ss6622a1.)

clinical features. A large review of Swedish patients found that 16% had neuroborreliosis, whereas only 7% had arthritis; a series from Austria reported that 24% of patients had neurologic manifestations, as compared with 2% with arthritis.[108,116] These higher rates of neuroborreliosis likely reflect infection with *B. garinii* or *B. bavariensis*.[117] Conversely, *B. afzelii* is detected more often in patients with the cutaneous manifestations of EM, and especially those with ACA.[118–121] This later association may explain why ACA is well known in Europe but rare in the United States. Interestingly, cutaneous manifestations may be generally more common among women in Europe, whereas noncutaneous manifestations are more common among men.[63,111] In a large Slovenian series, women accounted for 59% of patients with EM and 69% with ACA but only 39% of patients with neuroborreliosis and 25% with Lyme arthritis.[122]

Mortality

Death due to Lyme disease is rare. Among ~120,000 US patients with reported Lyme disease during 1995 to 2013, fewer than 1% died from any cause within a year of diagnosis, a rate that is actually less than the expected, age-adjusted all-cause mortality.[123] Nevertheless, the risk of death is appreciable among patients with Lyme carditis, and it is critical that clinicians be alert to this rare manifestation. In a series based on US national hospitalization records for the period 2003 to 2014, death occurred in 155 (1.6%) of 9729 patients hospitalized for conduction disorders attributed to Lyme disease.[124] Additional deaths may occur but go unrecognized, as suggested by cases discovered incidentally through examination of donated organs.[125] Tragically, deaths are also reported among patients receiving bizarre or unproven treatments for Lyme disease and among patients whose treatment of another condition was delayed due to misdiagnosis as Lyme disease.[126–129]

Risk Factors of Infection

Contact with infected ticks determines the risk of Lyme disease. In the northeastern United States, where homes are often situated in heavily tick-infested areas, exposure is thought to occur primarily in the peridomestic environment immediately around the home.[130] Contributing factors include the amount of forest cover and suitable tick habitat, landscaping practices that enhance tick survival (eg, failure to clear leaf litter), deer density, and outdoor activities such as gardening.[131–134] Specific yard items such as bird feeders, rock walls, or woodpiles have been suggested to increase the risk in some studies, presumably by attracting or harboring reservoir hosts.[131] One study in Connecticut found that tick bite was associated with the amount of time spent in one's own yard rather than public recreational areas.[135] In the North Central United States, where areas of highest risk are often lightly populated, weekend travel and recreation away from home may play a greater role in human infections.[136] Occupational risk is well documented among landscapers, gardeners, forestry workers, farmers, soldiers, hunters, hikers, and orienteers, both in the United States and overseas.[63,137–141]

Prevention and Chemoprophylaxis

Current methods for Lyme disease prevention include community interventions (eg, deer control), household interventions (yard pesticide treatments), and personal protective measures (eg, repellents, tick checks).[142,143] To date, none of these approaches has proven highly effective on its own, and a layered approach based on multiple methods is generally advised. Information on community and household interventions are described elsewhere; the focus here is on personal protective measures individuals can use to reduce their risk of Lyme or other tick-borne infections.[143–145]

Most commercially available insect repellents have ingredients with repellent or toxicant activity against ticks, as demonstrated in field or laboratory studies. These include products with N-diethyl-meta-toluamide, picaridin, ethyl-3-(N-n-butyl-N-acetyl) aminopropionate (IR3535), oil of lemon eucalyptus, p-methane-3,8-diol, 2-undecanone, and permethrin.[146] Observational studies evaluating real-world effectiveness in the general population have yielded mixed results. Repellent use has been found protective in a few studies but not in many others.[131,134,147,148] Interpretation of these studies is complicated by diverse study designs, lack of precision about repellent use, and the possibility that repellent use is intrinsically higher in those at greatest risk for tick bite. Use of protective clothing, such as light-colored clothing, long sleeves, long pants, and boots has been evaluated in multiple observational studies, again with mixed results.[131,133,134,147–149] Wearing uniforms factory-treated with permethrin has been shown to significantly reduce tick bites among outdoor workers in several randomized, placebo-controlled trials.[150,151] Permethrin can be used on clothing but should not be applied to skin.

Laboratory studies show that *I. scapularis* ticks must attach for more than 24 hours before they can transmit *B. burgdorferi*.[152] This suggests that daily checks to find and remove ticks could largely eliminate the risk of infection.[134,147] Unfortunately, nymphal ticks are small and difficult to detect, and most epidemiologic studies have not found evidence that tick checks are protective.[131,147–149] One notable exception is a Connecticut study by Connelly and colleagues demonstrating a protective effect of ticks checks performed within 36 hours of time spent outdoors (adjusted odds ratio of 0.55), as well as a strong protective effect of bathing within 2 hours of time spent outdoors (adjusted odds ratio of 0.4).[134] Prompt bathing may have special potential since it simultaneously presents an opportunity to find newly attached ticks, to wash off undetected ticks that have yet to attach, and to reduce exposure to ticks remaining on clothing. Daily tick checks are less likely to prevent infection with other *Ixodes*-associated pathogens, which are transmitted more rapidly, or to be effective with *I. ricinus* ticks, which can transmit *B. afzelii* after shorter periods of attachment.[2]

For people who discover an attached *Ixodes* tick, postexposure prophylaxis can reduce the risk of developing Lyme disease.[153–155] In a randomized, placebo-controlled study of 482 patients living in a highly endemic area of New York, treatment with a single 200 mg dose of doxycycline within 72 hours of tick removal reduced the development of EM at the tick-bite site by 87%, from 3.2% to 0.4%.[153] Approximately 30% of treated participants reported side effects, principally nausea or other gastrointestinal symptoms. These results were confirmed and extended in a recent open-label study conducted in the Netherlands, in which treatment with single dose doxycycline within 72 hours of removing an *I. ricinus* tick reduced the frequency of physician-diagnosed Lyme disease from 2.9% to 0.96%.[155] This European trial, in which participants were followed for up to 6 months, found no evidence of delayed disseminated disease to suggest prophylaxis obscured the clinical course without preventing infection. As seen in both studies, only a small percentage of participants developed illness, thus ~30 to 40 persons required prophylaxis to prevent a single case. This rate can potentially be improved by targeting patients for whom history or tick engorgement suggest the tick was attached for longer than 36 hours.[156,157] Current US recommendations hold that prophylaxis should only be given for a verified *I. scapularis* bite in a highly endemic area when the tick had been attached for greater than 36 hours.[115] Doxycycline prophylaxis has not been shown to prevent anaplasmosis.

Vaccination and Preexposure Prophylaxis

Vaccination, although not currently available, is the one of the few interventions empirically proven to prevent Lyme disease.[158] A vaccine targeting the OspA protein of *B. burgdorferi* was marketed in the United States in 1998 following clinical trials demonstrating ~75% efficacy.[159] The vaccine, LYMErix, was withdrawn from the market in 2002 for reasons variously attributed to poor sales, safety concerns, and inadequate support from the medical and public health community.[160] In 2021, a second-generation OspA vaccine entered phase II clinical trials in children and adults in Europe and the United States.[161,162] This multivalent vaccine stimulates antibodies against 6 different OspA serotypes, thereby providing coverage for common North American and European strains.[163] A small Osp A epitope that was present in LYMErix has been deleted from this vaccine as a precautionary measure, even though concerns that it might stimulate autoreactive antibodies have proven unfounded.[164]

Along with vaccine studies, research is underway to develop anti-OspA human monoclonal antibody for use as seasonal, single-dose, pre-exposure prophylaxis. Monoclonal antibodies have proven effective in preventing tick-transmitted *B. burgdorferi* infection in studies of mice and nonhuman primates.[165] As with all interventions, the impact of this or other interventions will depend heavily on uptake by those at risk and support by the medical and public health community.

DISCUSSION

The epidemiology of Lyme disease is complex, shaped by human behavior and local ecology. A detailed understanding can be challenging for busy clinicians, yet some epidemiologic knowledge is clinically useful.[166] Presenting symptoms of Lyme disease can be nonspecific, and a patient's exposure history strongly influences the prior probability of disease, which in turn determines the predictive value of clinical signs and diagnostic tests. It is critical that providers have a sense of the magnitude of risk—or lack of risk—in their practice area, as well as the risk associated with travel to other areas. In high-incidence areas, clinicians should be alert for cases of carditis and know the indications of postexposure prophylaxis.

An additional reason for awareness of Lyme disease epidemiology is the growing, malignant challenge of medical misinformation. Misinformation about Lyme disease is widespread in the general population, and patients often misinterpret their level of risk, believing the disease occurs everywhere in the United States, or that Lyme disease is a reasonable explanation for any set of symptoms.[167] The harms of misdiagnosis are real.[127]

Heath care providers can play a vital role in preventing Lyme disease by educating patients about their risk and in recommending prevention measures.[143] Although vaccination is not currently available, this or other forms of prophylaxis may soon reach the market, and clinicians will invariably influence their acceptance. In the meantime, patients at risk should be advised to use personal protective measures such as repellents, tick checks, and prompt bathing to reduce their risk. Although such measures are not highly effective at the population level, they have little downside and may be quite effective for the vigilant individual. Risk may be reduced further by treating clothing with permethrin. Tick abundance around homes and in recreational areas can be reduced by removing brush and leaf litter, creating buffer zones of wood chips or gravel between forests and lawn, excluding deer, and use of pesticides.[143–145]

In the 40 years since the cause of Lyme disease was discovered, an enormous amount has been learned about the diversity and distribution of *B. burgdorferi* sensu lato in nature and its relation to human illness. Many questions remain, and no doubt an even fuller picture will emerge in the coming decades. Perhaps, the most pressing challenge, however, is the ever-increasing number and distribution of cases. The ongoing emergence of Lyme disease underscores the urgent need for new and more effective interventions.

CLINICS CARE POINTS

- Epidemiologic factors, especially local incidence, should factor heavily when evaluating patients with possible signs and symptoms of Lyme disease.
- Health-care providers can prevent Lyme disease by educating patients to use repellent, check daily for ticks, and bath soon after exposure to tick habitat.
- Postexposure prophylaxis with doxycycline can be beneficial in select circumstances.
- New preventives, including a vaccine and monoclonal antibodies, are under development but will require clinician support to be adopted by the public.

DISCLAIMER

The findings and conclusions in this article are those of the author and do not necessarily represent the views of the Centers for Disease Control and Prevention.

ACKNOWLEDGMENTS

The author thanks the dedicated staff of the Bacterial Diseases Branch Epidemiology Team, CDC, for their comments and support. This article is derived in part from previous articles by the author.

REFERENCES

1. Steere AC, Coburn J, Glickstein L. The emergence of Lyme disease. J Clin Invest 2004;113(8):1093–101.

2. Piesman J, Gern L. Lyme borreliosis in Europe and North America. Parasitology 2004;129(Suppl):S191–220.
3. Strle F, Stantic-Pavlinic M. Lyme disease in Europe. N Engl J Med 1996; 334(12):803.
4. Stanek G, Strle F. Lyme borreliosis-from tick bite to diagnosis and treatment. FEMS Microbiol Rev 2018;42(3):233–58.
5. Rosenberg R, Lindsey NP, Fischer M, et al. Vital signs: trends in reported vec-torborne disease cases - United States and territories, 2004-2016. MMWR Morb Mortal Wkly Rep 2018;67(17):496–501.
6. Steere AC, Malawista SE, Hardin JA, et al. Erythema chronicum migrans and Lyme arthritis. The enlarging clinical spectrum. Ann Intern Med 1977;86(6): 685–98.
7. Matuschka FR, Ohlenbusch A, Eiffert H, et al. Antiquity of the Lyme-disease spirochaete in Europe. Lancet 1995;346(8986):1367.
8. Ginsberg HS, Hickling GJ, Burke RL, et al. Why Lyme disease is common in the northern US, but rare in the south: the roles of host choice, host-seeking behavior, and tick density. PLoS Biol 2021;19(1):e3001066.
9. Parte A, Sardà Carbasse J, Meier-Kolthoff J, et al. List of Prokaryotic names with Standing in Nomenclature (LPSN) moves to the DSMZ. Int J Syst Evol Microbiol 2020;70:5607–12.
10. Margos G, Fingerle V, Cutler S, Gofton A, Stevenson B, Estrada-Pena A. Contro-versies in bacterial taxonomy: The example of the genus *Borrelia*. Ticks Tick Borne Dis 2020;11(2):101335.
11. Lin T, Oliver JH Jr, Gao L, Kollars TM Jr, Clark KL. Genetic heterogeneity of *Borrelia burgdorferi* sensu lato in the southern United States based on restriction fragment length polymorphism and sequence analysis. J Clin Microbiol 2001; 39(7):2500–7.
12. Kingry L, Sheldon S, Oatman S, et al. Targeted Metagenomics for Clinical Detection and Discovery of Bacterial Tick-Borne Pathogens. J Clin Microbiol 2020;58(11):e00147-20.
13. Eisen L. Vector competence studies with hard ticks and *Borrelia burgdorferi* sensu lato spirochetes: a review. Ticks Tick Borne Dis 2020;11(3):101359.
14. Maggi RG, Reichelt S, Toliver M, Engber B. *Borrelia* species in *Ixodes affinis* and *Ixodes scapularis* ticks collected from the coastal plain of North Carolina. Ticks Tick Borne Dis 2010;1(4):168–71.
15. Ginsberg HS, Rulison EL, Azevedo A, et al. Comparison of survival patterns of northern and southern genotypes of the North American tick Ixodes scapularis (Acari: Ixodidae) under northern and southern conditions. Parasit Vectors 2014; 7:394.
16. Goddard J. A ten-year study of tick biting in Mississippi: implications for human disease transmission. J Agromedicine 2002;8(2):25–32.
17. Oliver JH, Gao L, Lin T. Comparison of the spirochete *Borrelia burgdorferi* s.l. isolated from the tick *Ixodes scapularis* in southeastern and northeastern United States. J Parasitol 2008;94(6):1351–6.
18. Smith RP Jr, Rand PW, Lacombe EH, Morris SR, Holmes DW, Caporale DA. Role of bird migration in the long-distance dispersal of *Ixodes dammini*, the vector of Lyme disease. J Infect Dis 1996;174(1):221–4.
19. Johnson SE, Swaminathan B, Moore P, Broome CV, Parvin M. *Borrelia burgdorferi*: survival in experimentally infected human blood processed for transfusion. J Infect Dis 1990;162(2):557–9.

20. McQuiston JH, Childs JE, Chamberland ME, Tabor E. Transmission of tick-borne agents of disease by blood transfusion: a review of known and potential risks in the United States. Transfusion 2000;40(3):274–84.

21. Woodrum JE, Oliver JH Jr. Investigation of venereal, transplacental, and contact transmission of the Lyme disease spirochete, *Borrelia burgdorferi*, in Syrian hamsters. J Parasitol 1999;85(3):426–30.

22. Moody KD, Barthold SW. Relative infectivity of *Borrelia burgdorferi* in Lewis rats by various routes of inoculation. Am J Trop Med Hyg 1991;44(2):135–9.

23. Schlesinger PA, Duray PH, Burke BA, Steere AC, Stillman MT. Maternal-fetal transmission of the Lyme disease spirochete, *Borrelia burgdorferi*. Ann Intern Med 1985;103(1):67–8.

24. Figueroa R, Bracero LA, Aguero-Rosenfeld M, Beneck D, Coleman J, Schwartz I. Confirmation of *Borrelia burgdorferi* spirochetes by polymerase chain reaction in placentas of women with reactive serology for Lyme antibodies. Gynecol Obstet Invest 1996;41(4):240–3.

25. Waddell LA, Greig J, Lindsay LR, Hinckley AF, Ogden NH. A systematic review on the impact of gestational Lyme disease in humans on the fetus and newborn. PLoS One 2018;13(11):e0207067.

26. Markowitz LE, Steere AC, Benach JL, Slade JD, Broome CV. Lyme disease during pregnancy. J Am Med Assoc 1986;255(24):3394–6.

27. Walsh CA, Mayer EW, Baxi LV. Lyme disease in pregnancy: case report and review of the literature. Obstet Gynecol Surv 2007;62(1):41–50.

28. CDC. Nationally Notifiable Diseases Surveillance System (NNDSS). Surveillance Case Definitions. Lyme disease (*Borrelia burgdorferi*). Available at: https://ndc. services.cdc.gov/conditions/lyme-disease/. Accessed January, 2022.

29. Kwit NA, Dietrich EA, Nelson C, et al. Notes from the field: high volume of lyme disease laboratory reporting in a low-Incidence State - Arkansas, 2015-2016. MMWR Morb Mortal Wkly Rep 2017;66(42):1156–7.

30. CDC. National Notifiable Diseases Surveillance System, 2019 Annual Tables of Infectious Disease Data. 2021. Available at: https://www.cdc.gov/nndss/data-statistics/infectious-tables/index.html. Accessed 9 December 2021.

31. Naleway AL, Belongia EA, Kazmierczak JJ, Greenlee RT, Davis JP. Lyme disease incidence in Wisconsin: a comparison of state-reported rates and rates from a population-based cohort. Am J Epidemiol 2002;155(12):1120–7.

32. Doyle TJ, Glynn MK, Groseclose SL. Completeness of notifiable infectious disease reporting in the United States: an analytical literature review. Am J Epidemiol 2002;155(9):866–74.

33. Hinckley AF, Connally NP, Meek JI, et al. Lyme disease testing by large commercial laboratories in the United States. Clin Infect Dis 2014;59(5):676–81.

34. Nelson CA, Saha S, Kugeler KJ, et al. Incidence of clinician-diagnosed lyme disease, United States, 2005-2010. *Emerg Infect Dis*. Sep 2015;21(9):1625–31.

35. Schwartz AM, Kugeler KJ, Nelson CA, Marx GE, Hinckley AF. Use of commercial claims data for evaluating trends in lyme disease diagnoses, United States, 2010-2018. Emerg Infect Dis 2021;27(2):499–507.

36. Kugeler KJ, Schwartz AM, Delorey MJ, Mead PS, Hinckley AF. Estimating the Frequency of Lyme Disease Diagnoses, United States, 2010-2018. Emerg Infect Dis 2021;27(2):616–9.

37. CDC. Notice to Readers: Final 2013 Reports of Nationally Notifiable Infectious Diseases. Morb Mortal Weekly Rep 2014;63(32):702–15.

38. Schwartz AM, Hinckley AF, Mead PS, Hook SA, Kugeler KJ. Surveillance for Lyme Disease - United States, 2008-2015. *MMWR Surveill Summ*. Nov 10 2017;66(22):1–12.

39. California Department of Public Health. Vector-Borne Disease Section Annual Report, 2020. Kjemtrup AM, Kramer V, editors. Scaramento, California, 2021. p. 1-29. Available at: https://www.cdph.ca.gov/Programs/CID/DCDC/Pages/VBDSAnnualReports.aspx.

40. Kugeler KJ, Farley GM, Forrester JD, Mead PS. Geographic Distribution and Expansion of Human Lyme Disease, United States. Emerg Infect Dis 2015; 21(8):1455–7.

41. Barbarin AM, Seagle SW, Creede S. Notes from the field: four cases of lyme disease at an outdoor wilderness camp - North Carolina, 2017 and 2019. MMWR Morb Mortal Wkly Rep 2020;69(4):114–5.

42. Mead P, Goel R, Kugeler K. Canine serology as adjunct to human Lyme disease surveillance. Emerg Infect Dis 2011;17(9):1710–2.

43. Bowman D, Little SE, Lorentzen L, Shields J, Sullivan MP, Carlin EP. Prevalence and geographic distribution of *Dirofilaria immitis, Borrelia burgdorferi, Ehrlichia canis*, and *Anaplasma phagocytophilum* in dogs in the United States: results of a national clinic-based serologic survey. Vet Parasitol 2009;160(1-2):138–48.

44. IDEXX. Sensitivity and specificity of the SNAP® 4Dx® Test Updated October 1, 2010. Available at: http://www.idexx.com/view/xhtml/en_us/smallanimal/inhouse/snap/4dx.jsf?selectedTab=Accuracy#tabs. Accessed 1 October 2010.

45. Duncan AW, Correa MT, Levine JF, Breitschwerdt EB. The dog as a sentinel for human infection: prevalence of *Borrelia burgdorferi* C6 antibodies in dogs from southeastern and mid-Atlantic States. Vector Borne Zoonotic Dis 2005;5(2): 101–9.

46. Millen K, Kugeler KJ, Hinckley AF, Lawaczeck EW, Mead PS. Elevated lyme disease seroprevalence among dogs in a nonendemic county: harbinger or artifact? Vector Borne Zoonotic Dis 2013;13(5):340–1.

47. Ogden NH, Maarouf A, Barker IK, et al. Climate change and the potential for range expansion of the Lyme disease vector *Ixodes scapularis* in Canada. Int J Parasitol 2006;36(1):63–70.

48. Ogden NH, Trudel L, Artsob H, et al. *Ixodes scapularis* ticks collected by passive surveillance in Canada: analysis of geographic distribution and infection with Lyme borreliosis agent *Borrelia burgdorferi*. J Med Entomol 2006;43(3): 600–9.

49. Public Health Agency of Canada. Lyme disease. Surveillance. 2021. Available at: http://www.phac-aspc.gc.ca/id-mi/lyme/surveillance-eng.php. Accessed 15 December 2021.

50. Herrin BH, Peregrine AS, Goring J, Beall MJ, Little SE. Canine infection with *Borrelia burgdorferi, Dirofilaria immitis, Anaplasma spp.* and *Ehrlichia spp.* in Canada, 2013-2014. Parasit Vectors 2017;10(1):244.

51. Colunga-Salas P, Sanchez-Montes S, Volkow P, Ruiz-Remigio A, Becker I. Lyme disease and relapsing fever in Mexico: An overview of human and wildlife infections. PLoS One 2020;15(9):e0238496.

52. Gordillo-Perez G, Vargas M, Solorzano-Santos F, et al. Demonstration of *Borrelia burgdorferi* sensu stricto infection in ticks from the northeast of Mexico. Clinical Microbiology and Infection 2009;15(5):496–8.

53. Faccini-Martinez AA. Call for caution to consider lyme neuroborreliosis as a frequent neurological disease in Mexico. Arch Med Res 2019;50(1):18.

54. Faccini-Martinez AA, Rosas AF. Is it proper to consider Lyme borreliosis as an autochthonous cause of cardiac disease in Mexico? J Electrocardiol 2020;58: 103–4.
55. Cicuttin GL, De Salvo MN, Venzal JM, Nava S. Borrelia spp. in ticks and birds from a protected urban area in Buenos Aires city, Argentina. Ticks Tick Borne Dis 2019;10(6):101282.
56. Dall'Agnol B, Michel T, Weck B, et al. *Borrelia burgdorferi* sensu lato in *Ixodes longiscutatus* ticks from Brazilian Pampa. Ticks Tick Borne Dis 2017;8(6): 928–32.
57. Munoz-Leal S, Ramirez DG, Luz HR, Faccini JLH, Labruna MB. "Candidatus *Borrelia ibitipoquensis*," a *Borrelia valaisiana*-Related Genospecies Character-ized from *Ixodes paranaensis* in Brazil. Microb Ecol 2020;80(3):682–9.
58. Carvalho LA, Maya L, Armua-Fernandez MT, et al. *Borrelia burgdorferi* sensu lato infecting *Ixodes auritulus* ticks in Uruguay. Exp Appl Acarol 2020;80(1): 109–25.
59. Ivanova LB, Tomova A, Gonzalez-Acuna D, et al. *Borrelia chilensis*, a new mem-ber of the *Borrelia burgdorferi* sensu lato complex that extends the range of this genospecies in the Southern Hemisphere. Environ Microbiol 2014;16(4): 1069–80.
60. de Oliveira SV, Faccini-Martinez AA, Cerutti Junior C. Lack of serological evi-dence for Lyme-like borreliosis in Brazil. Travel Med Infect Dis 2018;26:62–3.
61. European Centre for Disease Control. Tick Species Distribution Maps: *Ixodes ri-cinus/persultatus* - known distribution September 2021 2022. Available at: https://www.ecdc.europa.eu/en/disease-vectors/surveillance-and-disease-data/tick-maps. Accessed 2 Jan 2022.
62. Rauter C, Hartung T. Prevalence of *Borrelia burgdorferi* sensu lato genospecies in *Ixodes ricinus* ticks in Europe: a metaanalysis. *Applied* and Environmental Microbiology 2005;71(11):7203–16.
63. Hubalek Z. Epidemiology of lyme borreliosis. Curr Probl Dermatol 2009;37: 31–50.
64. Sykes RA, Makiello P. An estimate of Lyme borreliosis incidence in Western Eu-ropedagger. J Public Health (Oxf) 2017;39(1):74–81.
65. Rizzoli A, Hauffe H, Carpi G, et al. Lyme borreliosis in Europe. Euro Surveill 2011;16(27). https://doi.org/10.2807/ese.16.27.19906-en [pii=19906].
66. van den Wijngaard CC, Hofhuis A, Simoes M, et al. Surveillance perspective on Lyme borreliosis across the European Union and European Economic Area. Euro Surveill 2017;22(27):30569.
67. Lancet. Introducing EU-wide surveillance of Lyme neuroborreliosis. Lancet 2018;392(10146):452.
68. Vandekerckhove O, De Buck E, Van Wijngaerden E. Lyme disease in Western Europe: an emerging problem? A systematic review. Acta Clin Belg 2021; 76(3):244–52.
69. Lindgren E, Jaenson T. Lyme borreliosis in Europe: influences of climate and climate change, epidemiology, ecology and adaptation measures. World Health Organization Regional Office for Europe. Available at: http://www.euro.who. int/__data/assets/pdf_file/0006/96819/E89522.pdf. Accessed 1 October 2010.
70. Vandenesch A, Turbelin C, Couturier E, et al. Incidence and hospitalisation rates of Lyme borreliosis, France, 2004 to 2012. Euro Surveill 2014;19(34):20883.
71. Bennet L, Halling A, Berglund J. Increased incidence of Lyme borreliosis in southern Sweden following mild winters and during warm, humid summers. Eur J Clin Microbiol Infect Dis 2006;25(7):426–32.

72. Wilking H, Stark K. Trends in surveillance data of human Lyme borreliosis from six federal states in eastern Germany, 2009-2012. Ticks Tick Borne Dis 2014; 5(3):219–24.

73. Hofhuis A, Harms M, Bennema S, van den Wijngaard CC, van Pelt W. Physician reported incidence of early and late Lyme borreliosis. *Parasit Vectors*. M 2015; 8:161.

74. Enkelmann J, Bohmer M, Fingerle V, et al. Incidence of notified Lyme borreliosis in Germany, 2013-2017. Sci Rep 2018;8(1):14976.

75. Zbrzezniak J, Rosolak A, Paradowska-Stankiewicz I. Lyme disease in Poland in 2019. Przegl Epidemiol 2021;75(2):210–4.

76. Petruloniene A, Radzisauskiene D, Ambrozaitis A, Caplinskas S, Paulauskas A, Venalis A. Epidemiology of Lyme Disease in a Highly Endemic European Zone. Medicina (Kaunas) 2020;56(3):115.

77. Sajanti E, Virtanen M, Helve O, et al. Lyme Borreliosis in Finland, 1995-2014. Emerg Infect Dis 2017;23(8):1282–8.

78. Septfons A, Goronflot T, Jaulhac B, et al. Epidemiology of Lyme borreliosis through two surveillance systems: the national Sentinelles GP network and the national hospital discharge database, France, 2005 to 2016. Euro Surveill 2019;24(11). https://doi.org/10.2807/1560-7917.ES.2019.24.11.1800134.

79. Cairns V, Wallenhorst C, Rietbrock S, Martinez C. Incidence of Lyme disease in the UK: a population-based cohort study. BMJ Open 2019;9(7):e025916. https://doi.org/10.1136/bmjopen-2018-025916.

80. Tulloch JSP, Christley RM, Radford AD, et al. A descriptive epidemiological study of the incidence of newly diagnosed Lyme disease cases in a UK primary care cohort, 1998-2016. BMC Infect Dis 2020;20(1):285.

81. Mavin S, Watson EJ, Evans R. Distribution and presentation of Lyme borreliosis in Scotland - analysis of data from a national testing laboratory. J R Coll Physicians Edinb 2015;45(3):196–200.

82. Ermenlieva N, Tsankova G, Todorova TT. Epidemiological study of Lyme disease in Bulgaria. Cent Eur J Public Health 2019;27(3):235–8.

83. Smith R, Takkinen J. Lyme borreliosis: Europe-wide coordinated surveillance and action needed? Euro Surveill 2006;11(6):E060622 1.

84. Vigfusson HB, Hardarson HS, Ludviksson BR, Gudlaugsson O. [Lyme disease in Iceland - Epidemiology from 2011 to 2015]. Laeknabladid 2019;105(2):63–70.

85. Kurtenbach K, Hanincova K, Tsao JI, Margos G, Fish D, Ogden NH. Fundamental processes in the evolutionary ecology of Lyme borreliosis. Nat Rev Microbiol 2006;4(9):660–9.

86. Korenberg E, Gorelova N, Kovalevskii Y. Ecology of *Borrelia burgdorferi* sensu lato in Russia. In: Gray JSKO, Lane RS, Stanek G, editors. Lyme borreliosis: biology, epidemiology and control. New York: CABI Publishing; 2002. p. 175–200.

87. Masuzawa T. Terrestrial distribution of the Lyme borreliosis agent *Borrelia burgdorferi* sensu lato in East Asia. Jpn J Infect Dis 2004;57(6):229–35.

88. World Health Organization. Report of WHO workshop on Lyme borreliosis diagnosis and surveillance (who/cds/vph/95141-1), WHO. Geneva 1995;1–220.

89. von Fricken ME, Rolomjav L, Illar M, et al. Geographic Range of Lyme Borreliosis in Mongolia. Vector Borne Zoonotic Dis 2019;19(9):658–61.

90. Zhang F, Gong Z, Zhang J, Liu Z. Prevalence of *Borrelia burgdorferi* sensu lato in rodents from Gansu, northwestern China. BMC Microbiol 2010;10:157.

91. Wang Y, Li S, Wang Z, Zhang L, Cai Y, Liu Q. Prevalence and identification of *Borrelia burgdorferi* sensu lato genospecies in ticks from northeastern China. Vector Borne Zoonotic Dis 2019;19(5):309–15.
92. Fang LQ, Liu K, Li XL, et al. Emerging tick-borne infections in mainland China: an increasing public health threat. Lancet Infect Dis 2015;15(12):1467–79.
93. Zhang L, Zhu X, Hou X, et al. Prevalence and prediction of Lyme disease in Hainan province. PLoS Negl Trop Dis 2021;15(3):e0009158.
94. Wen S, Xu Q, Liu D, et al. A seroepidemiological investigation of Lyme disease in Qiongzhong County, Hainan Province in 2019-2020. Ann Palliat Med 2021; 10(4):4721–7.
95. Hashimoto S, Kawado M, Murakami Y, et al. Epidemics of vector-borne diseases observed in infectious disease surveillance in Japan, 2000-2005. J Epidemiol 2007;17 Suppl:S48–55.
96. Uesaka K, Maezawa M, Inokuma H. Serological survey of *Borrelia* infection of dogs in Sapporo, Japan, where *Borrelia garinii* infection was previously detected. J Vet Med Sci 2016;78(3):463–5.
97. Chao LL, Chen YJ, Shih CM. First detection and molecular identification of *Borrelia garinii* isolated from human skin in Taiwan. J Med Microbiol 2010;59(Pt 2): 254–7.
98. Kim CM, Yun NR, Kim DM. Case Report: The First Borrelia yangtzensis Infection in a Human in Korea. Am J Trop Med Hyg 2021;106(1):45–6.
99. Tay ST, Kamalanathan M, Rohani MY. *Borrelia burgdorferi* (strain *B. afzelii*) antibodies among Malaysian blood donors and patients. Southeast Asian J Trop Med Public Health 2002;33(4):787–93.
100. Lau ACC, Qiu Y, Moustafa MAM, et al. Detection of *Borrelia burgdorferi* sensu lato and relapsing fever *Borrelia* in feeding *Ixodes* ticks and rodents in Sarawak, Malaysia: ew geographical records of *Borrelia yangtzensis* and *Borrelia miyamotoi*. Pathogens 2020;9(10):846.
101. Khor CS, Hassan H, Mohd-Rahim NF, et al. Seroprevalence of *Borrelia burgdorferi* among the indigenous people (Orang Asli) of Peninsular Malaysia. J Infect Dev Ctries 2019;13(5):449–54.
102. Vinayaraj EV, Gupta N, Sreenath K, et al. Clinical and laboratory evidence of Lyme disease in North India, 2016-2019. Trav Med Infect Dis 2021;43:102134.
103. Brown JD. A description of 'Australian Lyme disease' epidemiology and impact: an analysis of submissions to an Australian senate inquiry. Intern Med J 2018; 48(4):422–6.
104. Frean JA, Isaacson M. Absence of Lyme borreliosis from Gauteng, South Africa. Trans R Soc Trop Med Hyg 1995;89(4):464.
105. Bacon RM, Kugeler KJ, Mead PS, Centers for Disease C, Prevention. Surveillance for Lyme disease–United States, 1992-2006. MMWR Surveill Summ 2008;57(10):1–9.
106. CDC. Lyme Disease. Data and Surveillance. Available at;. https://www.cdc.gov/lyme/datasurveillance/index.html?CDC_AA_refVal=https%3A%2F%2Fwww.cdc.gov%2Flyme%2Fstats%2Findex.html. Accessed 12/15/2021.
107. Falco RC, McKenna DF, Daniels TJ, et al. Temporal relation between *Ixodes scapularis* abundance and risk for Lyme disease associated with erythema migrans. Am J Epidemiol 1999;149(8):771–6.
108. Berglund J, Eitrem R, Ornstein K, et al. An epidemiologic study of Lyme disease in southern Sweden. N Engl J Med 1995;333(20):1319–27.

109. Alekseev AN, Dubinina HV. Abiotic parameters and diel and seasonal activity of *Borrelia*-infected and uninfected *Ixodes persulcatus* (Acarina: Ixodidae). J Med Entomol 2000;37(1):9–15.
110. Moore SM, Eisen RJ, Monaghan A, et al. Meteorological influences on the seasonality of Lyme disease in the United States. Am J Trop Med Hyg 2014;90(3):486–96.
111. Fulop B, Poggensee G. Epidemiological situation of Lyme borreliosis in germany: surveillance data from six Eastern German States, 2002 to 2006. Parasitol Res 2008;103(Suppl 1):S117–20.
112. Steere AC, Sikand VK. The presenting manifestations of Lyme disease and the outcomes of treatment. N Engl J Med 2003;348(24):2472–4.
113. Stanek G, Strle F. Lyme borreliosis. Lancet 2003;362(9396):1639–47.
114. Ogrinc K, Maraspin V, Lusa L, et al. Acrodermatitis chronica atrophicans: clinical and microbiological characteristics of a cohort of 693 Slovenian patients. J Intern Med 2021;290(2):335–48.
115. Lantos PM, Rumbaugh J, Bockenstedt LK, et al. Clinical Practice Guidelines by the Infectious Diseases Society of America (IDSA), American Academy of Neurology (AAN), and American College of Rheumatology (ACR): 2020 Guidelines for the Prevention, Diagnosis, and Treatment of Lyme Disease. Arthritis Rheum 2021;73(1):12–20.
116. Stanek G, Flamm H, Groh V, et al. Epidemiology of *Borrelia* infections in Austria. Zentralbl Bakteriol Mikrobiol Hyg A 1987;263(3):442–9.
117. Margos G, Wilske B, Sing A, et al. *Borrelia bavariensis sp. nov.* is widely distributed in Europe and Asia. Int J Syst Evol Microbiol 2013;63(Pt 11):4284–8.
118. Ruzic-Sabljic E, Lotric-Furlan S, Maraspin V, et al. Analysis of *Borrelia burgdorferi* sensu lato isolated from cerebrospinal fluid. APMIS 2001;109(10):707–13.
119. Ruzic-Sabljic E, Arnez M, Lotric-Furlan S, et al. Genotypic and phenotypic characterisation of *Borrelia burgdorferi* sensu lato strains isolated from human blood. J Med Microbiol 2001;50(10):896–901.
120. Busch U, Hizo-Teufel C, Bohmer R, et al. *Borrelia burgdorferi* sensu lato strains isolated from cutaneous Lyme borreliosis biopsies differentiated by pulsed-field gel electrophoresis. Scand J Infect Dis 1996;28(6):583–9.
121. Ornstein K, Berglund J, Nilsson I, et al. Characterization of Lyme borreliosis isolates from patients with erythema migrans and neuroborreliosis in southern Sweden. J Clin Microbiol 2001;39(4):1294–8.
122. Strle F, Wormser GP, Mead P, et al. Gender disparity between cutaneous and non-cutaneous manifestations of Lyme borreliosis. PLoS One 2013;8(5):e64110.
123. Forrester JD, Meiman J, Mullins J, et al. Notes from the field: update on Lyme carditis, groups at high risk, and frequency of associated sudden cardiac death–United States. MMWR Morb Mortal Wkly Rep 2014;63(43):982–3.
124. Uzomah UA, Rozen G, Mohammadreza Hosseini S, et al. Incidence of carditis and predictors of pacemaker implantation in patients hospitalized with Lyme disease. PLoS One 2021;16(11):e0259123.
125. CDC. Three sudden cardiac deaths associated with Lyme carditis - United States, November 2012-July 2013. Morb Mortal Wkly Rep 2013;62(49):993–6.
126. Patel R, Grogg KL, Edwards WD, et al. Death from inappropriate therapy for Lyme disease. Clin Infect Dis 2000;31(4):1107–9.
127. Lantos PM, Shapiro ED, Auwaerter PG, et al. Unorthodox alternative therapies marketed to treat Lyme disease. Clin Infect Dis 2015;60(12):1776–82.

128. Marzec NS, Nelson C, Waldron PR, et al. Serious bacterial infections acquired during treatment of patients given a diagnosis of chronic lyme disease - United States. MMWR Morb Mortal Wkly Rep 2017;66(23):607–9.
129. Strizova Z, Patek O, Vitova L, et al. Internet-based self-diagnosis of Lyme disease caused death in a young woman with systemic lupus erythematosus. Joint Bone Spine 2019;86(5):650–1.
130. Cromley EK, Cartter ML, Mrozinski RD, et al. Residential setting as a risk factor for Lyme disease in a hyperendemic region. Am J Epidemiol 1998;147(5):472–7.
131. Orloski KA, Campbell GL, Genese CA, et al. Emergence of Lyme disease in Hunterdon County, New Jersey, 1993: a case-control study of risk factors and evaluation of reporting patterns. Am J Epidemiol 1998;147(4):391–7.
132. Rand PW, Lubelczyk C, Lavigne GR, et al. Deer density and the abundance of *Ixodes scapularis* (Acari: Ixodidae). J Med Entomol 2003;40(2):179–84.
133. Smith G, Wileyto EP, Hopkins RB, et al. Risk factors for lyme disease in Chester County, Pennsylvania. Public Health Rep 2001;116(Suppl 1):146–56.
134. Connally NP, Durante AJ, Yousey-Hindes KM, et al. Peridomestic Lyme disease prevention: results of a population-based case-control study. Am J Prev Med 2009;37(3):201–6.
135. Mead P, Hook S, Niesobecki S, et al. Risk factors for tick exposure in suburban settings in the Northeastern United States. Ticks Tick Borne Dis 2018;9(2): 319–24.
136. Neitzel DF, Kemperman MM. Tick-borne diseases in Minnesota: an update. Minn Med 2012;95(8):41–4.
137. Kaya AD, Parlak AH, Ozturk CE, et al. Seroprevalence of *Borrelia burgdorferi* infection among forestry workers and farmers in Duzce, north-western Turkey. N Microbiol 2008;31(2):203–9.
138. Buczek A, Rudek A, Bartosik K, et al. Seroepidemiological study of Lyme borreliosis among forestry workers in southern Poland. Ann Agric Environ Med 2009; 16(2):257–61.
139. Bilski B. Occurrence of cases of borreliosis certified as an occupational disease in the province of Wielkopolska (Poland). Ann Agric Environ Med 2009;16(2): 211–7.
140. Nakama H, Muramatsu K, Uchikama K, et al. Possibility of Lyme disease as an occupational disease– seroepidemiological study of regional residents and forestry workers. Asia Pac J Public Health 1994;7(4):214–7.
141. Busova A, Dorko E, Feketeova E, et al. Association of seroprevalence and risk factors in Lyme disease. Cent Eur J Public Health 2018;26(Suppl):S61–6.
142. Poland GA. Prevention of Lyme disease: a review of the evidence. Mayo Clin Proc 2001;76(7):713–24.
143. Hayes EB, Piesman J. How can we prevent Lyme disease? N Engl J Med 2003; 348(24):2424–30.
144. Piesman J, Eisen L. Prevention of tick-borne diseases. Annu Rev Entomol 2008; 53:323–43.
145. The Tick Management Handbook: an integrated guide for homeowners, pest control operators, and public health officials for the prevention of tick-associated disease. Connecticut Agricultural Experiment Station; 2004. p. 72.
146. Eisen L, Dolan MC. Evidence for Personal Protective Measures to Reduce Human Contact With Blacklegged Ticks and for Environmentally Based Control Methods to Suppress Host-Seeking Blacklegged Ticks and Reduce Infection with Lyme Disease Spirochetes in Tick Vectors and Rodent Reservoirs. J Med Entomol 2016;53(5):1063–92. https://doi.org/10.1093/jme/tjw103.

147. Vazquez M, Muehlenbein C, Cartter M, et al. Effectiveness of personal protective measures to prevent Lyme disease. Emerg Infect Dis 2008;14(2):210–6.

148. Finch C, Al-Damluji MS, Krause PJ, et al. Integrated assessment of behavioral and environmental risk factors for Lyme disease infection on Block Island, Rhode Island. PLoS One 2014;9(1):e84758.

149. Phillips CB, Liang MH, Sangha O, et al. Lyme disease and preventive behaviors in residents of Nantucket Island, Massachusetts. Am J Prev Med 2001;20(3): 219–24.

150. Mitchell C, Dyer M, Lin FC, et al. Protective effectiveness of long-lasting permethrin impregnated clothing against tick bites in an endemic lyme disease setting: a randomized control trial among outdoor workers. J Med Entomol 2020; 57(5):1532–8.

151. Vaughn MF, Funkhouser SW, Lin FC, et al. Long-lasting permethrin impregnated uniforms: a randomized-controlled trial for tick bite prevention. Am J Prev Med 2014;46(5):473–80.

152. des Vignes F, Piesman J, Heffernan R, et al. Effect of tick removal on transmission of *Borrelia burgdorferi* and *Ehrlichia phagocytophila* by *Ixodes scapularis* nymphs. J Infect Dis 2001;183(5):773–8.

153. Nadelman RB, Nowakowski J, Fish D, et al. Prophylaxis with single-dose doxycycline for the prevention of Lyme disease after an *Ixodes scapularis* tick bite. N Engl J Med 2001;345(2):79–84.

154. Zhou G, Xu X, Zhang Y, et al. Antibiotic prophylaxis for prevention against Lyme disease following tick bite: an updated systematic review and meta-analysis. BMC Infect Dis 2021;21(1):1141.

155. Harms MG, Hofhuis A, Sprong H, et al. A single dose of doxycycline after an *Ixodes ricinus* tick bite to prevent Lyme borreliosis: an open-label randomized controlled trial. J Infect 2021;82(1):98–104.

156. Falco RC, Daniels TJ, Vinci V, et al. Assessment of duration of tick feeding by the scutal index reduces need for antibiotic prophylaxis after *Ixodes scapularis* tick bites. Clin Infect Dis 2018;67(4):614–6.

157. Pritt BS. Scutal index and its role in guiding prophylaxis for Lyme disease following tick bite. Clin Infect Dis 2018;67(4):617–8.

158. Poland GA, Jacobson RM. The prevention of Lyme disease with vaccine. Vaccine 2001;19(17–19):2303–8.

159. Wormser GP. A brief history of OspA vaccines including their impact on diagnostic testing for Lyme disease. Diagn Microbiol Infect Dis 2022;102(1): 115572.

160. Plotkin SA. Correcting a public health fiasco: The need for a new vaccine against Lyme disease. Clin Infect Dis 2011;52(Suppl 3):s271–5.

161. National Library of Medicine. Clinical Trials.Gov. VLA15 ongoing clinical trials. 2022. Available at: https://clinicaltrials.gov/ct2/results?term=vaccine&cond= Lyme+Disease. Accessed January 15, 2022.

162. Comstedt P, Schuler W, Meinke A, et al. The novel Lyme borreliosis vaccine VLA15 shows broad protection against *Borrelia* species expressing six different OspA serotypes. PLoS One 2017;12(9):e0184357.

163. Comstedt P, Hanner M, Schuler W, et al. Design and development of a novel vaccine for protection against Lyme borreliosis. PLoS One 2014;9(11):e113294.

164. Dattwyler RJ, Gomes-Solecki M. The year that shaped the outcome of the OspA vaccine for human Lyme disease. NPJ Vaccin 2022;7(1):10.

165. Schiller ZA, Rudolph MJ, Toomey JR, et al. Blocking *Borrelia burgdorferi* transmission from infected ticks to nonhuman primates with a human monoclonal antibody. J Clin Invest 2021;131(11):e144843.
166. Makhani N, Morris SK, Page AV, et al. A twist on lyme: the challenge of diagnosing european lyme neuroborreliosis. J Clin Microbiol 2010;10. https://doi.org/10.1128/JCM.01584-10. JCM.01584-10 [pii].
167. Cooper JD, Feder HM Jr. Inaccurate information about lyme disease on the internet. Pediatr Infect Dis J 2004;23(12):1105–8.

Early Lyme Disease (Erythema Migrans) and Its Mimics (Southern Tick-Associated Rash Illness and Tick-Associated Rash Illness)

Franc Strle, MD, PhD[a],*, Gary P. Wormser, MD[b]

KEYWORDS

- Erythema migrans • Lyme disease • Lyme borreliosis • Borrelia burgdorferi
- Tick-borne diseases

KEY POINTS

- The erythema migrans (EM) skin lesion is the most common clinical manifestation of Lyme disease.
- Approximately 50% of patients have symptoms at the site of the EM skin lesion.
- Constitutional symptoms are present in most US patients with EM and in approximately one-third of European patients.
- Diagnosis of typical EM is clinical.
- A 10 to 14-day course of an appropriate oral antibiotic is highly effective treatment.

HISTORY

Erythema migrans (EM) has an interesting history,[1,2] dating back to 1909 when Arvid Afzelius reported to the Swedish Dermatological Academy information about an expanding reddening of the skin, which he called "erythema migrans." In 1913, the Viennese dermatologist Benjamin Lipschütz published a case report on a skin rash that developed from a spot around a tick bite on the thigh, expanded slowly during a period of 7 months extending up to the shoulder, and finally healed spontaneously. He named this rash "erythema chronicum migrans." Lipschütz recognized the connection with the tick bite and suggested examination of tick saliva, which he assumed contained the cause of the observed skin disorder. Since the 1950s, dermatologists in Europe have successfully used penicillin for the treatment of erythema chronicum migrans, despite not knowing the cause. Hollström reported the outcome of the treatment of 16 patients

[a] University Medical Center Ljubljana, Japljeva 2, Ljubljana 1525, Slovenia; [b] New York Medical College, 40 Sunshine Cottage Road, Skyline Office, Valhalla, NY 10595, USA
* Correspondent author.
E-mail address: franc.strle@kclj.si

Infect Dis Clin N Am 36 (2022) 523–539
https://doi.org/10.1016/j.idc.2022.03.005
0891-5520/22/© 2022 Elsevier Inc. All rights reserved.

id.theclinics.com

with EM, including 1 patient who also had meningitis; he found penicillin superior to either bismuth or arsenic salt. He also mentioned that Carl Lennhoff of the dermatology hospital of Magdeburg University, Germany, and later from the Karolinska Institute in Stockholm, Sweden, had observed structures in a skin biopsy of an erythema chronicum migrans skin lesion that resembled spirochetes, pointing to the possibility that this disease may be caused by tick-associated spirochetes. The dermatologist Klaus Weber from Munich considered and excluded possible viral causes, as well as rickettsia and the etiologic agent of tularemia. He also discussed borreliae, which he ruled out due to the prevailing opinion among acarologists at that time that only soft ticks and not hard ticks, such as *Ixodes ricinus*, are carriers of borrelia. Nevertheless, the apparent effectiveness of antibiotics against the disorder suggested a bacterial cause, which was finally confirmed after the recognition of Lyme disease and its borrelial cause in the United States.[3] It later became clear that EM differs in the Untied States and Europe (**Table 1**), although there are many similarities.[4]

DEFINITION

Several definitions of EM have been proposed for different purposes. Best known among these are the definitions from the Centers for Disease Control and Prevention (CDC)[5] and the Infectious Diseases Society of America (IDSA)[6] in the United States and from the European Society for Clinical Microbiology and Infectious Disease study group in Europe.[7]

For purposes of surveillance in the United States, EM was defined as a skin lesion that typically begins as a red macule or papule and expands during a period of days to

Table 1
Erythema migrans: United States versus Europe

	United States	Europe
Tick vector	*I. scapularis* *I. pacificus*	*I. ricinus* *I. persulcatus*
Lyme borrelia	Mostly *B. burgdorferi* sensu stricto. *B. mayonii* may occur in the upper Midwestern United States	Mostly *B. afzelii* and *B. garinii* but several other species cause human disease including *B. burgdorferi* s.s., *B. bavariensis*, *B. spielmanii, and B. lusitaniae*
Speed of tick transmission of Lyme borrelia	Rarely before 36 h	*I. ricinus* may transmit *B. afzelii* within 24 h
Gender predominance	Most cases in men	Most cases occur in women
Coinfections	Risk depends on the geographic area. The most common coinfections are anaplasmosis and babesiosis	Risk depends on the geographic area. Tick-borne encephalitis virus is the most common coinfection
Erythema migrans mimic	Southern tick-associated rash illness following an *A. americanum* tick bite	None

Modified from Marques AR, Strle F, Wormser GP. Comparison of Lyme disease in the United States and Europe. Emerg Infect Dis 2021;27(8):2017–24.

weeks to form a large round lesion, often with partial central clearing. A single primary lesion must reach 5 cm or greater in size across its largest diameter. Secondary lesions also may occur. Annular erythematous lesions occurring within several hours of a tick bite represent hypersensitivity reactions rather than EM.[5]

According to the IDSA 2006 Lyme disease guidelines,[6] EM is a round or oval, expanding erythematous skin lesion that develops at the site of deposition of *Borrelia burgdorferi* by an *Ixodes* species tick. These skin lesions typically become apparent approximately 7 to 14 days (range, 3–30 days) after the tick has detached or was removed and should be at least 5 cm in largest diameter for a secure diagnosis. When there is more than 1 EM skin lesion, the secondary skin lesions are believed to arise by hematogenous dissemination from the site of primary infection. Secondary EM skin lesions can be less than 5 cm in largest diameter but similar to primary lesions, they may expand. In some patients with multiple EM skin lesions, the primary lesion cannot be identified with certainty.[6]

In Europe EM is defined as an expanding erythematous skin lesion, with or without central clearing, that developed days to weeks after a tick bite or exposure to ticks in a Lyme borreliosis endemic region and has a diameter of 5 cm or greater. If less than 5 cm in diameter, a history of a tick bite at that site, a delay in the appearance of at least 2 days, and an expanding rash at the bite site are required for the diagnosis of EM. Multiple EM is defined as the presence of 2 or more skin lesions, at least 1 of which fulfills the size criteria (≥5 cm) for a solitary EM.[7] The EM that appears at the site of the tick bite is defined as the primary EM. If no tick bite is recalled, the primary EM is defined as the lesion with longest duration, or in the case of the same or uncertain duration, the one with the largest diameter.

FREQUENCY

EM is by far the most common clinical manifestation of Lyme disease. In the United States, 70% of reported cases of Lyme disease in the period 2008 to 2019 had EM according to the CDC.[8] Data on signs/symptoms were available, however, for only 62% of 311,561 confirmed cases during that time period. Due to the way surveillance data are collected, patients who are seropositive, and typically have later clinical manifestations, may more likely be included in such surveillance data, and the percentages presented may therefore differ from what is typically seen in a "real world" setting.[8] Thus, the actual proportion of EM cases in the United States might be higher, at approximately 90%.[9]

Among 1471 patients found to have Lyme borreliosis in an epidemiologic study in Southern Sweden, EM was seen in 77% of cases.[10] In Slovenia, notification of Lyme borreliosis has been mandatory for 35 years, and during the past 20 years, the incidence of the disease has been more than 180 per 100,000 inhabitants, rising to 365 per 100,000 in 2018. During the second decade of notification, EM represented about 90% of reported cases, whereas during the last 15 years, the proportion of EM cases was 95% or greater.[11] This is consistent with the findings in Norway and Germany where 96% to 97% of reported Lyme borreliosis cases are EM.[12–14] The higher proportion of EM cases in recent years might be a consequence of fewer reported cases of extracutaneous manifestations of Lyme borreliosis due to more strict requirements for the diagnosis of extracutaneous manifestations and/or better and earlier recognition and treatment of early Lyme borreliosis.

TICK BITE

In the United States, only about 1 in 4 patients (14%–32%) with EM recall a previous tick bite at the site of the skin lesion.[15–18] In European studies, the proportion of patients recalling a tick bite is substantially higher and exceeds 50%.[13,16,18–20] Although differences in the tick species transmitting borrelia (*I. scapularis* and *I. pacificus* in North America; *I. ricinus* and *I. persulcatus* in Europe and Asia) may offer a potential explanation for the differences in the frequency of detection of tick bites, the reasons for this difference are not entirely clear. Nevertheless, patients with EM who do not recall a tick bite were bitten by an infected tick but were just not aware of the bite.

CAUSE

In North America, EM is caused by *B. burgdorferi* sensu stricto; however, in the mid-western United States, *B. mayonii* may also cause Lyme disease.[21] Reports from Europe, based on the characterization of borreliae isolated from skin, revealed that EM is most often caused by *B. afzelii* (up to 96%, most often 70%–90%), less frequently by *B. garinii* (up to 33%, most often 10%–20%), rarely by *B. burgdorferi* s.s. and only exceptionally by other *Borrelia* species such as *B. bissettii*, *B. spielmanii*, and as yet unidentifiable species.[22] Of 1972 borrelia skin isolates obtained from Slovenian patients with EM who were included in different prospective (predominantly treatment) studies, 1764 (89.5%) were typed as *B. afzelii*, 163 (8.3%) as *B. garinii*, 25 (1.3%) as *B. burgdorferi* s.s., 4 (0.2%) as *B. spielmanii*, whereas 16/1972 (0.8%) of the *Borrelia* species isolates remained unidentified.[19,23] The borrelia isolation rate was approximately 50% (44%–63%, depending on the study). In contrast, in a series of 82 patients with EM from Finland, 21.5% were skin culture positive (a rather low isolation rate), and all of the isolates were typed as *B. garinii*.[24] It seems, therefore, that the predominance of *B afzelii* is valid for western and central Europe but may not be for (eastern) Scandinavia, Eastern Europe, and Asia. It is of interest that in several studies the proportions of the main *Borrelia* species isolated from EM skin lesions did not completely match with the proportions found in the regional ticks.[22]

Information obtained predominantly by polymerase chain reaction testing,[25] but also from culture results,[26] indicates that an individual patient with an EM skin lesion may be simultaneously infected with more than one borrelia strain subtype of the same species and sometimes even with more than one *Borrelia* species.

HISTOLOGIC FINDINGS

Mild-to-moderate superficial perivascular infiltration of lymphocytes and some histiocytes is usually present and is sometimes accompanied by plasma cells, and rarely by neutrophils, in the dermis at the site of the EM lesion and also in the clinically normal appearing skin bordering the lesion. The epidermis is usually unaffected. Interstitial and deep perivascular infiltrates have also been described.[27]

PATHOGENESIS

Lyme borrelia (*B. burgdorferi* sensu lato) enter the skin during the blood meal of an infected *Ixodes* species tick. In the United States, transmission of *B. burgdorferi* s.s. by *I. scapularis* or *I. pacificus* is rare during the first 36 hours of attachment, whereas in Europe, transmission of *B. afzelii* by *I. ricinus* ticks may occur within 24 hours.[4]

The development of the EM skin lesion occurs as a result of cutaneous inflammation associated with the centrifugal spread of the spirochete from the bite site. The spirochete may also spread hematogenously to other skin locations, resulting in secondary EM skin lesions, or to nonskin sites, thereby leading to a variety of extracutaneous clinical manifestations. The likelihood of entry into the blood stream is affected by the strain of *B. burgdorferi* s.s. causing the infection. Unlike patients who are bacteremic with more conventional pathogens, patients with spirochetemia are rarely febrile. In one US study, only 5% of 93 spirochetemic patients were febrile when the blood culture was performed.[28] The absence of lipopolysaccharide within the borrelial cell wall might explain this observation.[29]

The host–pathogen interactions that occur in the skin probably have a critical role in determining the course and outcome of the infection. The presence of T cells and increased numbers of Langerhans cells suggest that cell-mediated immune mechanisms are involved in the initial host response to Lyme borrelia.[30] High levels of messenger RNA expression of the T cell-active chemokines (C-X-C) motif ligand 9(CXCL9) and CXCL10 and low levels of the B cell-active chemokine CXCL13 have been demonstrated in EM skin lesions, and cluster of differentiation 3 positive (CD3(+)) T cells have been visualized using immunohistologic methods.[31] The global transcriptional alterations in skin biopsy samples of EM lesions from untreated adult US patients with Lyme disease in comparison to controls have revealed more than 250 differentially regulated genes characterized by the induction of chemokines, cytokines, Toll-like receptors, antimicrobial peptides, monocytoid cell activation markers, and numerous genes annotated as interferon (IFN)-inducible. The IFN-inducible genes included 3 transcripts involved in tryptophan catabolism (Indoleamine-pyrrole 2,3-dioxygenase 1, IDO1; Kynurenine 3-Monooxygenase, KMO; Kynureninase, KYNU) that play a pivotal role in immune evasion by certain other microbial pathogens.[32]

CLINICAL CHARACTERISTICS

EM affects persons of all ages with a predominance of men in the United States and women in some European countries. Due to the close temporal association with tick bites, EM has a pronounced seasonal occurrence. In one study in adult European patients with *B. afzelii* isolated from skin, the median time from tick bite to rash onset was 17 days, whereas the median time in patients in the United States infected with *B. burgdorferi* s.s. was 11 days.[16] The erythema slowly enlarges and central clearing usually begins—in Europe typically by the end of the first week in adult patients but earlier in children—resulting in a ring-like lesion that spreads outward (spreading erythema). Lesions with central clearing are currently less often seen than previously, probably due to earlier recognition and treatment of EM. Nevertheless, although skin lesions that last longer and those with a larger diameter are more likely to have central clearing, some long-lasting or large EM lesions remain homogeneous in color. EM skin lesions are typically oval or round (**Fig. 1**) but can have an irregular shape. Their diameter may range from a few centimeters to more than a meter. In adult

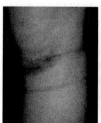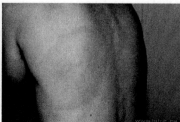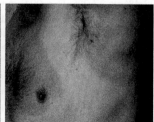

Fig. 1. Erythema migrans skin lesions from patients in Europe.

patients, EM is most often located on the lower extremities; in children, the upper part of the body is relatively more often involved.

Infrequently, lesions are purpuric, especially those located on the lower extremities. Vesicular, bullous, urticarial, and even linear patterns of EM exist, but they are rare and represent at most 5% of EM skin lesions.[6,9]

EM may be accompanied by local symptoms at the site of the skin lesion and/or by constitutional symptoms. About one-half of adult patients with EM report local symptoms, usually mild itching, rarely burning or pain.[16] Although the frequency of local symptoms at the EM skin site seems similar in the United States and Europe,[16,18] the proportion of patients with systemic symptoms is higher in the United States (up to 80%) than in Europe (20%–51%)[6,9,15,16] (**Table 2**). Constitutional symptoms, such as fatigue, malaise, headache, myalgia, and arthralgia, are usually intermittent and often vary in intensity. In adult European patients with EM, fever is uncommon, being present or recalled in fewer than 5%, whereas in the United States, it is recalled in up to one-third of patients.[15–19,22] Systemic symptoms are more frequent in patients with a positive blood culture for Lyme borreliae and are more common in patients with multiple EM. Although this is valid for both the United States and Europe, the proportion of patients with constitutional symptoms in each of these groups is much lower in Europe.[18,20]

In patients with multiple EM, the secondary lesions are similar in morphology to the primary EM skin lesion but lack the indurated center seen in primary lesions at the site of the tick bite. Secondary lesions are also smaller and are only exceptionally associated with local itching or pain. It seems that they are more frequent in children than in adults in Europe, and are apparently a more common finding in the United States (up to 50%) than in Europe (3%–8% of adult patients).[16,22] It is of interest that in European children with multiple EM, a mild, predominantly lymphocytic pleocytosis in cerebrospinal fluid was seen in 18% to 26% of patients, although none had clinical symptoms suggestive of central nervous system involvement and fewer than one-half of these patients reported systemic symptoms.[35]

In both Europe and the United States, most patients with EM are seronegative at the time of presentation. In patients with EM, abnormalities on routine laboratory tests (such as an elevated erythrocyte sedimentation rate [ESR], lymphopenia, and/or elevated liver enzyme levels) may be present. These abnormal laboratory test results are more often found in patients from the United States compared with Europe (**Table 3**) and are as a rule mild.[6,9,15–18,22]

There is a thought that the course of EM during pregnancy is similar to the course in the nonpregnant population; however, information on Lyme disease during pregnancy is limited. A recent European study that assessed and compared the course and outcome of EM in 304 pregnant women with that of age-matched nonpregnant women showed analogous findings for the most basic clinical and epidemiologic characteristics before treatment with antibiotics. An interesting exception was that pregnant women reported constitutional symptoms less frequently than non-pregnant women (22.4% vs 37.2%, $P < .001$), and that pregnant women diagnosed with EM later during pregnancy had a lower probability of reporting constitutional symptoms.[36] Because Lyme borrelia does not produce toxins or extracellular matrix-degrading proteases, most clinical manifestations result from inflammation generated by the host immune response to the spirochete.[29] Thus, fewer symptoms were interpreted to be associated with lower levels of inflammation due to downregulation of Th1 responses, most likely via the progesterone-mediated upregulation of Th2 cytokine production, resulting in a reduction in pathogenic inflammatory responses during gestation.[36]

Information on the course and outcome of Lyme borrelia infection in immunocompromised patients is limited. However, available published information indicates that

Table 2
Erythema migrans characteristics in borrelia culture positive patients: comparison of United States and Europe

Etiologic Agent	United States		Europe	p^d Bb vs Ba	p^d Bb vs Bg	p^d Ba vs Bg
	B. burgdorferi s.s.[a]	B. afzelii[b]	B. garinii[c]			
Recognized tick bite at skin site	52/212 (24.5%; 18.9%–30.9%)	402/660 (60.9%; 57.1%–64.7%)	179/282 (63.5%; 57.6%–69.1%)	<0.0001	<0.0001	0.5037
Central clearing	36/119 (30.3%; 22.2%–39.4%)	303/517 (58.6%; 54.2%–69.9%)	135/243 (55.6%; 49.1%–61.9%)	<0.0001	<0.0001	0.4744
Local symptoms at EM lesion	50/119 (42.0%; 33.0%–51.4%)	244/517 (47.2%; 42.8%–51.6%)	161/243 (66.3%; 59.9%–72.2%)	0.3570	<0.0001	<0.0001
Systemic symptoms	165/212 (77.8%; 71.6%–83.2%)	219/660 (33.2%; 29.6%–36.9%)	95/282 (33.7%; 28.2%–39.5%)	<0.0001	<0.0001	0.9399
Multiple EM	55/212 (25.9%; 20.2%–32.4%)	43/429 (10.0%; 7.4%–13.3%)	12/208 (5.8%; 3.0%–9.9%)	<0.0001	<0.0001	0.1005
Regional lymphadenopathy	80/212 (37.7%; 31.2%–44.6%)	9/203 (4.4%; 2.1%–8.3%)	4/155 (2.6%; 0.7%–6.5%)	<0.0001	<0.0001	0.5199
Temperature >38°C on physical examination	23/212 (10.8%; 7.0%–17.8%)	8/461 (1.7%; 0.8%–3.4%)	3/229 (1.3%; 0.3%–3.8%)	<0.0001	<0.0001	1.0000
Jarisch Herxheimer reaction	8/93 (8.6%; 3.8%–16.3%)	0/144 (0%; 0.0%–2.5%)	0/39 (0%; 0.0%–9.0%)	0.0004	0.1043	-

Data are given as ratio (%, 95% Confidence Interval).
Abbreviations: Ba, Borrelia afzelii; Bb, Borrelia burgdorferi sensu stricto; Bg, Borrelia garinii; EM, erythema migrans.
[a] Source: references 16 and 18.
[b] Source: references 16, 18, 20, and 33.
[c] Source: references 18, 20, 33, and 34.
[d] P values were determined using Yates corrected chi square test.
Data from Refs.[16,18,20,33,34]

Table 3
Selected routine laboratory test results for borrelia culture positive patients with erythema migrans: comparison of United States and Europe

Laboratory Finding	United States	Europe		p^d Bb vs Ba	p^d Bb vs Bg	p^d Ba vs Bg
	B. burgdorferi s.s.[a]	B.afzelii[b]	B. garinii[c]			
ESR >20 mm	70/196 (35.7%; 29.0%–42.9%)	51/624 (8.2%; 6.2%–10.6%)	29/242 (12.0%; 8.2%–16.8%)	<0.0001	<0.0001	0.1081
WBC >10 × 10⁹/L	1/91 (1.1%; 0.0%–6.0%)	13/560 (2.3%; 1.2%–3.9%)	3/158 (1.9%; 0.4%–5.5%)	0.7049	1.0000	1.0000
WBC<5 × 10⁹/L	10/91 (11.0%; 5.4%–19.3%)	32/559 (5.7%; 4.0%–8.0%)	12/158 (7.6%; 4.0%–12.9%)	0.0960	0.4985	0.4987
Lymphopenia <1 × 10⁹/L	26/92 (28.3%; 19.4%–38.6%)	12/144 (8.3%; 4.4%–14.1%)	3/39 (7.7%; 1.6%–20.9%)	<0.0001	0.0181	1.0000
Platelets < 140 × 10⁹/L	7/87 (8.0%; 3.3%–15.9%)	21/555 (3.8%; 2.4%–5.7%)	1/156 (0.6%; 0.0%–3.5%)	0.0862	0.0040	0.0622
ALT elevated	45/207 (21.7%; 16.3%–28.0%)	65/458 (14.2%; 11.1%–17.7%)	31/205 (15.1%; 10.5%–15.8%)	0.0207	0.1251	0.8454

Data are given as ratio (%, 95% Confidence Interval).

Abbreviations: ALT, alanine aminotransferase (normal: United States: ≤50 U/L; Slovenia: <0.74 μkat/L); Ba, *Borrelia afzelii*; Bb, *Borrelia burgdorferi sensu stricto*; Bg, *Borrelia garinii*; ESR, erythrocyte sedimentation rate (normal range was defined as follows: men: age ≤50 y, 0–15 mm/h, age >50 y, 0–20 mm/h; women, age ≤50 y, 0 to 20 mm/h, age greater than 50 y, 0 to 30 mm/h); WBC, white blood cell (normal: 4–10 × 10⁹/L).

[a] Source: references 16, 18, and 34.

[b] Source: references 16, 18, 20, and 33.

[c] Source: references 18, 20, 33, and 34.

[d] *P* values were determined using Yates corrected chi square test.

Data from Refs.[16,18,20,33,34]

the course and presentation of EM in immunocompromised patients is, in general, similar to that in immunocompetent individuals, with the exception that immunocompromised patients (especially those with B cell deficiency) seem to more often remain seronegative and may more often have multiple EM skin lesions or other signs of disseminated Lyme borreliosis.[37–39]

REINFECTION

Although the first case of reinfection with Lyme borrelia was most probably reported as early as 1958,[40] only limited data exist on reinfections. Patients who are treated for EM do not seem to develop an immunologic response that is adequate to protect against reinfection. Therefore, patients who had EM may become reinfected and develop another EM lesion at a different skin site. In the United States, reinfection has been well documented only in patients who were treated for early infection (nearly always EM) and not after later clinical manifestations of Lyme disease, and certainly not after Lyme arthritis.[41] In Europe, however, cases of EM that appeared at the site of a new tick bite in patients who had been treated for Lyme neuroborreliosis have been reported.[42] According to current information clinical manifestations of EM due to reinfection seem to be similar to those of a primary infection.[41,42]

DIAGNOSIS

Because EM skin lesions often do not have prominent local symptoms and because the lesion may occur on parts of the body that are difficult for the patient to visualize, a complete skin examination should be performed for any patient who might have early localized or disseminated Lyme disease.

EM is the only clinical manifestation sufficiently distinctive to allow a clinical diagnosis in the absence of a positive laboratory test. The 3 essential bases for diagnosis are as follows: 1) compatible information on the course of the skin lesion and 2) recognition of the characteristic appearance in 3) persons who live in or have recently traveled to areas endemic for Lyme disease.[6,7,22,43]

Serologic testing is not indicated for the diagnosis of typical EM and also not in routine follow-up of patients after treatment. For atypical lesions for which EM is in the differential diagnosis, antibody testing at presentation should be performed and if negative, repeated at least 2 to 3 weeks later.[44]

DIFFERENTIAL DIAGNOSIS

Even "typical" EM skin lesions may not be considered pathognomonic for Lyme disease, especially in the southern part of the United States, where the clinical entity called Southern tick-associated rash illness (STARI) exists.[43,45,46] STARI is associated with a very similar skin lesion to EM. STARI occurs, however, following the bite of a different tick species, Amblyomma americanum, and is not caused by Lyme borrelia. The cause of STARI has not been determined. A. americanum is most frequently found in the southeastern and southcentral US but its range is spreading to geographic areas where I scapularis bites are common, such as Long Island, NY. The potential for diagnostic confusion clearly exists in geographic areas, where both tick species coexist. However, a comparison of STARI cases diagnosed in Missouri with EM cases diagnosed in New York State revealed several differences, such as a higher proportion of recognized tick bites, shorter time from tick bite to the onset of the skin lesion, smaller and more often homogeneous skin lesions, and less frequent constitutional symptoms or stiff neck in patients with STARI (**Table 4**).[45] Furthermore, available,

Table 4
Comparison of selected variables of a case series of erythema migrans diagnosed in New York State with that of a case series of Southern tick-associated rash illness diagnosed in Missouri during the same time period

Variable	STARI Cases N = 21	Erythema Migrans Cases N = 101	P Value
Male sex; number (%)	13 (61.9)	72 (71.3)	.438
Recognized tick bite at lesion site; number (%)	18 (85.7)	20 (19.8)	<.001
Number of days from tick bite to lesion; mean ± SD	n = 18 6.1 ± 4.2	n = 19 10.4 ± 6.1	.011
Largest diameter of lesion in centimeters; mean ± SD	8.3 ± 2.2	16.4 ± 11.5	<.001
Number (%) with central clearing of skin lesion	16 (76.2)	16/74 (21.6)	<.001
Number (%) with systemic symptoms	4 (19.0)	77 (76.2)	<.001
Number (%) with multiple skin lesions	1 (4.8)	27 (26.7)	.042
Number (%) with regional lymphadenopathy	1 (4.8)	27 (26.7)	.042
Number (%) with fatigue	4 (19.0)	58 (57.4)	.002
Number (%) with joint pain	1 (4.8)	34 (33.7)	.007
Number (%) with stiff neck	0 (0)	35 (34.7)	<.001
Number (%) with concentration or memory problems	0 (0)	30 (29.7)	.002
Number (%) with headache	2 (9.5)	37 (36.6)	.019
Number (%) with an elevated erythrocyte sedimentation rate	2/15 (13.3)	40/96 (41.7)	.045

Data from Wormser GP, Masters E, Nowakowski J, et al. Prospective clinical evaluation of patients from Missouri and New York with erythema migrans-like skin lesions. Clin Infect Dis. 2005;41(7):958-965. https://doi.org/10.1086/432935.

but limited, data suggest that STARI can be distinguished from EM based on different serum metabolic profiles.[47]

STARI does not occur in Europe, presumably because the tick species *A. americanum* is not found in Europe. However, in Japan, a skin lesion resembling EM that developed at the site of an *A. testudinarium* tick bite, and was not caused by borreliae, was reported in 2014.[48] The lesion was named tick-associated rash illness (TARI). Three additional cases have been reported recently from Japan.[49] The cause of TARI is unclear but a hypothesis is that TARI is a type of allergic reaction.

In Lyme disease, there is typically a symptom-free interval of at least a few days from the tick bite to the onset of an EM skin lesion. When an erythematous skin lesion is present while an *Ixodes* tick is still attached, or which has developed within 48 h of detachment, this most likely represents a tick bite hypersensitivity reaction (ie, a noninfectious process), rather than EM. Tick bite hypersensitivity reactions are usually small (<5 cm in largest diameter), pruritic, and typically begin to disappear within 24 to 48 hours. In contrast, an early primary EM lesion usually increases in size over this time frame[6] and in untreated patients persists for a median time of approximately 4 weeks in the United States and even longer in Europe. To differentiate between the 2 processes, it may be useful to observe the skin site for 1 to 2 days without antibiotic therapy to see if the lesion is expanding.[6]

EM is sometimes misdiagnosed as a fungal infection and vice versa, especially when lesions are present in inguinal or axillary regions. Bacterial cellulitis rarely occurs at the most frequent skin sites for EM and would not be expected to demonstrate central clearing or a target-like appearance. EM, unlike erythema multiforme, does not involve the mucous membranes, palms, or soles.[6,29,30,43,50,51]

Other considerations in the differential diagnosis of EM that usually can be readily distinguished include pityriasis rosea, nummular eczema, granuloma annulare, contact dermatitis, urticaria, fixed drug eruption, reaction to an insect bite, and pseudolymphoma.

COINFECTIONS

Ixodes ticks can carry multiple pathogens, and a single tick bite may result in transmission of 2 or more infectious agents. In the United States, pathogens potentially transmitted by *I. scapularis* to humans include *B. burgdorferi* s.s., *B. mayonii*, *B. miyamotoi*, *Anaplasma phagocytophilum*, *Babesia microti*, *Ehrlichia muris eauclairensis*, and the deer tick virus subtype of Powassan virus.[4] The frequency of coinfections depends on the prevalence of the infectious agents in ticks, which tend to vary in different geographic areas. In the United States, *A. phagocytophilum* and *B. microti* are the most frequent coinfections in patients with Lyme disease. In Europe, in addition to Lyme borrelia, *I. ricinus/persulcatus* can transmit tick-borne encephalitis virus, *A. phagocytophilum*, species of the bacterial genus *Rickettsia*, *B. miyamotoi*, and *Babesia* protozoans. Tick-borne encephalitis virus is well recognized as a cause of co-infection in patients with Lyme disease in Europe.[4] However, according to some reports, clinically manifested coinfections in patients with EM are rare.[52,53] More data on the frequency of coinfections in both the United States and Europe are needed.

TREATMENT

EM eventually heals spontaneously without antibiotic treatment. The main reason to treat such patients is to shorten the duration of the skin manifestation and associated symptoms and to prevent the development of later complications, especially Lyme neuroborreliosis and Lyme arthritis; Lyme arthritis has occurred in approximately 60% of untreated patients in the United States.[54]

For treatment of EM, antibiotics with high *in vitro* activity against Lyme borrelia and with demonstrated efficacy in rigorous clinical trials should be used. Lyme borrelia are susceptible to tetracyclines, most penicillins, and many second-generation and third-generation cephalosporins but are resistant to certain fluoroquinolones, rifampin, and first-generation cephalosporins. For EM, oral doxycycline, amoxicillin, and cefuroxime axetil are each highly effective and are the preferred agents in the United States;[50] in Europe, in addition to these agents, phenoxymethylpenicillin is recommended[51] (**Table 5**). Macrolides such as azithromycin are somewhat less effective and are therefore recommended as a second-line therapy. Under most circumstances, oral therapy is effective and preferred over intravenous therapy due to equivalent efficacies, better tolerability, and lower cost.[6,22,50,51]

Patients with EM are treated with either a 10-day course of doxycycline or a 14-day course of amoxicillin, cefuroxime axetil, or phenoxymethylpenicillin rather than longer treatment courses (see **Table 5**). If azithromycin is used, the indicated duration is 5 to 10 days, with a 7-day course preferred in the United States, whereas in Europe a 5-day course in often used.[29,50,51]

Within 24 hours of initiation of antimicrobial therapy, some patients (according to early reports up to 15% of patients) treated for EM will experience a Jarisch-

Table 5
Treatment of erythema migrans[a]

Drug	Route	Dosage for Adults	Dosage for Children	Duration, Days (Range)[b]	Contraindications, Restrictions
Preferred					
Doxycycline	Oral	100 mg twice daily or 200 mg once daily	4.4 mg/kg/day in divided doses every 12 hours (maximum 100 mg per dose)	10	Allergy Children <8 y old[c] Pregnancy, Breast Feeding
Amoxicillin	Oral	500 mg 3 times daily	50 mg/kg/day in 3 divided doses (maximum 500 mg per dose)	14	Allergy
Cefuroxime axetil	Oral	500 mg twice daily	30 mg/kg/day in divided doses every 12 hours (maximum 500 mg per dose)	14	Allergy
Phenoxymethylpenicillin	Oral	$0.5–1.0 \times 10^6$ IU[d] 3 times daily	$0.1–0.15 \times 10^6$ IU[d]/kg/day in 3 divided doses (maximum 1×10^6 IU[d] per dose)	14	Allergy; only recommended for use in Europe, not the United States
Alternative					
Azithromycin[e]	Oral	500 mg once daily[f]	10 mg/kg once daily (maximum 500 mg per dose)	7 (range: 5–10)	Allergy

Abbreviation: IU, International Units (1 mg is approximately 1600 IU).

[a] Recommendations apply to patients either with a single erythema migrans skin lesion or with multiple lesions.

[b] Ranges are given where different durations have been studied, and the optimal duration remains uncertain.

[c] There is increasing favorable information on the safety of short courses of doxycycline in young children; however, the risk to benefit ratio of using this antibiotic in young children with erythema migrans probably still does not favor the usage of doxycycline for the treatment of erythema migrans.

[d] A diversity of doses of phenoxymethylpenicillin is used in different geographic areas in Europe. There is no general agreement on the appropriate dosage and no clinical trials that compare the different regimens in use.

[e] Because of concerns for lower efficacy, macrolide antibiotics including azithromycin are considered second-line agents, and should be reserved for patients for whom other antibiotic classes are contraindicated.

[f] In some European countries, the total dosage for adult patients is 3g (first day: 500 mg twice daily; days 2–5: 500 mg once daily).

Modified from Lantos PM, Rumbaugh J, Bockenstedt LK, et al. Clinical Practice Guidelines by the Infectious Diseases Society of America (IDSA), American Academy of Neurology (AAN), and American College of Rheumatology (ACR): 2020 Guidelines for the Prevention, Diagnosis, and Treatment of Lyme Disease. Arthritis Care Res (Hoboken). 2021;73(1):1-9. https://doi.org/10.1002/acr.24495; and Stanek G, Strle F. Lyme borreliosis - from tick bite to diagnosis and treatment. FEMS Microbiol Rev. 2018;42(3):233–258. https://doi.org/10.1093/femsre/fux047; with permissions.

Herxheimer-like reaction[43] characterized by an increase in the size or intensity of erythema in the skin lesion and more severe systemic symptoms.

Doxycycline is the only first-line agent proven to be effective against *A. phagocytophilum* coinfection. Doxycycline, however, may cause photosensitivity, which is a concern because early Lyme disease occurs most commonly during the summer months. When EM cannot be reliably distinguished from community-acquired bacterial cellulitis, cefuroxime axetil may be used because this antimicrobial is likely to be effective against both types of infection.[6,29,30,50]

In the United States, antibiotic treatment of Lyme disease in pregnant women is the same as for nonpregnant patients, except that doxycycline is not recommended, whereas some authorities in Europe recommend intravenous ceftriaxone for the treatment of EM, as well as other manifestations of Lyme disease, in pregnant women.[36,50]

According to European experiences, the choice of antibiotic, the dosages, and duration of the treatment of EM in immunocompromised patients may, in general, be the same as for immunocompetent patients.[37–39] Close follow-up, however, is desirable, especially in patients with EM who have an underlying hematological malignancy because in some of the published case series such patients more often had signs of disseminated Lyme borreliosis and more frequently needed antibiotic retreatment than sex-matched, age-matched, and antibiotic treatment-matched immunocompetent persons with EM; however, the final outcome was excellent in both groups.[38,39]

OUTCOME

Regardless of the antimicrobial regimen, complete response to treatment may be delayed beyond the treatment duration. In patients with EM, fever, if present, should resolve within 48 hours. Other symptoms, such as fatigue or arthralgia, tend to improve but not invariably resolve within the treatment time frame, lasting for more than 3 months in one-quarter of patients in the United States;[55] in Europe the large majority (83%) of adult patients return to their pre-EM health status by the 2 month time point.[19] A European study on adult patients with EM treated with either doxycycline or cefuroxime axetil revealed that constitutional symptoms that newly developed or worsened since the onset of the EM and had no other known medical explanation were present in 33.3% (95/285) of patients at the baseline visit, in 4.6% (9/194) of the patients at 6 months and in 2.2% at 12 months (5/230).[56]

In the United States, the mean duration of the EM skin lesion after the onset of treatment with recommended antibiotics has been reported to be 5 to 6 days.[57] The assessment of 1220 adult patients with EM from Slovenia revealed that the median time to resolution of EM after starting antibiotic treatment was 7 days. In 11 (0.9%) patients, EM was still visible at 2 months after initiation of antibiotic therapy.[19]

Objective treatment failures based on the appearance of a new EM skin lesion or development of an extracutaneous manifestation are very rare. Nevertheless, patients with objective signs of relapse or those who develop an extracutaneous manifestation of Lyme borreliosis may need a second course of treatment. In one European study, only 2/1220 (0.2%) patients with EM developed a new objective manifestation of Lyme borreliosis (meningitis in one and multiple EM in another); both complications developed within 14 days after beginning antibiotic treatment. There was no relapse of the EM skin lesion during the first year after antibiotic treatment.[19] A review of 19 US and European studies revealed that Lyme neuroborreliosis developed in 14/1850 (0.8%) patients treated for EM with oral antibiotics.[58] Similarly, microbiologic treatment failure is also very rare: according to one European report *B. burgdorferi* s. l. was isolated from only one posttreatment rebiopsy of 610 pretreatment skin culture-positive EM patients but even in this single case, reinfection could not be excluded.[19]

SUMMARY

EM is by far the most common clinical manifestation of Lyme disease. Diagnosis is clinical in a patient bitten by, or exposed to, ticks in a Lyme disease endemic region. A 10 to 14 day course of treatment with a recommended oral antibiotic shortens the duration of the skin lesion and prevents the development of extracutaneous manifestations of Lyme disease in the large majority of patients. In the United States, patients with EM more often have concomitant systemic symptoms than in Europe.

CLINICS CARE POINTS

- The presence of an erythema migrans like skin lesion is not pathognomonic for Lyme disease.
- A similar skin lesion is found in both STARI and TARI.
- Any skin lesion at the bite site of an *Amblyomma* tick species is not from Lyme disease.

DISCLOSURE

G.P. Wormser reports receiving research grants from the Institute for Systems Biology and Pfizer, Inc. He has been an expert witness in malpractice cases involving Lyme disease and is an unpaid board member of the American Lyme Disease Foundation. He is coowner of US Patent No. 11230728 entitled: Differentiation of Lyme disease and Southern Tick-associated rash illness; issue Date: 1/25/22. F. Strle served on the scientific advisory board for Roche on Lyme disease serologic diagnostics, on the scientific advisory board for Pfizer on Lyme disease vaccine, received research support from the Slovenian Research Agency [grant numbers P3-0296, J3-1744, and J3-8195] and is an unpaid member of the steering committee of the ESCMID Study Group on Lyme Borreliosis/ESGBOR.

REFERENCES

1. Weber K, Pfister HW. History. In: Weber K, Burgdorfer W, editors. Aspects of Lyme borreliosis. Berlin: Springer-Verlag; 1993. p. 1–20.
2. Stanek G, Strle F. The history, epidemiology, clinical manifestations and treatment of Lyme borreliosis. In: Hunfeld KP, et al, editors. Lyme borreliosis. Berlin: Springer; 2022. in press.
3. Burgdorfer W, Barbour AG, Hayes SF, et al. Lyme disease-a tick-borne spirochetosis? Science 1982;216(4552):1317–9.
4. Marques AR, Strle F, Wormser GP. Comparison of Lyme disease in the United States and Europe. Emerg Infect Dis 2021;27(8):2017–24.
5. Case Anon. definitions for infectious conditions under public health surveillance: Lyme disease (revisited 9/96). MMWR Morb Mortal Wkly Rep 1997;46(suppl RR-10):20–1.
6. Wormser GP, Dattwyler RJ, Shapiro ED, et al. The clinical assessment, treatment, and prevention of Lyme disease, human granulocytic anaplasmosis, and babesiosis: clinical practice guidelines by the Infectious Diseases Society of America. IDSA2006 Practice Guideline. Clin Infect Dis 2006;43(9):1089–134.

7. Stanek G, Fingerle V, Hunfeld KP, et al. Lyme borreliosis: clinical case definitions for diagnosis and management in Europe. Clin Microbiol Infect 2011;17(1):69–79.

8. CDC. Lyme disease - relative frequency of clinical features among confirmed cases-United States, 2008–2019 2021. Available at: https://www.cdc.gov/lyme/stats/graphs.html. Accessed February 24, 2022.

9. Nadelman RB. Erythema migrans. Infect Dis Clin North Am 2015;29(2):211–39.

10. Berglund J, Eitrem R, Ornstein K, et al. An epidemiologic study of Lyme disease in southern Sweden. N Engl J Med 1995;333:1319–27.

11. Anon: epidemiologic surveillance of infectious diseases in Slovenia in 2018. Ljubljana, Slovenia: Institute of Public Health of the Republic of Slovenia; 2019 (in Slovene).

12. Böhmer MM, Ens K, Böhm S, et al. Epidemiological surveillance of Lyme borreliosis in Bavaria, Germany, 2013-2020. Microorganisms 2021;9(9):1872.

13. Enkelmann J, Böhmer M, Fingerle V, et al. Incidence of notified Lyme borreliosis in Germany, 2013–2017. Sci Rep 2018;8(1):14976.

14. Eliassen KE, Berild D, Reiso H, et al. Incidence and antibiotic treatment of erythema migrans in Norway 2005–2009. Ticks Tick Borne Dis 2017;8(1):1–8.

15. Nadelman RB, Nowakowski J, Forseter G, et al. The clinical spectrum of early Lyme borreliosis in patients with culture-confirmed erythema migrans. Am J Med 1996;100:502–8.

16. Strle F, Nadelman RB, Cimperman J, et al. Comparison of culture-confirmed erythema migrans caused by *Borrelia burgdorferi* sensu stricto in New York State and *Borrelia afzelii* in Slovenia. Ann Intern Med 1999;130:32–6.

17. Smith RP, Schoen RT, Rahn DW, et al. Clinical characteristics and treatment outcome of early Lyme disease in patients with microbiologically confirmed erythema migrans. Ann Intern Med 2002;136:421–8.

18. Maraspin V, Bogovič P, Ogrinc K, et al. Are differences in presentation of early Lyme borreliosis in Europe and North America a consequence of a more frequent spirochetemia in American patients? J Clin Med 2021;10(7):1448.

19. Boršič K, Blagus R, Cerar T, et al. Clinical course, serologic response, and long-term outcome in elderly patients with early Lyme borreliosis. J Clin Med 2018; 7(12):506.

20. Maraspin V, Ogrinc K, Rojko T, et al. Characteristics of spirochetemic patients with a solitary erythema migrans skin lesion in Europe. PLoS One 2021;16(4): e0250198.

21. Pritt BS, Mead PS, Johnson DKH, et al. Identification of a novel pathogenic Borrelia species causing Lyme borreliosis with unusually high spirochaetaemia: a descriptive study. Lancet Infect Dis 2016;16(5):556–64.

22. Strle F, Stanek G. Clinical manifestations and diagnosis of Lyme borreliosis. Curr Probl Dermatol 2009;37:51–110.

23. Ružić-Sabljić E, Maraspin V, Lotrič-Furlan S, et al. Characterization of *Borrelia burgdorferi* sensu lato strains isolated from human material in Slovenia. Wien Klin Wochenschr 2002;114:544–50.

24. Oksi J, Marttila H, Soini H, et al. Early dissemination of *Borrelia burgdorferi* without generalized symptoms in patients with erythema migrans. APMIS 2001; 109:581–8.

25. Seinost G, Golde WT, Berger BW, et al. Infection with multiple strains of *Borrelia burgdorferi* sensu stricto in patients with Lyme disease. Arch Dermatol 1999;135: 1329–33.

26. Ruzic-Sabljic E, Arnez M, Logar M, et al. Comparison *of Borrelia burgdorferi* sensu lato strains isolated from specimens obtained simultaneously from two

different sites of infection in individual patients. J Clin Microbiol 2005;43: 2194–200.

27. De Koning J, Duray PH. Histopathology of human Lyme borreliosis. In: Weber K, Burgdorfer W, editors. Aspects of Lyme borreliosis. Berlin: Springer-Verlag; 1993. p. 70–92.

28. Wormser GP, McKenna D, Carlin J, et al. Hematogenous dissemination in early Lyme disease. Ann Intern Med 2005;142(9):751–5.

29. Steere AC, Strle F, Wormser GP, et al. Lyme borreliosis. Nat Rev Dis Primers 2016; 2:16090.

30. Stanek G, Strle F. Lyme borreliosis. Lancet 2003;362:1639–47.

31. Mullegger RR, Means TK, Shin JJ, et al. Chemokine signatures in the skin disorders of Lyme borreliosis in Europe: predominance of CXCL9 and CXCL10 in erythema migrans and acrodermatitis and CXCL13 in lymphocytoma. Infect Immun 2007;75:4621–8.

32. Marques A, Schwartz I, Wormser GP, et al. Transcriptome assessment of erythema migrans skin lesions in patients with early Lyme disease reveals predominant interferon signaling. J Infect Dis 2017;217(1):158–67.

33. Logar M, Ružić-Sabljić E, Maraspin V, et al. Comparison of erythema migrans caused by Borrelia afzelii and Borrelia garinii. Infection 2003;31:404–9.

34. Strle F, Ružić-Sabljić E, Logar M, et al. Comparison of erythema migrans caused by Borrelia burgdorferi and Borrelia garinii. Vector Borne Zoonotic Dis 2011; 11(9):1253–8.

35. Arnez M, Pleterski-Rigler D, Luznik-Bufon T, et al. Children with multiple erythema migrans: are there any pre-treatment symptoms and/or signs suggestive for central nervous system involvement? Wien Klin Wochenschr 2002;114:524–9.

36. Maraspin V, Lusa L, Blejec T, et al. Course and outcome of erythema migrans in pregnant women. J Clin Med 2020;9(8):2364.

37. Furst B, Glatz M, Kerl H, et al. The impact of immunosuppression on erythema migrans. A retrospective study of clinical presentation, response to treatment and production of Borrelia antibodies in 33 patients. Clin Exp Dermatol 2006; 31:509–14.

38. Maraspin V, Cimperman J, Lotric-Furlan S, et al. Erythema migrans in solid-organ transplant recipients. Clin Infect Dis 2006;42:1751–4.

39. Maraspin V, Ružić-Sabljić E, Lusa L, et al. Course and outcome of early Lyme borreliosis in patients with hematological malignancies. Clin Infect Dis 2015;61(3): 427–31.

40. Hollström E. Penicillin treatment of erythema chronicum migrans Afzelius. Acta Derm Venereol (Stockh) 1958;38:285–9.

41. Nadelman RB, Hanincová K, Mukherjee P, et al. Differentiation of reinfection from relapse in recurrent Lyme disease. N Engl J Med 2012;367(20):1883–90.

42. Weber K, Pfister HW, Reimers CD. Clinical features of Lyme borreliosis. In: Weber K, Burgdorfer W, editors. Aspects of Lyme borreliosis. Berlin: Springer-Verlag; 1993. p. 93–104.

43. Tibbles CD, Edlow JA. Does this patient have erythema migrans? JAMA 2007; 297(23):2617–27.

44. Pitrak D, Nguyen CT, Cifu AS. Diagnosis of Lyme disease. JAMA 2022;327(7): 676–7.

45. Wormser GP, Masters E, Nowakowski J, et al. Prospective clinical evaluation of patients from Missouri and New York with erythema migrans-like skin lesions. Clin Infect Dis 2005;41(7):958–65.

46. Philipp MT, Masters E, Wormser GP, et al. Serologic evaluation of patients from Missouri with erythema migrans-like skin lesions with the C6 Lyme test. Clin Vaccin Immunol 2006;13(10):1170–1.
47. Molins CR, Ashton LV, Wormser GP, et al. Metabolic differentiation of early Lyme disease from southern tick-associated rash illness (STARI). Sci Transl Med 2017; 9(403):eaal2717.
48. Natsuaki M, Takada N, Kawabata H, et al. Case of tick-associated rash illness caused by Amblyomma testudinarium. J Dermatol 2014;41(9):834–6.
49. Moriyama Y, Kutsuna S, Toda Y, et al. Three cases diagnosed not Lyme disease but "tick-associated rash illness (TARI)" in Japan. J Infect Chemother 2021;27(4): 650–2.
50. Lantos PM, Rumbaugh J, Bockenstedt LK, et al. Clinical Practice Guidelines by the Infectious Diseases Society of America (IDSA), American Academy of Neurology (AAN), and American College of Rheumatology (ACR): 2020 Guidelines for the prevention, diagnosis and treatment of Lyme disease. Clin Infect Dis 2021;72(1):e1–48.
51. Stanek G, Strle F. Lyme borreliosis-from tick bite to diagnosis and treatment. FEMS Microbiol Rev 2018;42(3):233–58.
52. Strle F, Bogovič P, Cimperman J, et al. Are patients with erythema migrans who have leukopenia and/or thrombocytopenia coinfected with Anaplasma phagocytophilum or tick-borne encephalitis virus? PLoS One 2014;9(7):e103188.
53. Eliassen KE, Ocias LF, Krogfelt KA, et al. Tick-transmitted co-infections among erythema migrans patients in a general practice setting in Norway: a clinical and laboratory follow-up study. BMC Infect Dis 2021;21(1):1044.
54. Steere AC, Schoen RT, Taylor E. The clinical evolution of Lyme arthritis. Ann Intern Med 1987;107:725–31.
55. Wormser GP, Ramanathan R, Nowakowski J, et al. Duration of antibiotic therapy for early Lyme disease. A randomized, double-blind, placebo-controlled trial. Ann Intern Med 2003;138(9):697–704.
56. Cerar D, Cerar T, Ruzić-Sabljić E, et al. Subjective symptoms after treatment of early Lyme disease. Am J Med 2010;123(1):79–86.
57. Steere AC, Hutchinson GJ, Rahn DW, et al. Treatment of the Early Manifestations of Lyme disease. Ann Intern Med 1983;99(1):22–6.
58. Strle F, Stupica D, Bogovič P, et al. Is the risk of early neurologic Lyme borreliosis reduced by preferentially treating patients with erythema migrans with doxycycline? Diagn Microbiol Infect Dis 2018;91(2):156–60.

Early Disseminated Lyme Disease

Cranial Neuropathy, Meningitis, and Polyradiculopathy

Tyler Crissinger, MD*, Kelly Baldwin, MD

KEYWORDS

- Neuroborreliosis • Lyme meningitis • Lyme disease • Bell's palsy
- Bannwarth syndrome

KEY POINTS

- Neuroborreliosis as a manifestation of early disseminated Lyme disease should be suspected in patients with tick exposure or those living in an endemic area that present with cranial neuropathies, meningitis, or acute painful polyradiculopathy.
- Laboratory confirmation of neuroborreliosis should begin with two-tiered serologic testing for antibodies serum serology for *Borrelia burgdorferi*, but may also include cerebrospinal fluid (CSF) analysis demonstrating a lymphocytic pleocytosis and abnormal Lyme antibody index.
- Treatment of neuroborreliosis consists of 14 to 21 days of oral doxycycline or intravenous (IV) ceftriaxone.
- Treatment with oral doxycycline is equally effective as IV ceftriaxone for early disseminated Lyme disease presenting as meningitis, cranial neuropathy, or polyradiculopathy.

BACKGROUND

Among the presentations of early disseminated Lyme disease, neuroborreliosis is a manifestation that can be dramatic while also somewhat elusive for clinicians unfamiliar with common presenting syndromes. As many as 15% of cases of untreated Lyme disease may progress to neurologic involvement, affecting both the peripheral and central nervous system. Clinical knowledge of the three most common syndromes (cranial neuropathy, meningitis, and polyradiculopathy) is essential for clinicians practicing in Lyme endemic areas and allows for more efficient diagnosis and treatment. An organized clinical and diagnostic approach is helpful to ensure appropriate treatment is not delayed due to diagnostic uncertainty.

Maine Medical Center, 22 Bramhall St., Portland, ME, 04101, USA
* Corresponding author.
E-mail address: Tyler.Crissinger@mainehealth.org

Infect Dis Clin N Am 36 (2022) 541–551
https://doi.org/10.1016/j.idc.2022.02.006
0891-5520/22/© 2022 Elsevier Inc. All rights reserved.

CLINICAL PRESENTATION

Acute neurologic presentations of Lyme disease may affect the peripheral or central nervous system to cause characteristic clinical syndromes. The most common manifestations are cranial neuropathy, meningitis, and polyradiculopathy. These were originally described as a clinical triad that occurred together, although any of these can also occur in isolation.[1] The most common presentation of neurologic disease is a combination of mild meningitis, and one or more cranial neuropathies.[2,3] Neurologic manifestations can occur as early as 1 to 2 weeks after exposure to a tick, but are also seen as subacute presentation weeks to months later.[2–9] A history of a recent rash or systemic illness with arthralgias, myalgias, and/or fever is common but not universal.[10–12] Patients often do not recall having had a tick bite, and 20% of patients with Lyme disease may not have had erythema migrans as an early sign.[13] In nonendemic areas for Lyme disease, a travel history may provide necessary epidemiologic evidence for possible exposure to *Borrelia burgdorferi* infection. It is important to emphasize that patients may, indeed, present with isolated neurologic complaints such as facial weakness or limb weakness without a history of systemic symptoms or meningeal irritation.

Cranial Neuropathy

Facial nerve (CN VII) palsy is a common presenting symptom of neuroborreliosis. In fact, of the patients who develop cranial neuropathy, 80% will have cranial nerve VII involvement, and in 25% of those it is bilateral.[14,15] Typically, this will be a peripheral facial nerve palsy, or Bell's palsy, with weakness in muscles of the upper and lower face. Neuroimaging evidence of CN VII inflammation can sometimes be demonstrated where the nerve exits the pons (see case 1 later in discussion), or there may be presumed irritation of the nerve along its course through the subarachnoid space, as there is often evidence of a lymphocytic pleocytosis in the cerebrospinal fluid (CSF). Although isolated CN VII palsy is most commonly seen, there can be involvement of other cranial nerves, whether alone, or in combination, such as an optic (CN II) neuropathy with visual acuity impairment, CN III, IV, or VI manifesting as diplopia, cranial nerve V causing atypical facial pain or paresthesias, or CN VIII causing hearing impairment and vertigo.[2,4,5] Any clinical presentation of multiple cranial neuropathies in a Lyme-endemic area should prompt a rapid workup for neuroborreliosis. Although there is an increase in cases during spring and summer months, patients often present in fall and early winter as temperatures rise.[16]

CASE 1

A 91-year-old man with a history of hypertension (HTN), hyperlipidemia (HLD), and type-2 diabetes mellitus (T2DM) presented to the emergency department with 4 days of progressive right upper and lower facial weakness. The patient reported complete paralysis of his face, with difficulty eating and drinking, and associated slurred speech. On further questioning, the patient also reported persistent binocular diplopia, and right eyelid ptosis that occurred 2 weeks prior. He denied any change in mentation, numbness, weakness, pain, fever, rash, arthralgia, or headache. Neurologic examination was consistent with a right facial nerve palsy, and right pupil-sparing cranial nerve 3 palsy.

Data

- Serum ELISA Positive, Western Blot negative

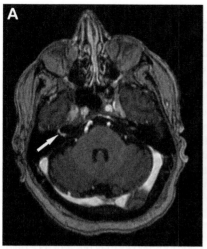 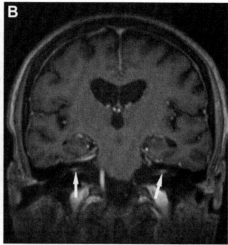

Fig. 1. (*A, B*) MRI brain with gadolinium revealing bilateral cranial nerve VII enhancement (*arrows*).

- MRI Brain with gadolinium demonstrates bilateral cranial nerve 7 enhancement (**Fig. 1**A, B)
- Lumbar Puncture: 120/mm3 WBC (85% lymphocytes, 5% polymorphonucleocytes (PMN), 10% monocytes), 32/mm3 RBC, Protein 210 mg/dL, Glucose 85 mg/dL
- Bacterial and Fungal Culture, Cryptococcal antigen, and Cytology were negative.

Clinical Course: The patient was treated with Doxycycline 100 mg orally twice daily for 14 days and had complete resolution of neurologic symptoms at 3-month follow-up

Commentary: This case illustrates presumed acute neurologic Lyme disease manifested by multiple cranial neuropathies. Though initially puzzling given the patient's lack of history of tick bite, erythema migrans rash or systemic symptoms, and lack of 2 tiered test confirmation, the onset of bilateral CN VII nerve involvement with lymphocytic meningitis in a patient living in an endemic area, especially when coupled with the subsequent response to antibiotics is highly suggestive of *B burgdorferi* infection. Few other diagnoses are associated with bilateral CN VII palsies (see John J. Halperin's article, "Nervous System Lyme Disease – Facts and Fallacies," in this issue). It is important for clinicians to recognize that early in the course of Lyme disease (<3 weeks) it is possible to have a falsely negative serum Lyme Western blot or other confirmatory tests due to the time required for the development of measurable antibody.[17] Lumbar puncture is not routinely recommended in patients with Lyme disease and isolated 7th nerve palsy, but may be helpful in patients presenting with multiple cranial neuropathies. CSF analysis can confirm the suspicion of neuroborreliosis by demonstrating lymphocytic meningitis with an elevated antibody index and is also helpful in ruling out neoplastic or inflammatory etiologies. Appropriate antibiotic treatment should not be delayed in presumed acute neurologic Lyme disease even when serum testing is negative (see **Fig. 4**).

Meningitis

Bacterial meningitis classically presents with acute onset fever, nuchal rigidity, headache, vomiting, photophobia, and altered mentation. Lyme meningitis (and meningitis associated with other spirochetal etiologies such as syphilis and leptospirosis) characteristically differs from most other causes of acute bacterial meningitis, in that the typical presentation is of a less severe isolated headache of subacute onset. Neck pain or stiffness is common but meningismus is typically mild.[1] The onset of Lyme meningitis is typically less acute than bacterial or viral meningitis, evolving over days rather than hours.[17] Rarely, Lyme meningitis can also present with fever, photophobia, and systemic symptoms.[3–7] Clinical features of viral meningitis, especially in the pediatric population, overlap with those due to Lyme disease. Though clinical decision rules to distinguish the two entities have been developed, a recent emergency department-based study underscored the difficulty of identification of Lyme meningitis on clinical findings alone.[11] Lyme meningitis without other findings is sometimes considered a rare presentation of neuroborreliosis in adults, in part because patients will typically seek medical evaluation only when they also demonstrate concomitant cranial neuropathies and polyradiculopathy.[1,3,5,13]

Polyradiculopathy

Thought to be much more common in Europe, neuroborreliosis may present as a painful, usually asymmetric or unilateral polyradiculopathy. When combined with lymphocytic pleocytosis it was termed Bannwarth syndrome.[3,18,19] Patients may describe burning, lightning-like, shooting pains down one or multiple limbs, and may have associated weakness, numbness, or loss of reflexes. This can involve multiple dermatomes, and when polyradiculopathy involves the thoracic nerve roots, pain can be difficult to distinguish from abdominal or thoracic pathologies. This condition is likely underdiagnosed in the United States, and can sometimes coincide with mononeuritis multiplex, another peripheral nervous system manifestation of neuroborreliosis which is the occurrence of multiple mononeuropathies, often mimicking a polyneuropathy.[19,20] It is important for clinicians to be aware that Lyme polyradiculopathy is a nonlength dependent presentation that can closely mimic Guillain–Barre syndrome (GBS) with severe back pain, ascending weakness, and areflexia with sparing of the sensory system. In Lyme endemic areas, a GBS-like presentation should always provoke serum and CSF analysis for mimics such as early disseminated Lyme disease.[20–22] With accurate diagnoses and appropriate early treatment, prognosis for polyradiculopathy is excellent.[23,24]

CASE 2

A 65-year-old men with T2DM presented with 2 weeks of shooting electrical-like pains down his right arm and bilateral legs. The pain started as dull and aching, but soon progressed to severe lightning-bolt sensations of pain radiating from his neck to his right fingertips and from his lower back down both legs to his toes. He reported associated right hand and bilateral feet cramping. The patient presented to the emergency department because over the previous 2 days he began developing significant weakness in his legs, with inability to stand or walk. This started with difficulty getting up from a seated position or standing up from his bed, but rapidly progressed into losing the use of either leg. The patient denied any cranial nerve, bladder or bowel involvement, or sensory loss. Neurologic examination was significant for right intrinsic hand muscle weakness and profound bilateral LE weakness with 1/5 proximally and 3/5 strength distally with diffuse areflexia.

- Serum Lyme ELISA Positive, and Western Blot positive with 2 IgM bands p41 p23, 1 IgG band p41

- Lumbar Puncture: 96/mm3 WBC (98% lymphocytes, 2% monocytes), 10/mm3 RBC, Protein 130 mg/dL, Glucose 72 mg/dL
  - ○ Bacterial and Fungal Culture, Cryptococcal antigen, and Cytology were negative
  - ○ Lyme CSF Antibody Index positive indicating intrathecal antibody synthesis
- MRI Lumbar Spine with and without gadolinium demonstrated avid enhancement of the cauda equina (**Fig. 2**A, B).

Clinical Course: The patient was initially treated with IV ceftriaxone for several days and was subsequently transitioned to oral Doxycycline 100 mg BID for 14 days. The patient underwent repeated MRI and lumbar puncture at 3-month follow-up which were both normal. After several months of rehabilitation, the patient's weakness improved significantly, and at 6 months he was ambulating independently.

Commentary: This case illustrates the classic presentation of polyradiculopathy with CSF lymphocytosis secondary to Lyme disease, a condition called Bannwarth Syndrome. While sensory radiculopathy is usually most prominent, limb weakness can also occur. Rarely, acute Lyme disease may mimic GBS with ascending weakness, pain, and areflexia.[23] In the case of GBS, there would be albuminocytologic dissociation (high protein with normal cell count) rather than a lymphocytic pleocytosis as shown here.

CASE 3

An 80-year-old man with a history of HTN, HLD, T2DM, coronary artery disease (CAD) with pacemaker placement, and prostate cancer who presented to the hospital with progressive neurologic symptoms including diplopia, facial droop, dysphagia, and right arm and hand weakness. Approximately 1 month before presentation, the patient had gradual onset of binocular diplopia followed by developing a left upper and lower facial droop 1 week later. He sought treatment at a local clinic where he was initially treated for idiopathic Bell's palsy with acyclovir and steroids. Although there was some initial improvement in the facial droop, over the next 3 weeks the patient developed symptoms of headache, neck pain, and subsequently dysphagia and dysarthria leading to poor oral intake. The patient sought medical treatment in the emergency

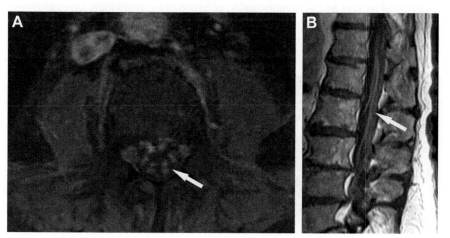

Fig. 2. (*A, B*) MRI lumbar spine with gadolinium showing enhancement of lumbar nerve roots (*arrows*).

department several weeks later when he began to experience right arm and hand weakness with associated shooting pain. Neurologic examination revealed moderate dysarthria without aphasia. Cranial nerve examination was significant for left upper and lower facial paresis with the inability to close the left eye. Motor examination demonstrated distal weakness of right upper extremity with 3/5 strength wrist extension and 2/5 interossei. Reflexes were diminished throughout without upper motor neuron findings.

- Serum Lyme ELISA Positive. Western Blot Positive: IGM Immunoblot positive 3 bands (p41 p39 p23), IGG Immunoblot negative 4 bands (p41,p39,p23,p18)
- Lumbar Puncture: 155/mm3 WBC (90% lymphocytes, 2% PMN, 8% monocyte), 92/mm3 RBC Protein 178 mg/dL, Glucose 91 mg/dL
    - Lyme CSF Antibody Index positive indicating intrathecal antibody synthesis
    - Cytology negative, CSF Cryptococcal Antigen Negative
    - Serum Quantiferon Negative
- MRI Brain with and without gadolinium demonstrated grossly abnormal enhancement of bilateral facial nerves, left greater than right, as well as abnormal contrast enhancement of bilateral trigeminal and oculomotor nerves (**Fig. 3**A, B)

Clinical Course: This patient was admitted for 1 week before a presumptive diagnosis was made. On receipt of a confirmatory Western blot and supportive CSF findings, he was started on IV ceftriaxone. On hospital day 13 the patient suffered a cardiac arrest without successful return of circulation. The cause of death was deemed to be cardiac arrhythmia with pacemaker failure.

Commentary: Patients presenting with symptoms of meningitis, multiple cranial neuropathies, and polyradiculopathy localizes to pathology in the subarachnoid space or brainstem. The initial differential of this case was broad and included infectious (specifically Lyme disease, syphilis, fungal, or tuberculosis), autoimmune (including neurosarcoidosis), and neoplastic etiologies (such as leptomeningeal carcinomatosis or lymphoma). Brain MRI supported the initial localization of the subarachnoid space with the enhancement of multiple cranial neuropathies. Lumbar puncture revealed lymphocytic chronic meningitis. After extensive serum and CSF testing, the diagnosis was established as Lyme meningitis, polyradiculitis, and cranial neuritis. This was specifically supported by a positive peripheral Lyme disease ELISA with confirmatory Western blot as well as the demonstration of lymphocytic meningitis with intrathecal synthesis of Lyme antibodies. Given the sudden and unexpected nature of death, one may consider how Lyme carditis could have played a role in the ultimate cardiac

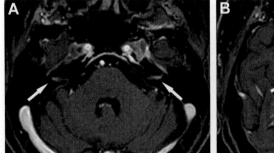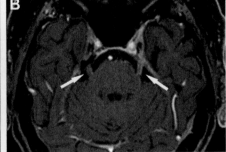

Fig. 3. MRI brain with gadolinium demonstrating enhancement of cranial nerve VII (*arrow, A*), and cranial nerve V (*arrow, B*).

death (see Richard V. Shen and Carol A. McCarthy's article, "Cardiac Manifestations of Lyme Disease," in this issue).

DIAGNOSTIC APPROACH, CLINICAL, LABORATORY, AND IMAGING
Diagnosis

A diagnostic approach to neuroborreliosis should be organized in a stepwise fashion to avoid false positives or delayed diagnosis and to facilitate prompt treatment. In many, but not all cases, there is a history of the presence of other findings suggestive of Lyme disease. With a history of plausible exposure to ticks infected with *B burgdorferi* (see Paul Mead's article, "Epidemiology of Lyme Disease," in this issue), the Infectious Disease Society of America (IDSA) guidelines recommend a two-tiered serum serology testing as the first step, whereby an ELISA test is then confirmed with Western Blot or second ELISA (Modified 2 tier test) to accurately diagnose acute Lyme disease infection.[8] Neurologic manifestations such as those noted above typically occur several weeks after the initial infection, thus at the time of presentation most of these patients will have positive Lyme serology.[3–8] This is not always the case, however, as there can be early manifestations of neuroborreliosis within 1 to 2 weeks of onset of symptoms.[1,3,4] Therefore, in a patient in an endemic area or with recent exposure, and a presentation consistent with neuroborreliosis, empiric treatment is often reasonable even in the absence of positive serum serology. Retesting with serum serology in 3 to 6 weeks will show strongly positive titers,[4,5] but if confirmation is needed sooner, one can pursue a lumbar puncture to demonstrate typical CSF features of lymphocytic pleocytosis with elevated protein and assess Lyme antibody index. This is a measurement of IgG in the CSF as compared with the serum. A level greater than 1 is highly specific to indicate intrathecal production of immunoglobulin against Lyme, and confirms the diagnosis of neuroborreliosis. The sensitivity of antibody index is greater than 85% in 2 small North American studies,[25–27] but a negative CSF antibody index value does not exclude the diagnosis. This titer can remain elevated for years even after successful treatment so is not useful for following the effect of therapy, or for retesting in case of repeat presentation.[26,27] CSF testing for Lyme PCR is generally not helpful, with sensitivity around 5% to 17%.[28–30] CXCL13 is a chemokine which has been suggested to be a potential biomarker for neuroborreliosis, but this is also elevated in other conditions, and standardized thresholds, and interpretive criteria have not been established; therefore, use of this marker is not yet recommended for routine clinical use.[31–33] If neuroimaging is obtained in a patient with meningitis or cranial neuropathy, there may be leptomeningeal or cranial nerve enhancement, respectively.[34] An appropriate diagnostic approach for neuroborreliosis is summarized in **Fig. 4**.

Treatment

Recommended treatment of most cases of early disseminated neuroborreliosis is oral doxycycline. In several studies from Europe, oral therapy has been found to be as effective as intravenous (IV) therapy such as ceftriaxone.[35,36] However, the choice of oral doxycycline or IV ceftriaxone, cefotaxime, and penicillin is dependent on clinical factors such as allergy or medication intolerance, access to parenteral treatment, and patient preference. IV ceftriaxone therapy is often chosen as initial therapy in hospitalized patients or in rare case of parenchymal disease.[8,37] Dose and duration of treatment are listed in **Table 1**. Alternative antibiotics may include amoxicillin, azithromycin, cefuroxime, cefotaxime, or penicillin G, but these choices have not been shown to have equal efficacy for neurologic disease.[8] If a facial nerve palsy is thought to be due to Lyme disease, corticosteroids are not currently recommended

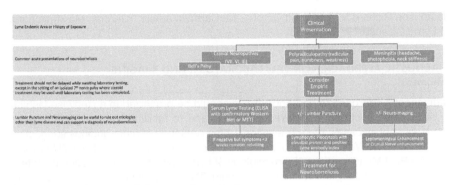

Fig. 4. Diagnostic approach for neuroborreliosis.

as efficacy has not been demonstrated. Important to note, there is efficacy of steroid use in patients with acute onset isolated CN VII palsy due to other causes.[38,39]

Pediatric Considerations

Presentations of neuroborreliosis in children are similar to those in adults, with the exception of reported cases of increased intracranial pressure in some pediatric cases (see also Carol A McCarthy and colleagues' article, "Lyme Disease in Children," in this issue). The diagnosis can be difficult when neurologic symptoms are subtle or accompanied by various systemic complaints. Common symptoms in children affected with neuroborreliosis include headache, fatigue, and neck pain, although if a typical cranial nerve palsy such as CN VII is present, there should be a high index of suspicion for neuroborreliosis.[40] In Europe, lymphocytic meningitis and facial palsy are the most frequent manifestations of neuroborreliosis in children.[40] Neuroborreliosis may account for around 5% of pediatric patients with facial palsy,[13] but this number may be substantially higher for a child in a Lyme endemic area. The presence of bilateral facial nerve palsies is unusual unless due to neuroborreliosis.[4,5,40] Radicular symptoms are rare in children. As noted above, pediatric Lyme meningitis can cause an elevation in intracranial pressure and can mimic idiopathic intracranial HTN.[2] Care should be given to treating elevations in intracranial pressure while also treating the underlying infection.[3,7] The diagnostic approach for children should mirror that of adults, with testing of serum serology followed by CSF testing if clinically indicated. Treatment is also with doxycycline or ceftriaxone for pediatric patients, but the dosing is weight-based (see **Table 1**).[8] Doxycycline is equally effective as in adults and has been shown not to have a significant risk of tooth staining as older tetracyclines, especially with short courses.[41,42]

Outcomes

With adequate treatment of neuroborreliosis, outcomes are excellent.[3,43] While some studies have shown up to 28% of patients may have some residual symptoms, most

Table 1
Treatment recommendations for neuroborreliosis

Drug	Route	Dose	Duration
Doxycycline	Oral	Adults: 100–200 mg daily; Children: 4.4 mg/kg divided twice daily	14–21 d
Ceftriaxone	IV	Adults: 2 g once daily; Children: 50–75 mg/kg once daily (maximum 2 g per dose)	14–21 d

long-term studies have found no effect on mortality, overall health, or educational and social function.[17,44] The amount of those with long-term symptoms thought to be sequelae of Lyme disease have been found to be similar to controls, and many of these may have been unmasked preexisting comorbidities that are unrelated to Lyme infection.[45,46]

SUMMARY

Early disseminated Lyme disease that involves the nervous system commonly presents as cranial neuropathy, meningitis, and polyradiculopathy, although many times in combination. Diagnosis can be made by using an algorithmic approach with serum testing, and in early or complex cases with the aid of CSF or neuroimaging data. Pediatric presentations may additionally include elevations in intracranial pressure that may require additional intervention. With prompt treatment using oral doxycycline or IV ceftriaxone, prognosis is excellent, even for severe manifestations.

CLINICS CARE POINTS

- In Lyme endemic areas or after suspected tick exposure, a presentation of facial palsy, lymphocytic meningitis, polyradiculopathy, or combination of these, should raise suspicion for neuroborreliosis.

- Diagnosis of neuroborreliosis should proceed in a stepwise manner beginning with two-tiered serum serology, and followed by CSF testing to measure IgG index if needed to confirm.

- Treatment of neuroborreliosis consists of 14 to 21 days of oral doxycycline or IV ceftriaxone.

DISCLOSURE

There are no commercial, or financial conflicts of interest, or funding sources for the authors.

REFERENCES

1. Pachner AR, Steere AC. The triad of neurologic manifestations of Lyme disease: meningitis, cranial neuritis, and radiculoneuritis. Neurology 1985;35(1):47–53.
2. Eppes SC, Nelson DK, Lewis LL, et al. Characterization of Lyme meningitis and comparison with viral meningitis in children. Pediatrics 1999;103:957–60.
3. Halperin JJ. Nervous system Lyme disease. In: Biller J, Ferro JM, editors. Handbook of clinical neurology. Neurologic aspects of systemic disease part III121. Elsevier; 2014. p. 1473–83.
4. Halperin JJ. Neuroborreliosis Neurosyphilis. Continuum (Minneap Minn) 2018; 24(5):1439–58.
5. Rauer S, Kastenbauer S, Fingerle V, et al. Lyme neuroborreliosis. Dtsch Arztebl Int 2018;115(45):751–6.
6. Halperin JJ. Lyme disease: a multisystem infection that affects the nervous system. Continuum (Minneap Minn) 2012;18(6, Infectious Disease):1338–50.
7. Halperin JJ. Neuroborreliosis. Neurol Clin 2018;36(4):821–30.
8. Lantos PM, Rumbaugh J, Bockenstedt LK, et al. Clinical Practice Guidelines by the Infectious Diseases Society of America, American Academy of Neurology, and American College of Rheumatology: 2020 guidelines for the prevention, diagnosis, and treatment of lyme disease. Neurology 2021;96(6):262–73.

9. Bingham PM, Galetta SL, Athreya Balu, et al. Neurologic Manifestations in Children with Lyme Disease. Pediatrics 1995;96(6):1053–6.

10. Cohn KA, Thompson AD, Shah SS, et al. Validation of a clinical prediction rule to distinguish Lyme meningitis from aseptic meningitis. Pediatrics 2012;129(1): e46–53.

11. Nigrovic LE, Bennett JE, Balamuth F, et al. Accuracy of Clinician Suspicion of Lyme Disease in the Emergency Department. Pediatrics 2017;140(6):e20171975.

12. Kullberg BJ, Vrijmoeth HD, van de Schoor F, et al. Lyme borreliosis: diagnosis and management. BMJ 2020;369:m1041.

13. Steere AC, Sikand VK. The presenting manifestations of Lyme disease and the outcomes of treatment. N Engl J Med 2003;348(24):2472–4.

14. Halperin JJ. Facial nerve palsy associated with Lyme disease. Muscle Nerve 2003;28(4):516–7.

15. Bierman SM, van Kooten B, Vermeeren YM, et al. Incidence and characteristics of Lyme neuroborreliosis in adult patients with facial palsy in an endemic area in the Netherlands. Epidemiol Infect 2019;147:e160.

16. Kindler W, Wolf H, Thier K, et al. Peripheral facial palsy as an initial symptom of Lyme neuroborreliosis in an Austrian endemic area. Wien Klin Wochenschr 2016;128(21–22):837–40.

17. Knudtzen FC, Andersen NS, Jensen TG, et al. Characteristics and Clinical Outcome of Lyme Neuroborreliosis in a High Endemic Area, 1995–2014: A Retrospective Cohort Study in Denmark. Clin Infect Dis 2017;65(9):1489–95.

18. Tuerlinckx D, Bodart E, Jamart J, et al. Prediction of Lyme Meningitis based on a logistic regression model using clinical and cerebrospinal fluid analysis: a European study. Pediatr Infect Dis 2009;28(5):394–7.

19. Halperin JJ, Luft BJ, Volkman DJ, et al. Lyme neuroborreliosis. Peripheral nervous system manifestations. Brain 1990;113(pt 4):1207–21.

20. Reik L, Steere AC, Bartenhagen NH, et al. Neurologic abnormalities of Lyme disease. Medicine 1979;58(4):281–94.

21. Halperin JJ. Lyme disease and the peripheral nervous system. Muscle Nerve 2003;28(2):133–43.

22. Shah A, O'Horo JC, Wilson JW, et al. An Unusual Cluster of Neuroinvasive Lyme Disease Cases Presenting With Bannwarth Syndrome in the Midwest United States. Open Forum Infect Dis 2017;5(1):ofx276.

23. Muley SA, Parry GJ. Antibiotic responsive demyelinating neuropathy related to Lyme disease. Neurology 2006;74(11):935.

24. Ogrinc K, Lusa L, Lotrič-Furlan S, et al. Course and Outcome of Early European Lyme Neuroborreliosis (Bannwarth Syndrome): Clinical and Laboratory Findings. Clin Infect Dis 2016;63(3):346–53.

25. Steere AC, Berardi VP, Weeks KE, et al. Evaluation of the intrathecal antibody response to Borrelia burgdorferi as a diagnostic test for Lyme neuroborreliosis. J Infect Dis 1990;161:1203–9.

26. Halperin JJ, Volkman DJ, Wu P. Central nervous system abnormalities in Lyme neuroborreliosis. Neurology 1991;41(10):1571–82.

27. Dumler JS. Molecular diagnosis of Lyme disease: review and meta-analysis. Mol Diag 2001;6:1–11.

28. Avery RA, Frank G, Eppes SC. Diagnostic utility of Borrelia burgdorferi cerebrospinal fluid polymerase chain reaction in children with Lyme meningitis. Pediatr Infect Dis J 2005;24:705–8.

29. Cerar T, Ogrinc K, Cimperman J, et al. Validation of cultivation and PCR methods for diagnosis of Lyme neuroborreliosis. J Clin Microbiol 2008;46:3375–9.

30. Eckman EA, Pacheco-Quinto J, Herdt AR, et al. Neuroimmunomodulators in neuroborreliosis and Lyme encephalopathy. Clin Infect Dis 2018;67:80–8.
31. Schmidt C, Plate A, Angele B, et al. A prospective study on the role of CXCL13 in Lyme neuroborreliosis. Neurology 2011;76:1051–8.
32. Cerar T, Ogrinc K, Lotric-Furlan S, et al. Diagnostic value of cytokines and chemokines in Lyme neuroborreliosis. Clin Vaccin Immunol 2013;20:1578–84.
33. Angel TE, Jacobs JM, Smith RP, et al. Cerebrospinal fluid proteome of patients with acute Lyme disease. J Proteome Res 2012;11(10):4814–22.
34. Lindland ES, Solheim AM, Andreassen S, et al. Imaging in Lyme neuroborreliosis. Insights Imaging 2018;9(5):833–44.
35. Bremell D, Dotevall L. Oral doxycycline for Lyme neuroborreliosis with symptoms of encephalitis, myelitis, vasculitis or intracranial hypertension. Eur J Neurol 2014; 21(9):1162–7.
36. Karlsson M, Hammers-Berggren S, Lindquist L, et al. Comparison of intravenous penicillin G and oral doxycycline for treatment of Lyme neuroborreliosis. Neurology 1994;44(7):1203–7.
37. Halperin JJ, Shapiro ED, Logigian EL, et al. Practice parameter: treatment of nervous system Lyme disease (an evidence-based review): report of the Quality Standards Subcommittee of the American Academy of Neurology. Neurology 2007;69(1):91–102.
38. Jowett N, Gaudin RA, Banks CA, et al. Steroid use in Lyme disease-associated facial palsy is associated with worse long-term outcomes. Laryngoscope 2017; 127(6):1451–8.
39. Avellan S, Bremell D. Adjunctive Corticosteroids for Lyme Neuroborreliosis Peripheral Facial Palsy-A Prospective Study With Historical Controls. Clin Infect Dis 2021;73(7):1211–5.
40. Kozak S, Kaminiów K, Kozak K, et al. Lyme Neuroborreliosis in Children. Brain Sci 2021;11(6):758.
41. Volovitz B, Shkap R, Amir J, et al. Absence of tooth staining with doxycycline treatment in young children. Clin Pediatr (Phila) 2007;46(2):121–6.
42. Pöyhönen H, Nurmi M, Peltola V, et al. Dental staining after doxycycline use in children. J Antimicrob Chemother 2017;72(10):2887–90.
43. Garcia-Monco JC, Benach JL. Lyme neuroborreliosis: clinical outcomes, controversy, pathogenesis, and polymicrobial infections. Ann Neurol 2019;85(1):21–31.
44. Obel N, Dessau RB, Krogfelt KA, et al. Long term survival, health, social functioning, and education in patients with European Lyme neuroborreliosis: nationwide population based cohort study. BMJ 2018;361:k1998.
45. Seltzer EG, Gerber MA, Cartter ML, et al. Long-term outcomes of persons with Lyme disease. JAMA 2000;283(5):609–16.
46. Wills AB, Spaulding AB, Adjemian J, et al. Long-term Follow-up of Patients with Lyme Disease: Longitudinal Analysis of Clinical and Quality-of-life Measures. Clin Infect Dis 2016;62(12):1546–51.

Cardiac Manifestations of Lyme Disease

Richard V. Shen, MD[a],*, Carol A. McCarthy, MD[b]

KEYWORDS

- Lyme • Carditis • Cardiac • Atrioventricular block • Heart block

KEY POINTS

- The most common manifestation of Lyme carditis is atrioventricular heart block, but other findings include other arrhythmias and structural manifestations such as myopericarditis.
- Antibiotics (ie, ceftriaxone, doxycycline), are considered effective therapy for Lyme carditis. Adjunctive therapies include cardiac pacing.
- Lyme carditis is generally self-limited with a good prognosis, but rare deaths do occur.
- Early recognition and treatment of Lyme disease are critical for the prevention of Lyme carditis.

INTRODUCTION

Cardiac manifestations of Lyme disease, caused by *Borrelia burgdorferi* sensu stricto in North America, broadly referred to as Lyme carditis, were initially described in 1980 by Steere, and colleagues[1,2] This entity is associated with early disseminated Lyme disease, typically within 2 to 6 weeks of onset of erythema migrans. Steere's initial series of 20 patients, mostly young adult men, were noted to have fluctuating AV heart block and, in some, a diffuse cardiac involvement with left ventricular dysfunction. While some patients received antibiotic treatment, cardiac involvement seemed to resolve regardless of treatment. Subsequent case series, both in children and adults, support the observations that Lyme carditis is usually a self-limited inflammatory process.[1,3–5] Despite the generally benign prognosis, several well-documented cases of untreated Lyme carditis resulted in fatalities, underscoring the importance of early recognition and treatment.

In 1990, the Centers for Disease Control suggested a standard case definition for Lyme carditis as patients with Lyme disease and "acute onset of high-grade atrioventricular conduction defects that resolve in days to weeks and are sometimes

[a] Division of Infectious Diseases, Southcoast Physicians Group, 363 Highland Avenue, Fall River, MA 02720, USA; [b] Division of Pediatric Infectious Diseases, Department of Pediatrics, Barbara Bush Children's Hospital at Maine Medical Center, 887 Congress Street, Suite 310, Portland, ME 04102, USA
* Corresponding author.
E-mail address: shenr@southcoast.org

Infect Dis Clin N Am 36 (2022) 553–561
https://doi.org/10.1016/j.idc.2022.03.001
0891-5520/22/© 2022 Elsevier Inc. All rights reserved.

id.theclinics.com

associated with myocarditis."[6] This definition assumes serologic criteria for Lyme disease are met.

The most common manifestation of cardiac Lyme disease is an acute atrioventricular block, which can be of any degree, and may fluctuate rapidly from first-degree block to Mobitz type 2 or complete heart block. Other reported electrocardiogram findings include T wave abnormalities, ST-segment changes, and prolonged QT intervals.[4,7,8] There have been some case reports of atrial fibrillation.[9] Cardiomyopathy, myocarditis, pericarditis, and cardiomegaly also occur, but these are reported much less frequently than conduction disturbances.[8] One case report documents *B. burgdorferi* in endocardial vegetation suggestive of bacterial endocarditis.[10,11] Abscesses, cardiac or otherwise, have not been reported as a manifestation of cardiac Lyme disease.

Lyme carditis occurs in about 1% of persons with early Lyme disease, and as it is a consequence of disseminated infection, its development may be prevented with early treatment. Therefore, the recognition of early Lyme disease is essential for the prevention of this potentially life-threatening complication.

PATHOPHYSIOLOGY

Lyme carditis follows *B. burgdorferi* infiltration of cardiac tissue and associated curvilinear ("road map") interstitial lymphocytic inflammation involving any anatomic area of the heart.[12–15] Autopsy studies of several patients who had died of Lyme carditis demonstrate similar microscopic findings, along with spirochetes that were usually aligned with collagen fibers.[13–15] There have been limited reports of endomyocardial biopsies that have also demonstrated spirochetes.[16]

This tissue invasion and resultant inflammation can interfere with the heart's conduction system, leading to heart block or other conduction abnormalities. Electrophysiologic studies implicate blocks above the bundle of His, but multiple levels of heart block have been demonstrated.[17,18] More diffuse inflammation outside the conduction system may lead to myocarditis or pericarditis. Myocyte necrosis has rarely been observed, even in fatal cases, consistent with the concept that long-lasting myocardial damage is not expected from this infection.

EPIDEMIOLOGY AND RISK FACTORS

According to the CDC, Lyme carditis is estimated to affect approximately 1% of people with Lyme disease.[19–21] Earlier studies have suggested an incidence ranging from 4% to 10%, but with early recognition and treatment of patients with erythema migrans rashes, incidence has fallen.[1,4,7,22,23] Early diagnosis and treatment of Lyme disease before dissemination may prevent carditis from developing or progressing.[24] *Borrelia spp.* in Europe and Asia can also cause carditis, but the frequency seems to be lower, from 0.3% to 4%.[12,23] The reason for this difference in frequency is unclear but may be related to differing virulence or cardiac tropism in North American and Eurasian *B. spp.*

In North America, Lyme carditis occurs in endemic areas of Lyme disease, that is, the Northeast, northern Midwest, and parts of the Western states. In Canada, the endemic areas include the eastern provinces, mostly in the southern portions. Warming climates and range expansion of blacklegged ticks are increasing the geographic and seasonal pattern of risk exposure to *B. burgdorferi*.

Case series have consistently documented a male predominance in Lyme carditis in general and particularly in the development of complete heart block.[25] A report of 33 pediatric Lyme carditis cases were 64% male and a combined adult and pediatric series of 30 patients from one medical center were 90% male.[4,5] A large European case series of 105 adults noted a "3:1" male predominance, as had Steere's original report.[1,17] Complete heart block has been almost exclusively limited to males in these series and case reports.[25] Reasons for this are unclear, and could potentially be due to a biologic difference in cardiac tissue inflammatory response, stage of disease progression at diagnosis, or other ascertainment or study bias. A similar but less marked phenomenon of male predominance has been reported in viral myocarditis, also without clear explanation.

CLINICAL PRESENTATION
Lyme Carditis and Early Disseminated Lyme Disease

Lyme carditis is a complication of early disseminated disease, typically manifesting in the acute to the subacute phase of Lyme disease, during the second to sixth week of the disease. This is the case for both pediatric and adult patients, and can be in conjunction with localized or disseminated erythema migrans rashes, though a rash is not always seen or reported.[1,4,22] Other findings consistent with early Lyme disease are usually present, such as fever, headache and meningitis, neck pain, and arthralgias.

Cardiac Presentation

Cardiac symptoms, if present, depend on the specific heart manifestation. For instance, with heart block, these symptoms may include presyncope, syncope, or dizziness. Chest pain and dyspnea may accompany myopericarditis. Cardiomyopathies may present with peripheral edema, shortness of breath, or other signs and symptoms of heart failure. These symptoms would be indications for further evaluation, that is, electrocardiograms and, if indicated, echocardiography. Current IDSA guidelines do not recommend routine electrocardiograms in the evaluation of patients with early Lyme disease in the absence of signs or symptoms that indicate possible cardiac involvement.[26] This is based on the observation that although nonspecific changes in the electrocardiogram are common in early Lyme disease, there is no difference in these findings from normal controls.[26] It is important to note that patients with early Lyme disease should be specifically asked about the presence of cardiac symptoms and that the risk of Lyme carditis may be higher in patients with disseminated erythema migrans or other manifestations of disseminated Lyme disease.[4]

Heart block is the most frequent manifestation of Lyme carditis and ranges from very mild first-degree heart block to more severe second- and third-degree atrioventricular block. The degree of atrioventricular block can rapidly progress or worsen. Third-degree heart block is commonly noted in hospital-based series, but usually resolves within a week.[25] Severe disease includes cases with significant PR prolongation greater than 300 milliseconds, second- and/or third-degree AV blocks, and those with more diffuse cardiac involvement that is, myocarditis of pericarditis.[26] Cases with severe disease or at risk of progression to severe disease usually require cardiac monitoring.

Natural History and Outcomes

Early case series noted that conduction disturbances and other manifestations of Lyme carditis usually resolve spontaneously.[1] There are no controlled antibiotic treatment trials, but observational series suggest that antibiotic treatment hastens resolution. Improvement can be rapid, with one study finding a median time for PR interval improvement to less than 300 ms to be about 4 days, but this time period can extend to over a week.[1,4,5] Relapse following standard treatment has not been reported. It is unknown if prior Lyme disease or carditis affects the future risk of Lyme carditis.

Though rare, there have been reports of deaths associated with Lyme carditis, with the CDC noting 11 fatal cases reported worldwide from 1985 to 2019.[14,15,19,27] Many of these are attributed to sudden cardiac arrest. Others are associated with coincident events, whereby the exact cause of death cannot be determined. There has been at least one report of a patient who died soon after an episode of Lyme carditis, which was treated appropriately and had documented improvement with residual mild first-degree heart block at discharge. Unfortunately, details for this specific death are sparse.[5]

ATYPICAL AND RARE PRESENTATIONS
Lyme Endocarditis

In North America, there has thus far been one reported case of Lyme endocarditis.[10,11] This case involved a patient with mitral valve vegetations with negative blood and valve tissue cultures. Lyme endocarditis was diagnosed based on 16S rRNA signature nucleotide analysis testing ("universal PCR") of the valve tissue, which detected *B. burgdorferi*. The diagnosis was further supported by serologic testing consistent with acute Lyme disease by CDC criteria. The patient was treated with 6 weeks of ceftriaxone with reported good clinical outcomes. There have also been 2 case reports of Lyme endocarditis, or at least cardiac valve involvement, in Europe with other *B spp*. Overall, Lyme endocarditis is an extremely rare entity.

Chronic Dilated Cardiomyopathy

In a few European studies, Lyme disease has been proposed as a cause of chronic dilated cardiomyopathy.[1] *B. burgdorferi sensu lato* was detected by PCR in endomyocardial biopsies from several cases with dilated cardiomyopathy.[28] In a North American study of dilated cardiomyopathy in an area endemic for Lyme disease, there was no difference in seropositivity to *B. burgdorferi* between patients with known ischemic cardiomyopathy and those with no known cause.[29] Other studies have reported *B. burgdorferi* cultured in endomyocardial biopsies or a higher than expected seropositivity in dilated cardiomyopathy cases.[30–32] No significant clinical improvement with ceftriaxone treatment was noted in cases seropositive for *B. burgdorferi* in this series or several others.[31–33] A few European case reports of improvement associated with ceftriaxone treatment have led to ongoing discussion, but at this time a possible association of chronic dilated cardiomyopathy and Lyme disease remains speculative.[34]

EVALUATION AND DIAGNOSTICS

The diagnosis of Lyme carditis can be challenging at times, but in essence is based on the recent onset of cardiac manifestations, typically heart block, in conjunction with clinical or serologic evidence of Lyme disease.[19,35] The diagnosis of Lyme disease can be made based on the presence of erythema migrans, or with other suggestive symptoms coupled with serologic testing, which currently consists of a two-tiered testing with an initial Lyme antibody screening test and then subsequent Western blot or other orthogonal confirmatory testing.[26,35] The latter is usually positive at presentation with Lyme carditis, though false negative serology can occur in the first few weeks of Lyme disease.

Dizziness, presyncope, or irregular heartbeats are indications to obtain an electrocardiogram in patients with suspected Lyme disease. As atrioventricular block is the most common cardiac manifestation, the electrocardiogram is an important diagnostic tool.[7,26] Other conduction abnormalities may occur, but are much less frequently reported and may be difficult to attribute to Lyme disease by themselves.[1,9,22]

If there is acute onset of an otherwise unexplained acute myocarditis or pericarditis in a patient with potential exposure, serology for Lyme disease testing is advised. If this testing is consistent with recent Lyme disease and the clinical scenario is suggestive, a diagnosis of Lyme carditis may be considered.[26] Lyme disease-associated pericarditis or myocarditis is usually of mild severity with an excellent outcome, though transient cardiac decompensation has been reported.[4]

Preexisting arrhythmia, cardiomyopathy, or other chronic cardiac conditions are very unlikely to represent sequelae of cardiac Lyme disease. Seropositivity in the setting of a chronic cardiac condition may be due to prior or recent, but unrelated exposure. In the absence of a high clinical probability of Lyme disease, false-positive serologies are common (see Takaaki Kobayashi and Paul G. Auwaerter's article, "Diagnostic Testing for Lyme Disease," in this issue).

It is important to emphasize that the time of onset of cardiac findings is important in informing a diagnosis. Most cases present as a manifestation of early disseminated Lyme disease. Even though it is an early manifestation, seropositivity for antibodies to *B. burgdorferi* is present in most of the cases. Patients who have had symptoms for a month or more are almost uniformly seropositive. Lack of a positive serologic test after this duration of symptoms should cast doubt on a diagnosis of Lyme carditis.

OTHER DIAGNOSTICS

Inflammatory markers, such as sedimentation rate or C-reactive protein, are not specific and do not have a routine role in the management of Lyme carditis. Troponins or other markers of cardiac stress might be elevated in cases of Lyme myopericarditis, but are also nonspecific markers of cardiac injury.

Imaging studies such as echocardiograms or cardiac magnetic resonance imaging can be useful in certain circumstances. For instance, imaging studies may aid in diagnosing myocardial involvement in a patient with Lyme disease without more typical conduction abnormalities on EKG. However, pursuit of these studies depends on the individual patient's situation and the clinical suspicion for non–conduction-related cardiac manifestations.

DIFFERENTIAL DIAGNOSIS

Other infectious etiologies of new onset of atrioventricular heart block or myopericarditis include bacterial endocarditis, syphilis, cardiac abscess, viral or bacterial myopericarditis, and acute rheumatic fever. Noninfectious etiologies that may explain a recently acquired heart block or myopericarditis may include ischemia, rheumatic or autoimmune conditions, infiltrative myocardial diseases such as amyloidosis or sarcoidosis, or intrinsic and degenerative conduction system abnormalities.

TREATMENT

The mainstay of treatment of Lyme carditis, as per 2020 IDSA guidelines, is interim cardiac monitoring and intensive care support as needed, and antibiotic therapy.[26]

Antibiotics

For milder cases treated as outpatients, oral antibiotics are preferred, with doxycycline being the first-line option. Alternative oral antibiotics include amoxicillin and cefuroxime.[26]

In more severe cases, intravenous ceftriaxone is recommended as initial therapy. Ceftriaxone is typically continued until there is improvement, such as the resolution of heart block or improvement to the point that further monitoring is not needed. In the case of atrioventricular heart block, improvement of a PR interval to less than 300 milliseconds would a reasonable point to transition to oral therapy. Of course, what constitutes improvement depends on the specific cardiac manifestation, clinical scenario, and patient symptoms. At the point of improvement and cardiac stability, transition to oral antibiotics offers less potential toxicity and is usually recommended.[26]

Of note, there is limited case report data to suggest the use of oral doxycycline alone as an option to treat even severe carditis. As an example, a case of Lyme carditis with complete heart block, which was initially misinterpreted as first-degree heart block, resolved with doxycycline alone.[36] It is not known whether other manifestations of carditis can be treated with oral agents alone.

The currently recommended antibiotic duration is 14 to 21 days.[26]

Cardiac Monitoring

Particularly in severe cases, continuous electrocardiographic monitoring may be necessary.[26] This can inform the need for temporary cardiac pacing, and also is useful to monitor response to antibiotics.

Cardiac Pacing

If indicated, temporary artificial cardiac pacing may be required in severe cases of Lyme carditis and can be lifesaving. The indications for artificial pacing are the same as for other causes of advanced atrioventricular or nodal blocks. Typically it is reserved for high degree heart blocks or for highly symptomatic or unstable patients.[37] If pacing is necessary, the duration of pacing can be variable but generally can be discontinued after improvement in the underlying conduction disturbance. Usually, atrioventricular conduction blocks due to Lyme carditis improve within 1 week, often in several days with antibiotics.[5] Thus, temporary pacing is almost always sufficient. There have been case reports of a need for permanent pacing, but these reports are rare and may have been required due to a coexisting cardiac condition.[38]

DISCUSSION

Lyme carditis is an infrequent but serious complication of untreated Lyme disease, usually occurring within the first few weeks of infection. Treatment at the onset of erythema migrans rashes or other early manifestations of Lyme disease may prevent the development of Lyme carditis.

A recent case series suggests that even in an area endemic to Lyme disease, there may still be gaps in the recognition and diagnosis of the disease.[5] In that series, most patients had seen an outpatient provider before developing symptoms of Lyme carditis, but only a minority were diagnosed with or suspected to have Lyme disease (41%), and even fewer were started on appropriate antibiotics (12%).[5] Missed or delayed diagnosis and treatment of Lyme disease would then increase the risk of Lyme carditis and other complications. Emphasizing education for frontline medical providers in endemic areas is needed to overcome this gap.

The paucity of data and studies surrounding risk factors for Lyme carditis presents further hurdles for preventing and understanding this complication of Lyme disease. Clinical observations of Lyme carditis consist of case reports and series, and one autopsy series.[22] The information on pediatric patients is even more limited; the largest published cases series in children (n = 33) includes only 14 with advanced heart block.[4] Another more recent series examined both adults and children, examining 10 pediatric and 20 adult cases.[5] There were no substantial differences seen between adult and pediatric outcomes.

Though there are effective antibiotics for treating Lyme carditis and managing its effects, the data are more observational than experimental.[26] The generally good prognosis and the relative rarity of Lyme carditis limit the feasibility of clinical trials to determine optimal therapies and antibiotic duration.

SUMMARY

Lyme carditis is an uncommon manifestation of Lyme disease. The vast majority of cases will present with an atrioventricular or nodal conduction block of varying degrees, but other findings occur less often. Lyme carditis typically has a good prognosis, especially when appropriately treated. However, there is still a chance of significant morbidity and rarely, mortality.

Experience over the decades has provided effective antibiotic options for Lyme carditis, but there are no controlled clinical trials to inform optimal management.

As with any disease, prevention is key. For this, earlier recognition and treatment of Lyme disease, which stops progression to Lyme carditis, is critical.

CLINICS CARE POINTS

- Lyme carditis is a manifestation of early disseminated Lyme disease, with heart block as the most common manifestation. However, the range of cardiac findings can be broad.
- Diagnosis of cardiac Lyme is based on a clinical or serologic diagnosis of acute Lyme disease, along with compatible acute cardiac manifestations.
- Effective treatment consists of 14 to 21 days of antibiotics. Mild or outpatient cases may be treated with oral antibiotics. More severe cases generally receive intravenous antibiotics, at least until substantial improvement occurs.
- Cardiac pacing, if needed, is generally temporary. Permanent pacing is a rare exception.
- Cardiac manifestations are either self-limited or completely resolve with appropriate antibiotics. However, rare deaths have been reported.
- Lyme carditis, and other Lyme disease complications, can be prevented with early recognition and treatment of Lyme disease.

DISCLOSURE

None of the authors of this article have any relevant commercial or financial conflicts of interest. The authors did not receive funding for this article.

REFERENCES

1. Steere AC, Batsford WP, Weinberg M, et al. Lyme carditis: cardiac abnormalities of lyme disease. Ann Intern Med 1980;93(1_Part_1):8–16.
2. Steere AC. Lyme disease. N Engl J Med 1989;321(9):586–96.
3. van der Linde MR, Crijns HJ, Lie KI. Transient complete AV block in Lyme disease. Electrophysiologic Observations. Chest 1989;96(1):219–21.
4. Costello JM, Alexander ME, Greco KM, et al. Lyme carditis in children: presentation, predictive factors, and clinical course. Pediatrics 2009;123(5):e835–41.

5. Shen RV, McCarthy CA, Smith RP. Lyme carditis in hospitalized children and adults, a case series. Open Forum Infect Dis 2021;8(7):ofab140.

6. Wharton M, Chorba TL, Vogt RL, et al. Case definitions for public health surveillance. MMWR Recomm Rep 1990;39(Rr-13):1–43.

7. Cox J, Krajden M. Cardiovascular manifestations of Lyme disease. Am Heart J 1991;122(5):1449–55.

8. McAlister HF, Klementowicz PT, Andrews C, et al. Lyme carditis: an important cause of reversible heart block. Ann Intern Med 1989;110(5):339–45.

9. Zainal A, Hanafi A, Nadkarni N, et al. Lyme carditis presenting as atrial fibrillation. BMJ Case Rep 2019;12(4).

10. Fatima B, Sohail MR, Schaff HV. Lyme disease-an unusual cause of a mitral valve endocarditis. Mayo Clin Proc Innov Qual Outcomes 2018;2(4):398–401.

11. Paim AC, Baddour LM, Pritt BS, et al. Lyme Endocarditis. Am J Med 2018;131(9): 1126–9.

12. Scheffold N, Herkommer B, Kandolf R, et al. Lyme carditis–diagnosis, treatment and prognosis. Dtsch Arztebl Int 2015;112(12):202–8.

13. Duray PH. Histopathology of clinical phases of human Lyme disease. Rheum Dis Clin North Am 1989;15(4):691–710.

14. Cary NR, Fox B, Wright DJ, et al. Fatal Lyme carditis and endodermal heterotopia of the atrioventricular node. Postgrad Med J 1990;66(772):134–6.

15. Muehlenbachs A, Bollweg BC, Schulz TJ, et al. Cardiac tropism of borrelia burgdorferi: an autopsy study of sudden cardiac death associated with lyme carditis. Am J Pathol 2016;186(5):1195–205.

16. de Koning J, Hoogkamp-Korstanje JA, van der Linde MR, et al. Demonstration of spirochetes in cardiac biopsies of patients with Lyme disease. J Infect Dis 1989; 160(1):150–3.

17. van der Linde MR. Lyme carditis: clinical characteristics of 105 cases. Scand J Infect Dis Suppl 1991;77:81–4.

18. Sigal LH. Early disseminated Lyme disease: cardiac manifestations. Am J Med 1995;98(4a):25S–8S [discussion: 28S-29S].

19. CDC. Lyme carditis | Lyme disease. CDC; 2020. Available at: https://www.cdc. gov/lyme/treatment/lymecarditis.html. Accessed November 12, 2021.

20. CDC. Lyme disease data tables | Lyme Disease. CDC; 2019. Available at: https:// www.cdc.gov/lyme/stats/tables.html#modalIdString_CDCTable_1. Accessed March 22, 2020.

21. CDC. Lyme Disease Cases by Symptoms. 2016. Available at: www.cdc.gov/lyme/ stats/graphs.html. Accessed March 22, 2020.

22. Robinson ML, Kobayashi T, Higgins Y, et al. Lyme carditis. Infect Dis Clin North Am 2015;29(2):255–68.

23. Fish AE, Pride YB, Pinto DS. Lyme carditis. Infect Dis Clin North Am 2008;22(2): 275–88, vi.

24. Kowalski TJ, Tata S, Berth W, et al. Antibiotic treatment duration and long-term outcomes of patients with early lyme disease from a lyme disease-hyperendemic area. Clin Infect Dis 2010;50(4):512–20.

25. Forrester JD, Mead P. Third-degree heart block associated with lyme carditis: review of published cases. Clin Infect Dis 2014;59(7):996–1000.

26. Lantos PM, Rumbaugh J, Bockenstedt LK, et al. Clinical Practice Guidelines by the Infectious Diseases Society of America (IDSA), American Academy of Neurology (AAN), and American College of Rheumatology (ACR): 2020 Guidelines for the Prevention, Diagnosis and Treatment of Lyme Disease. Clin Infect Dis 2021;72(1):1–8.

27. CDC. Three sudden cardiac deaths associated with Lyme carditis - United States. MMWR 2013;62:993–6.
28. Kubánek M, Šramko M, Berenová D, et al. Detection of Borrelia burgdorferi sensu lato in endomyocardial biopsy specimens in individuals with recent-onset dilated cardiomyopathy. Eur J Heart Fail 2012;14(6):588–96.
29. Sonnesyn SW, Diehl SC, Johnson RC, et al. A prospective study of the seroprevalence of Borrelia burgdorferi infection in patients with severe heart failure. Am J Cardiol 1995;76(1):97–100.
30. Stanek G, Klein J, Bittner R, et al. Isolation of Borrelia burgdorferi from the myocardium of a patient with longstanding cardiomyopathy. N Engl J Med 1990;322(4):249–52.
31. Stanek G, Klein J, Bittner R, et al. Borrelia burgdorferi as an etiologic agent in chronic heart failure? Scand J Infect Dis Supplementum 1991;77:85–7.
32. Bergler-Klein J, Glogar D, Stanek G. Clinical outcome of Borrelia burgdorferi related dilated cardiomyopathy after antibiotic treatment 1992;340(8814):317–8.
33. Piccirillo BJ, Pride YB. Reading between the Lyme: is Borrelia burgdorferi a cause of dilated cardiomyopathy? The debate continues. Eur J Heart Fail 2012; 14(6):567–8.
34. Gasser R, Dusleag J, Fruhwald F, et al. Early antimicrobial treatment of dilated cardiomyopathy associated with Borrelia burgdorferi. Lancet 1992; 340(8825):982.
35. CDC. Notice to readers: recommendations for test performance and interpretation from the Second National Conference on Serologic Diagnosis of Lyme Disease. MMWR Morb Mortal Wkly Rep 1995;44:590–1.
36. Burns M, Robben P, Venkataraman R. Lyme carditis with complete heart block successfully treated with oral doxycycline. USA: Military Medicine; 2021.
37. Gammage MD. Temporary cardiac pacing. Heart 2000;83(6):715–20.
38. Artigao R, Torres G, Guerrero A, et al. Irreversible complete heart block in lyme disease. Am J Med 1991;90(4):531–3.

Lyme Arthritis

Sheila L. Arvikar, MD*, Allen C. Steere, MD

KEYWORDS

- Lyme disease • *Borrelia burgdorferi* • Lyme arthritis • Postinfectious arthritis
- Postantibiotic arthritis • Inflammatory arthritis

KEY POINTS

- Lyme arthritis (LA) is a late disease manifestation, usually beginning months after the tick bite.
- Patients have intermittent or persistent attacks of joint swelling and pain, in one or a few large joints, especially the knee, without prominent systemic manifestations.
- The diagnosis is supported by 2-tier serologic testing for *B. burgdorferi* by ELISA and IgG Western blotting.
- Initial treatment is a 30-day course of oral doxycycline or amoxicillin. For patients with minimal or no response to oral treatment, IV therapy with ceftriaxone is recommended.
- A minority of patients may have persistent synovitis for months or several years after oral and IV antibiotic therapy, which may be caused by excessive inflammatory immune responses and is treated with anti-inflammatory agents, DMARDs, or synovectomy.

INTRODUCTION
Epidemiology

Lyme arthritis (LA) was originally recognized because of an outbreak of monoarticular and oligoarticular arthritis in children in Lyme, Connecticut in the 1970s.[1] It then became apparent that Lyme disease was a complex multisystem illness affecting primarily the skin, nervous system, heart or joints.[2] Before the use of antibiotic therapy for the treatment of the disease, about 60% of untreated patients developed LA, a late disease manifestation.[3] In recent years, 30,000 to 40,000 cases of Lyme disease have been reported annually to the Centers for Disease Control and Prevention (CDC), and in a third of reported cases, arthritis was a manifestation of the disease.[4] However, CDC estimates suggest the actual number of patients diagnosed with Lyme disease annually may be 10-fold higher.[5] There is a male predominance (60% cases) among reported LA cases.[4] Although Lyme disease may affect individuals of any age, there is a bimodal age distribution with middle-aged adults and children being most

Center for Immunology and Inflammatory Diseases, Massachusetts General Hospital, CNY149 Room 8301, 149 13th Street, Charlestown, MA 02129, USA
* Corresponding author.
E-mail address: sarvikar@mgh.harvard.edu

Infect Dis Clin N Am 36 (2022) 563–577
https://doi.org/10.1016/j.idc.2022.03.006
0891-5520/22/© 2022 Elsevier Inc. All rights reserved.

affected; 35% of reported LA cases between 2008 and 2015 were in the 10 to 14-year-old age group.[4]

The infection is transmitted primarily by nymphal *Ixodes scapularis* ticks, which quest in the late spring and early summer.[6] However, LA can present at any time of the year. Most of the cases occur in the Northeastern, Mid-Atlantic, and upper-Midwestern areas of the United States.[4]

In the United States, *Borrelia burgdorferi* is the sole cause of Lyme disease, and arthritis is the primary disseminated disease manifestation. In contrast, in Europe where *Borrelia afzelii* and *Borrelia garinii* are the major agents of Lyme borreliosis, acrodermatitis, and neuroborreliosis, respectively, are more frequent manifestations than arthritis.[7] Subtypes of *B. burgdorferi* also differ in pathogenicity.[8,9] OspC type A (RST1) strains, which account for 30% to 50% of the infection in the northeastern US,[8,9] but only 3% in mid-Western states,[10] are particularly virulent and arthritogenic. These strains are thought to have played an important role in the emergence of the Lyme disease epidemic in the northeastern US in the late 20th century.[11]

Pathogenesis

B. burgdorferi often disseminates to joints, tendons, or bursae early in the infection.[6] Although this event may be asymptomatic, transient or migratory arthralgias may occur at that time. LA, a late disease manifestation, usually occurs months later. Why there is a delay in the onset of arthritis following the initial infection is unclear. However, one explanation may be that the spirochete initially evades immune clearance by residing in relatively avascular structures such as tendons and later invades synovial tissue.[12] LA is accompanied by intense innate and adaptive immune responses, particularly Th1 responses in synovial mononuclear cells to *B. burgdorferi* antigens, producing large amounts of IFN-γ.[13] The adaptive immune response leads to the production of specific antibodies, which opsonize the organism, facilitating phagocytosis and effective spirochetal killing.

With appropriate oral and, if necessary, IV antibiotic therapy, spirochetes are eradicated, and joint inflammation resolves in the great majority of patients. However, in a small percentage of patients (<10%), synovial inflammation persists for months or several years despite receiving oral and intravenous antibiotic therapy for 2 or 3 months, called postinfectious or postantibiotic arthritis (previously antibiotic-refractory arthritis).[14] Steroid use before antibiotic treatment may be associated with a refractory outcome.[14,15] In children, older age, longer duration of arthritis before diagnosis, and poor initial response to antibiotics are risk factors for this outcome.[16]

The synovial lesion in patients with postinfectious LA is similar to that of other chronic inflammatory arthritides, such as rheumatoid arthritis, with marked synovial fibroblast proliferation, fibrosis, and infiltration of mononuclear cells (**Fig. 1**). However, there is more evidence of vascular damage in postinfectious LA, with obliterative microvascular lesions seen in approximately 50% of patients, which is a unique feature of LA synovia.[17] A combination of pathogen and host-associated factors (**Box 1**) contribute to postinfectious LA.[18]

Postantibiotic LA is associated with infection with highly inflammatory strains of *B. burgdorferi* (RST 1 strains) commonly found in the northeastern United States. However, persistent infection in the postantibiotic period does not appear to play role in this outcome. Polymerase chain reaction (PCR) testing of synovial fluid for *B. burgdorferi* DNA, which is often positive before treatment, is usually negative by the conclusion of antibiotic treatment, and both culture and PCR testing of synovial tissue have been uniformly negative from synovectomy specimens obtained months to years after antibiotic therapy.[19] Although active infection has resolved, spirochetal

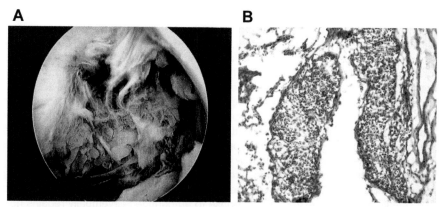

Fig. 1. Postantibiotic Lyme arthritis synovium. (*A*) An image of postantibiotic Lyme arthritis at arthroscopic synovectomy is shown, demonstrating vascular proliferation and synovial hypertrophy. (*B*) The histology of synovial tissue is shown in a patient postantibiotic Lyme arthritis highlighting 2 villi with dense inflammatory infiltrate along the synovial lining and sublining layer. The section is stained with hematoxylin and eosin and shown at 20X magnification.

remnants may play a role in driving continued inflammation in the postinfectious period. In MyD88 −/− mice, which have high pathogen loads, spirochetal antigens are retained on cartilage surfaces.[20] *B. burgdorferi* peptidoglycan, a cell wall component that is difficult to clear, has been found in synovial fluid of patients with LA and has been shown to trigger arthritis in BALB/c mice.[21]

However, the critical factor in postinfectious LA seems to be an excessive, maladaptive host inflammatory response during the infection, and failure to down-regulate inflammatory responses appropriately after spirochetal killing.[22] The excessive proinflammatory response prevents tissue repair and return to homeostasis following spirochetal killing and results in vascular damage, autoimmune responses, cell-mediated cytotoxicity, and fibrosis. A hallmark feature of postinfectious LA is exceptionally elevated IFN-γ levels which persist in the postinfectious period, accompanied by inadequate levels of the anti-inflammatory cytokine IL-10.[18] Patients with a TLR1 polymorphism (1805 GG), which is found in half of the European Caucasian population, are at risk for excessively elevated IFN-γ levels in joints when infected with

---

Box 1
Factors associated with postantibiotic lyme arthritis

Pathogen
- Infection with highly inflammatory RST-1 type strain[9]
- Possible retained spirochetal antigens such as peptidoglycan[12,20,21]

Genetic
- Certain HLA-DR alleles[24]
- TLR1-1805 GG polymorphism[23]

Immunologic
- Excessive inflammatory response with high amounts of IFN-gamma[18]
- Inadequate amounts of the anti-inflammatory cytokine IL-10[18]
- Decreased ratio of Treg/Teff cells among synovial fluid mononuclear cells[26,27]
- Lyme-associated autoantibodies[27–30]

B. burgdorferi RST1 strains.[23] Similarly, specific HLA-DR alleles, such as DRB1:0401 that bind an epitope of *B. burgdorferi* outer-surface protein A (OspA), may also predispose to elevated IFN-γ levels.[24] Further, immune dysregulation may result from an imbalance in Th-1 effector-T regulatory cells, as some cells which are ordinarily regulatory T cells secrete large amounts of IFN-γ.[25,26] In addition, patients with postinfectious LA may have Lyme-disease-associated autoantibodies to vascular antigens, such as endothelial cell growth factor, apolipoprotein B-100, or annexin A2, or toan extracellular matix protein, matrix metalloproteinase-10, which may further contribute to pathology.[27–29] IgG4 Lyme disease autoantibody titers correlate with magnitude of obliterative microvascular lesions and fibrosis in synovial tissue.[30]

Despite heightened immune reactivity, postinfectious arthritis eventually resolves. Thus, it seems that spirochetal killing, either by the immune system or with the assistance of antibiotic therapy, removes the innate immune "danger" signals. Without these signals, the adaptive immune response to autoantigens eventually regains homeostasis, and arthritis resolves. This process may be facilitated by therapy with disease-modifying antirheumatic drugs (DMARDs).

CLINICAL PRESENTATION

During the 1970s before the cause of the disease was known, the natural history of LA was elucidated in a study of 55 nonantibiotic-treated patients who were followed prospectively from the onset of erythema migrans (EM), the initial skin lesion, through the period of arthritis.[3] Clinical features of the infection in these patients included the following:

- Arthritis began from 4 days to 2 years (mean, 6 months) after the EM skin lesion.
- Patients had intermittent or persistent attacks of joint swelling and pain, primarily in one or a few large joints, especially the knee, during a period of several years.[3] However, particularly in earlier episodes, other large or small joints, the temporomandibular joint, or periarticular sites (bursa, tendons) were sometimes affected.
- Generally fewer than 5 joints were affected at one time.
- Knee joints were often very swollen, but not particularly painful, and ruptured Baker's cysts were common.
- By the time arthritis was present, systemic manifestations (fever or other constitutional symptoms) were uncommon.

In present times, early Lyme disease is often recognized and treated with antibiotics, preventing the development of arthritis. Therefore, LA now occurs primarily in patients with asymptomatic early infection in whom arthritis is the presenting manifestation of the disease. Thus, the diagnosis should be considered in patients from endemic areas presenting with monoarticular or oligoarticular arthritis, whether or not there is an history of an antecedent tick bite, flu-like illness, or EM rash.

Patients with LA typically lack fever or prominent systemic symptoms. Since acute neurologic involvement, meningitis, facial palsy, radiculoneuropathy or carditis occurs with early disseminated infection, they are rarely seen concurrently in patients with LA. However, in rare cases, patients with LA may have concurrent sensory polyneuropathy or radiculoneuropathy.

Differential Diagnosis

In addition to serologic testing, clinical features may distinguish LA from other entities (**Table 1**). A common concern is mechanical injury in an active individual, and therefore, orthopedists are often the first specialist to see patients with LA. However, the

Table 1
Differential diagnosis of Lyme arthritis

Diagnosis	Distinguishing Clinical Features	Helpful Laboratory Tests
Septic arthritis	Significant pain with range of motion, fever	Synovial fluid culture
Gonococcal arthritis	Tenosynovitis, fever, pustular rash	Synovial fluid culture
Crystalline arthritis	Significant pain with range of motion, history of podagra	Synovial fluid crystals
Rheumatoid arthritis	Symmetric polyarthritis (5 or more joints involved),	RF and CCP
Juvenile idiopathic arthritis	May have polyarthritis, enthesitis, psoriasis	ANA, RF, CCP
Reactive arthritis	Preceding gastrointestinal, genitourinary, or respiratory infection, enthesitis, eye involvement, rashes	HLA-B27
Ankylosing spondylitis, Psoriatic arthritis, or other spondyloarthropathy	Axial (spine, sacroiliac joint) symptoms, psoriasis, enthesitis,	HLA-B27
Fibromyalgia	Diffuse pain, lack of synovitis	ESR/CRP (normal)
Posttreatment Lyme disease syndrome	Nonspecific pain, fatigue, and neurocognitive symptoms, lack of synovitis	ESR/CRP (normal)
Autoimmune/Inflammatory arthritis triggered by Lyme	History of treated Lyme disease, polyarthritis, psoriasis, spondyloarthropathy features, axial involvement	RF/CCP antibodies, HLA-B27, *B. burgdorferi* antibodies (low titer)

clinical picture of LA is most like reactive arthritis in adults or oligoarticular juvenile idiopathic arthritis in children, and serologic testing is essential to distinguish LA from these entities. Children may have a more acute presentation, with higher synovial WBC counts, which may suggest a diagnosis of acute septic arthritis.[31–33] However, LA typically causes only minimal-to-moderate pain with passive range of motion, and involvement of more than one joint (currently or by history) may help to distinguish LA from septic bacterial arthritis.[31–33] LA rarely, if ever, causes chronic, symmetric polyarthritis, which helps to distinguish LA from rheumatoid arthritis and lupus. Fibromyalgia is sometimes misdiagnosed as "chronic" Lyme disease, but patients with fibromyalgia generally have diffuse pain, and they lack objective evidence of joint inflammation. However, a subset of patients, usually following early Lyme disease, may experience persistent pain, fatigue, and neurocognitive symptoms after appropriate antibiotic treatment, known as posttreatment Lyme disease syndrome (PTLDS).[34] The clinical picture in these patients is like that seen in fibromyalgia. Patients with PTLDS do not have objective synovitis as is seen in patients with LA.

Other autoimmune or autoinflammatory arthritides, such as rheumatoid arthritis, reactive arthritis, or psoriatic arthritis may develop within months after Lyme disease.[35] Although these events may be coincidental, it is possible that latent autoimmunity may be triggered by adjuvant or other immune effects of spirochetal infection. As antibody responses to *B. burgdorferi* following antibiotic-treated LA typically persist for many years, positive serologic results can present a diagnostic challenge if these patients subsequently develop another type of arthritis.[36]

PHYSICAL EXAMINATION

Patients with LA typically have the following features on physical examination:

- Monoarthritis or oligoarthritis most commonly affects the knees, but other large or small joints may be affected, such as an ankle, shoulder, elbow, or wrist.
- Affected knees may have very large effusions with warmth, but in contrast with typical bacterial (eg, staphylococcal) septic arthritis, they are not particularly painful with the range of motion or weight-bearing. Baker's cysts may be present in the knees given the large size of effusions, and rupture of cysts is common.
- Fever is usually not present.

A photograph of typical knee swelling in LA is shown in **Fig. 2**.

IMAGING AND ADDITIONAL TESTING
Serologic Testing for Lyme Disease

The mainstay in diagnosing LA is serologic testing. In the US, the CDC currently recommends a two-test approach in which samples are first tested for antibodies to *B. burgdorferi* by enzyme-linked immunosorbent assay (ELISA) and those with equivocal or positive results are subsequently tested by a second assay, traditionally Western blotting (WB), with findings interpreted according to the CDC criteria.[37] Recently, the FDA approved the use of a second enzyme immunoassay (EIA) as an acceptable alternative to the Western blot, referred to as modified 2-tier testing.[38] However, for LA, the standard method involving an EIA followed by a Western blot provides more information and is preferred by the authors.

In contrast with early infection, when some patients may be seronegative, all patients with LA, have positive serologic results for IgG antibodies to *B. burgdorferi*, with the expansion of the response to many spirochetal proteins.[39] Using microarrays, patients with LA have been shown to have IgG reactivity to as many as 89 spirochetal proteins.[40] Serologic testing should be performed only in serum, as Western blots of synovial fluid are not accurate.[41]

In addition to IgG antibody responses to *B. burgdorferi*, patients with LA may also have low-titer IgM reactivity with the spirochete. On the other hand, a positive IgM response alone in a patient with arthritis is likely to be a false-positive response or one indicative of previous, antibiotic-treated early Lyme disease in a patient who now has another type of arthritis. Therefore, positive IgM antibody responses alone should not be used to support the diagnosis of LA. After spirochetal killing with antibiotics, antispirochetal antibody titers decline gradually, but both the IgG and IgM responses in patients with past LA may remain positive for years,[36] which seems to be an indicator of immune memory rather than active infection. We have not observed reinfection in patients with the expanded immune response generated in patients with LA. Therefore, a persistent, expanded IgG antibody response seems to be protective against reinfection, whereas the limited antibody response seen in patients with EM is not.

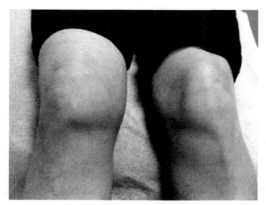

Fig. 2. Lyme arthritis. A swollen knee of a patient with Lyme arthritis is shown.

Synovial Fluid Polymerase Chain Reaction for B. burgdorferi

Although reported in a few patients,[42] it is exceedingly difficult to culture *B. burgdorferi* from synovial fluid in patients with LA. This is presumably due to the fact that joint fluid, with its many inflammatory mediators, is a hostile environment. In spiked cultures, adding small amounts of joint fluid results in rapid killing of spirochetes.[17] In contrast, PCR testing of synovial fluid for *B. burgdorferi* DNA often yields positive results before antibiotic therapy (range, 40%–96%),[19,43] and usually becomes negative following antibiotic treatment.[14] However, spirochetal DNA may persist for at least weeks after spirochetal killing, which limits its use as a test for active infection. Moreover, PCR testing has not been standardized for routine clinical use. Therefore, in most cases, the appropriate clinical picture and a positive serologic result are sufficient for the diagnosis of LA, and PCR testing is an optional test to further support the diagnosis.

Synovial Fluid Analysis, Imaging, and Other Tests

On presentation, joint aspiration is usually conducted for diagnostic purposes to rule out the presence of other arthritides such as crystalline arthropathy or staphylococcal septic arthritis. Joint fluid white cell counts are usually in an inflammatory range (10,000–25,000 cells/mm^3), but cell counts as low as 500 or as high as 100,000 cells/mm^3 have been reported.[3] Although tests for rheumatoid factor or antinuclear antibodies typically yield negative results, antinuclear antibodies in low titer may be detected. Peripheral white blood cell (WBC) counts are usually within the normal range, but inflammatory markers, such as ESR and CRP, may be elevated. An algorithm using elevated absolute neutrophil count >10,000 and ESR>40 mm/h, helped to distinguish septic monoarthritis from LA in pediatric patients in an endemic area.[44]

In patients with LA, plain films, MRI scanning, or ultrasound typically show nonspecific joint effusions. With MRI and ultrasound studies synovial thickening and inflammation may be apparent. In adult patients, imaging studies may show coincidental degenerative changes or chronic mechanical injuries, but these abnormalities would not be expected to cause significant synovitis or inflammation. Typical synovitis by ultrasound in an LA patient is shown in **Fig. 3**. LA is not rapidly erosive, but with longer arthritis durations, joint damage can be seen in radiographic studies.[45,46] Imaging is not required for diagnosis, but may be useful in following response to treatment and determining the extent of residual synovitis. In our clinic, we particularly use

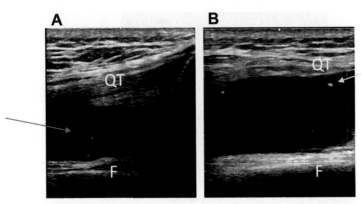

Fig. 3. Ultrasound image of Lyme arthritis. Longitudinal suprapatellar view (along long axis of quadriceps tendon) of left knee is shown. (*A*) Anechoic effusion is noted by blue arrow. Proximal continuation is shown in B, with large effusion distending suprapatellar recess, synovitis (gray material), and Doppler signal (*yellow arrow*). F, femur; QT, quadriceps tendon. (*Courtesy of* Minna Kohler, MD, Boston, MA).

musculoskeletal ultrasound for this purpose. Finally, MRI scanning may be useful in the planning of synovectomy by determining the extent of synovitis within the joint.

Treatment

Treatment of LA is based on several small, double-blind, or randomized studies and observational studies (summarized in **Table 2**). The efficacy of antibiotics was first demonstrated in a double-blind, placebo-controlled trial of IM benzathine penicillin, 2.4 million units weekly for 3 weeks versus placebo. In that study, 7 of 20 antibiotic-treated patients (35%) had complete resolution of arthritis, whereas all 20 placebo-treated patients continued to have arthritis.[47] Subsequently, 11 of 20 patients (55%) treated with IV penicillin, 20 million U daily in 6 divided doses for 10 days, had resolution of arthritis.[47] It was then reported that IV ceftriaxone, 2 g daily, was effective in 90% of patients who were given 2 to 4 weeks of therapy.[48] In a later randomized trial, treatment with 30 days of doxycycline, 100 mg twice daily, or amoxicillin, 500 mg four times daily, also led to the resolution of arthritis in 90% of patients.[49]

According to current recommendations from the Infectious Diseases Society of America American Academy of Neurology, and American College of Rheumatology,[50] patients with LA should be treated initially with a 28-day course of oral antibiotic, doxycycline, 100 mg twice daily, or amoxicillin, 500 mg three times daily. In patients who are unable to take either of these oral agents, cefuroxime axetil, 500 mg twice daily, may be an acceptable alternative. This medication was shown to be equivalent to treatment with doxycycline or amoxicillin in patients with EM,[51] but has not been studied systematically in patients with LA. Unless there are concomitant neurologic abnormalities, oral regimens are the initial treatment of choice as such therapy is safer and more cost-effective.

In our experience, some patients do require longer courses of antibiotic therapy for effective treatment of LA.[14] Thus, if there is mild residual joint swelling after a 28-day course of oral antibiotics, we repeat the oral antibiotic regimen for another 28 days. However, for patients with minimal response and continued moderate-to-severe joint swelling after a 28-day course of oral antibiotics, it is recommended to treat with IV antibiotics which may have better tissue penetration, rather than the second course

Table 2
Prospective studies of antibiotic therapy in lyme arthritis

Author	Year	Trial Type/Treatment	Patients	Outcomes
Steere et al.[47]	1985	Double-blind, placebo-controlled trial of intramuscular benzathine penicillin (PCN) for 3 wk vs placebo Additional 20 patients received IV PCN 20 million units/d for 10 d	40 with Lyme arthritis 20 with Lyme arthritis	7/20 (35%) PCN-treated patients had complete response vs 0/20 in placebo arm ($P = 0.02$) 11/20 (55%) had complete resolution
Dattwyler et al.[48]	1988	Randomized to IV treatment with PCN (10 d) or ceftriaxone (CTX) (14 d) Additional nonrandomized cohort treated with CTX 2 or 4g	23 patients with late Lyme (16 with arthritis) 31 patients (23 with arthritis)	5/10 responded to PCN vs 12/13 responded to CTX 27/31 patients responded to CTX Overall >90% response to CTX
Steere et al.[49]	1994	Randomized trial of doxycycline or amoxicillin plus probenecid for 30 d, Or 2 wk of IV CTX for patients with persistent arthritis 3 mo after oral antibiotics or PCN	50 with Lyme arthritis	18/20 patients receiving doxycycline and 16/18 receiving amoxicillin had a complete response by 3 mo 5 patients later developed neuroborreliosis. 0/16 patients treated with IV CTX had resolution with 3 mo.
Dattwyler et al.[52]	2005	Randomized trial of CTX, 14 vs 28 d regimen	143 patients with late Lyme disease	5 failures out of 80 patients in 14-d group, but 0 failures out of 63patients in the 28-d group ($P = 0.07$). Increased adverse events in the 28-d group ($P = 0.02$)
Oksi et al.[54]	2007	Double-blind randomized placebo-controlled trial of adjunct oral antibiotic therapy (amoxicillin) vs placebo for 100 d following 3 wk of IV CTX	107 patients with definite disseminated Lyme disease, including 45 with arthritis	Excellent/good response in 49/53 in the amoxicillin group and 47/54 in placebo-treated groups (NS). 37/45 patients with Lyme arthritis had excellent or good responses.

Abbreviations: CTX, ceftriaxone; IV, intravenous; PCN, Penicillin.

of oral antibiotics. Typically, we treat with IV ceftriaxone, 2gm/d. Although there is a trend toward greater efficacy with 4 weeks compared with 2 weeks of antibiotics, there is also a greater frequency of adverse events.[52] Thus, our practice is to prescribe a 4-week course of IV therapy, but to monitor the patient closely and to stop treatment if complications occur.

Even in patients with minimal or no improvement with oral doxycycline, we typically observe moderate improvement or even complete resolution of arthritis with IV therapy. Moreover, even in those with persistent joint inflammation, the synovitis tends to change after IV therapy with decreased size of effusions but increased synovial tissue hypertrophy and continued inflammation. Courses longer than 30 days of IV antibiotics seem not to be beneficial and may be associated with greater adverse effects.[53] Additionally, a double-blind, randomized, placebo-controlled study of patients in Europe did not find a benefit of additional oral amoxicillin therapy following treatment with IV ceftriaxone.[54] While bacterial "persisters" have been observed in culture and in some animal studies, it is not clear that alternative antibiotic regimens targeting spirochetal persisters would be beneficial in postantibiotic syndromes.[22]

Adjunctive Therapy

During antibiotic treatment, nonsteroidal antiinflammatory agents (NSAIDs), such as ibuprofen or naproxen, may be used for pain. We do not use oral or intraarticular corticosteroids before or during antibiotic treatment, as these drugs may permit greater growth of spirochetes[55] and may be associated with a worse outcome.[14,15] Moreover, we use them only sparingly after antibiotic treatment. When joints are inflamed, reduction of activity is important. If patients are limping, we advise crutch walking. Children may be more likely to regain normal function within 4 weeks after the initiation of antibiotic treatment,[32] but especially in adults, inflamed joints typically lead to quadriceps atrophy. Therefore, following the completion of antibiotic treatment and resolution of joint inflammation, formal physical therapy is often needed.

Therapy for Postantibiotic Arthritis

The algorithm that we use for the diagnosis and treatment of LA and postantibiotic arthritis is shown in **Fig. 4**.[14] If synovitis persists following 2 or more months of oral antibiotics and 1 month of IV antibiotics, we use a similar approach to that used in the treatment of other forms of chronic inflammatory arthritis, including rheumatoid arthritis and reactive arthritis. The agents used include NSAIDs, such as ibuprofen or naproxen, and DMARDs, typically methotrexate (MTX), depending on the severity of arthritis. Although there have been no formal trials with these agents, in practice, they reduce the severity of inflammation and have not resulted in breakthrough cases of active infection. We generally do not give oral corticosteroids. The role of intraarticular steroids following antibiotic treatment is unclear, though some studies in children have found benefit.[56,57] In our experience, intraarticular injections of corticosteroids may have clinical utility as bridge therapy when starting DMARDs, but alone do not usually lead to sustained improvement.

In more recent years, with greater experience using more potent DMARD agents, we have developed an enhanced treatment strategy, now more commonly choosing low-dose MTX, typically 15 to 20 mg/wk, over hydroxychloroquine as the initial DMARD, and reserving hydroxychloroquine, typically 400 mg daily, for cases with milder synovitis. Moreover, in a few patients who had incomplete responses to MTX or in those with contraindications to MTX, we have used TNF inhibitors, generally injectable forms such as etanercept or adalimumab.[14] The onset of action of MTX and other DMARDs can be slow, but we generally see a significant response in 1 to

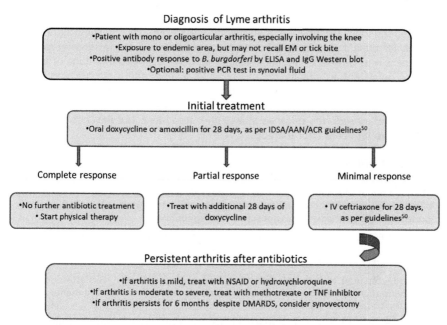

Fig. 4. Algorithm for the diagnosis and treatment of Lyme arthritis. AAN, American Academy of Neurology; ACR, American College of Rheumatology; DMARDs, disease-modifying antirheumatic drugs; ELISA, enzyme-linked immunosorbant assay; EM, erythema migrans; IDSA, Infectious Disease Society of America; IV, intravenous; NSAID, nonsteroidal anti-inflammatory drug; PCR, polymerase chain reaction.

3 months. As postantibiotic arthritis eventually resolves in all patients with LA,[14] long courses of DMARD therapy are generally not needed. We typically prescribe these medications for only 6 to 12 months rather than indefinitely as in the treatment of patients with rheumatoid arthritis. If the response to a DMARD agent is incomplete and if the arthritis is limited to one joint, primarily the knee, arthroscopic synovectomy is an option.[58]

Finally, though postantibiotic LA is the major postinfectious complication, we occasionally see patients with diffuse pain, neurocognitive or fatigue symptoms of PTLDS following LA. In addition, we occasionally see patients with LA who subsequently develop other forms of inflammatory arthritis.[35]

SUMMARY

In the United States, arthritis is the major late manifestation of Lyme disease, usually beginning months after the tick bite. However, because of greater recognition and treatment of early disease which prevents later arthritis, a history of EM or other early disease manifestations is now often lacking in patients with LA. Patients have intermittent or persistent attacks of joint swelling and pain, primarily in one or a few large joints, often the knee, during a period of months to several years, with few systemic manifestations. The diagnosis is established by two-tier serologic testing for *B. burgdorferi* by ELISA and IgG Western blotting, which typically shows strong responses to many spirochetal proteins with many bands present. PCR testing of synovial fluid for *B. burgdorferi* DNA is often positive before antibiotic therapy, but the test is not a reliable indicator of spirochetal eradication following antibiotic treatment. The recommended initial treatment is a 30-day course of oral doxycycline or amoxicillin. However, for patients with minimal or no response to oral therapy, IV ceftriaxone for 2 to 4 weeks may be needed for successful treatment. A small percentage of patients may have persistent arthritis for months or several years after both oral and IV antibiotic therapy, which may be treated successfully with anti-inflammatory agents, DMARDs, or synovectomy, depending on the severity of arthritis. The antibody response to *B. burgdorferi* declines slowly after treatment, but the test typically remains positive for years after therapy.

CLINICS CARE POINTS

- The diagnosis of LA is based on a positive IgG antibody response in blood. IgM positivity may also be present, but it is not required for the diagnosis. IgM positivity alone, without the presence of IgG antibodies, does not support a diagnosis of LA.

- A positive PCR test in synovial fluid is an optional test but is not required for the diagnosis of LA. PCR testing may remain positive for weeks or longer after spirochetal killing and is not a reliable marker for active infection.

- Antibody responses to *B. burgdorferi* may remain positive for many years after successful treatment of LA. Resolution of the serologic response cannot be used as criteria for successful treatment of the infection.

- The diagnosis of LA should be considered in patients from endemic areas presenting with monoarticular or oligoarticular arthritis, whether or not there is any history of an antecedent tick bite or EM rash.

- LA is most commonly a mono or oligoarticular arthritis affecting one or both knees and does not manifest as symmetric polyarthritis such as rheumatoid arthritis.

- Patients with postantibiotic LA respond well to DMARD therapy without recurrence of infection.

DISCLOSURE

The authors declare no conflicts of interest related to this article. Dr A.C. Steere is supported by NIH grants R01-AI-101175 and R01-AI-144365, the Mathers Foundation, and the Eshe Fund. Dr S.L. Arvikar has received support from the Global Lyme Alliance.

REFERENCES

1. Steere AC, Malawista SE, Snydman DR, et al. Lyme arthritis: an epidemic of oligoarticular arthritis in children and adults in three Connecticut communities. Arthritis Rheum 1977;20(1):7–17.
2. Steere AC, Malawista SE, Hardin JA, et al. Erythema chronicum migrans and Lyme arthritis. the enlarging clinical spectrum. Ann Intern Med 1977;86(6): 685–98.
3. Steere AC, Schoen RT, Taylor E. The clinical evolution of Lyme arthritis. Ann Intern Med 1987;107(5):725–31 *Key article.
4. Schwartz AM, Hickley AF, Mead PS, et al. Surveillance for Lyme disease—United States, 2008-2015. MMWR Surveill Summ 2017;66:1–12.
5. Kugeler KJ, Schwartz AM, Delory M, et al. Estimating the frequency of Lyme disease diagnoses – United States, 1020-2018. Emerg Infect Dis 2021;27:616–9.
6. Steere AC. Lyme disease. N Engl J Med 1989;321(9):586–96 *Key article.

7. Steere AC, Strle F, Wormser GP, et al. Lyme borreliosis. Nat Rev Dis Primers 2016; 15(2):16090.

8. Wormser GP, Brisson D, Liveris D, et al. *Borrelia burgdorferi* genotype predicts the capacity for hematogenous dissemination during early Lyme disease. J Infect Dis 2008;198(9):1358–64.

9. Jones KL, McHugh GA, Glickstein LJ, et al. Analysis of *Borrelia burgdorferi* genotypes in patients with Lyme arthritis: High frequency of ribosomal RNA intergenic spacer type 1 strains in antibiotic-refractory arthritis. Arthritis Rheum 2009;60(7): 2174–82.

10. Hanincova K, Mukherjee P, Ogden NH, et al. Multilocus sequence typing of *Borrelia burgdorferi* suggests existence of lineages with differential pathogenic properties in humans. PLoS One 2013;8(9):e73066.

11. Hoen AG, Margos G, Bent SJ, et al. Phylogeography of *Borrelia burgdorferi* in the eastern United States reflects multiple independent Lyme disease emergence events. Proc Natl Acad Sci USA 2009;106(35):15013–8.

12. Wormser GP, Nadelman RB, Schwartz I. The amber theory of Lyme arthritis: initial description and clinical implications. Clin Rheumatol 2012;31(6):989–94.

13. Steere AC, Coburn J, Glickstein L. The emergence of Lyme disease. J Clin Invest 2004;113(8):1093–101.

14. Steere AC, Angelis SM. Therapy for Lyme arthritis: strategies for the treatment of antibiotic-refractory arthritis. Arthritis Rheum 2006;54(10):3079–86 *Key article.

15. Bentas W, Karch H, Huppertz HI. Lyme arthritis in children and adolescents: outcome 12 months after initiation of antibiotic therapy. J Rheumatol 2000; 27(8):2025–30.

16. Horton DB, Taxter AJ, Davidow AL, et al. Pediatric antibiotic-refractory Lyme arthritis: a multicenter case-control study. J Rheumatol 2019;46(8):943–51.

17. Lochhead RB, Arvikar SL, Aversa JM, et al. Robust interferon signature and suppressed tissue repair gene expression in synovial tissue from patients with post-infectious, Borrelia burgdorferi-induced Lyme arthritis. Cell Microbiol 2019;21(2): e12954.

18. Lochhead RB, Strle K, Arvikar SL, et al. Lyme arthritis: linking infection, inflammation and autoimmunity. Nat Rev Rheumatol 2021;17(8):449–61 *Key article.

19. Li X, McHugh G, Damle N, et al. Burden and viability of *Borrelia burgdorferi* in skin or joints of patients with erythema migrans or Lyme arthritis. Arthritis Rheum 2011;63(8):2238–47.

20. Bockenstedt LK, Gonzalez DG, Haberman AM, et al. Spirochete antigens persist near cartilage after murine Lyme borreliosis therapy. J Clin Invest 2012;122(7): 2652–60.

21. Jutras BL, Lochhead RB, Kloos ZA, et al. *Borrelia burgdorferi* peptidoglycan is a persistent antigen in patients with Lyme arthritis. Proc Natl Acad Sci USA 2019; 116(27):13498–507.

22. Steere AC. Posttreatment Lyme disease syndromes: distinct pathogenesis caused by maladaptive host responses. J Clin Invest 2020;130(5):2148–51.

23. Strle K, Shin JJ, Glickstein LJ, et al. Association of a toll-like receptor 1 polymorphism with heightened Th1 inflammatory responses and antibiotic-refractory Lyme arthritis. Arthritis Rheum 2012;64(5):1497–507.

24. Steere AC, Drouin EE, Glickstein LJ. Relationship between immunity to *Borrelia burgdorferi* outer-surface protein A (OspA) and Lyme arthritis. Clin Infect Dis 2011;52(S3):S259–65.

25. Shen S, Shin JJ, Strle K, et al. Treg cell numbers and function in patients with antibiotic-refractory or antibiotic-responsive Lyme arthritis. Arthritis Rheum 2010;62(7):2127–37.

26. Vudattu NK, Strle K, Steere AC, et al. Dysregulation of CD4+CD25(high) T cells in the synovial fluid of patients with antibiotic-refractory Lyme arthritis. Arthritis Rheum 2013;65(6):1643–53.

27. Drouin EE, Seward RJ, Strle K, et al. A novel human autoantigen, endothelial cell growth factor, is a target of T and B cell responses in patients with Lyme disease. Arthritis Rheum 2013;65(1):186–96.

28. Londoño D, Cadavid D, Drouin EE, et al. Antibodies to endothelial cell growth factor and obliterative microvascular lesions in the synovium of patients with antibiotic-refractory Lyme arthritis. Arthritis Rheumatol 2014;66(8):2124–33.

29. Crowley JT, Strle K, Drouin EE, et al. Matrix metalloproteinase-10 is a target of T and B cell responses that correlate with synovial pathology in patients with antibiotic-refractory Lyme arthritis. J Autoimmun 2016;69:24–37.

30. Sulka KB, Strle K, Crowley JT, et al. Correlation of Lyme disease-associated IgG4 autoantibodies with synovial pathology in antibiotic-refractory Lyme arthritis. Arthritis Rheumatol 2018;70(11):1835–46.

31. Aiyer A, Hennrikus W, Walrath J, et al. Lyme arthritis of the pediatric lower extremity in the setting of polyarticular disease. J Child Orthop 2014;8(4):359–65.

32. Daikh BE, Emerson FE, Smith RP, et al. Lyme arthritis: a comparison of presentation, synovial fluid analysis, and treatment course in children and adults. Arthritis Care Res 2013;65(12):1986–90.

33. Deanehan JK, Kimia AA, Tan Tanny SP, et al. Distinguishing Lyme from septic knee monoarthritis in Lyme disease-endemic areas. Arthritis Rheumatol 2014; 66(8):2124–33.

34. Aucott JN. Posttreatment Lyme disease syndrome. Infect Dis Clin North Am 2015; 29(2):309–23.

35. Arvikar SL, Crowley JT, Sulka KB, et al. Autoimmune arthritides, rheumatoid arthritis, psoriatic arthritis, or peripheral spondyloarthritis following lyme disease. Arthritis Rheumatol 2017;69(1):194–202.

36. Kalish RA, McHugh G, Granquist J, et al. Persistence of immunoglobulin M or immunoglobulin G antibody responses to Borrelia burgdorferi 10-20 years after active Lyme disease. Clin Infect Dis 2001;33(6):780–5.

37. Centers for Disease Control and Prevention. Recommendations for test performance and interpretation from the second international conference on serologic diagnosis of lyme disease. MMWR Morb Mortal Wkly Rep 1995;44(31):590–1.

38. Mead P, Petersen J, Hinckley A. Updated CDC recommendation for serologic diagnosis of lyme disease. MMWR Morb Mortal Wkly Rep 2019;68(32):703.

39. Steere AC, McHugh G, Damle N, et al. Prospective study of serologic tests for Lyme disease. Clin Infect Dis 2008;47(2):188–95.

40. Barbour AG, Jasinskas A, Kayala MK, et al. A genome-wide proteome array reveals a limited set of immunogens in natural infections of humans and white-footed mice with Borrelia Burgdorferi. Infect Immun 2008;76(8):3374–89.

41. Barclay SS, Melia MT, Auwaerter PG. Misdiagnosis of late-onset Lyme arthritis by inappropriate use of Borrelia burgdorferi immunoblot testing with synovial fluid. Clin Vaccin Immunol 2012;19(11):1806–9.

42. Snydman DR, Schenkein DP, Berardi VP, et al. Borrelia burgdorferi in joint fluid in chronic Lyme arthritis. Ann Intern Med 1986;104(6):798.

43. Nocton JJ, Dressler F, Rutledge BJ, et al. Detection of *Borrelia burgdorferi* DNA by polymerase chain reaction in synovial fluid in Lyme arthritis. N Engl J Med 1994;330(4):229–34.

44. Grant DS, Neville DN, Levas M, et al. Validation of septic knee monoarthritis prediction rule in a lyme disease endemic area. Pediatr Emerg Care 2022;38(2): e881–5, for Pedi Lyme Net.

45. Lawson JP, Steere AC. Lyme arthritis: radiologic findings. Radiology 1985;154(1): 37–43.

46. Miller JB, Albayda J, Aucott JN. The value of musculoskeletal ultrasound for evaluation of postinfectious lyme arthritis. J Clin Rheumatol 2022;28(2):e605–8. https://doi.org/10.1097/RHU.0000000000001732. Epub ahead of print.

47. Steere AC, Green J, Schoen RT, et al. Successful parenteral penicillin therapy of established Lyme arthritis. N Engl J Med 1985;312(14):869.

48. Dattwyler RJ, Halperin JJ, Volkman DJ, et al. Treatment of late Lyme borreliosis–randomised comparison of ceftriaxone and penicillin. Lancet 1988;1(1896): 1191–4.

49. Steere AC, Levin RE, Molloy PJ, et al. Treatment of lyme arthritis. Arthritis Rheum 1994;37(6):878–88.

50. Lantos PM, Rumbaugh J, Bockenstedt LK, et al. Clinical practice guidelines by the infectious diseases society of America (IDSA), American Academy of neurology (AAN), and American college of rheumatology (ACR): 2020 guidelines for the prevention, diagnosis and treatment of lyme disease. Clin Infect Dis 2021; 72(1):1–8 *Key article. PMID: 33483734.

51. Nadelman RB, Luger SW, Frank E, et al. Comparison of cefuroxime axetil and doxycycline in the treatment of early Lyme disease. Ann Intern Med 1992; 117(4):273–80.

52. Dattwyler RJ, Wormser GP, Rush TJ, et al. A comparison of two treatment regimens of ceftriaxone in late Lyme disease. Wien Klin Wochenschr 2005; 117(11–12):393–7.

53. Fallon BA, Keilp JG, Corbera KM, et al. A randomized, placebo-controlled trial of repeated IV antibiotic therapy for Lyme encephalopathy. Neurology 2008;70(13): 992–1003.

54. Oksi J, Nikoskelainen J, Hiekkanen H, et al. Duration of antibiotic treatment in disseminated Lyme borreliosis: a double-blind, randomized, placebo-controlled, multicenter clinical study. Eur J Clin Microbiol Infect Dis 2007;26(8): 571–81.

55. Pachner AR, Delaney E, O'Neill T. Neuroborreliosis in the nonhuman primate: *Borrelia burgdorferi* persists in the central nervous system. Ann Neurol 1995;38(4): 667–9.

56. Nimmrich S, Becker I, Horneff G. Intraarticular corticosteroids in refractory childhood Lyme arthritis. Rheumatol Int 2014;34(7):987–94.

57. Horton DB, Taxter AJ, Davidow AL, et al. Intraarticular glucocorticoid injection as second-line treatment for lyme arthritis in children. J Rheumatol 2019;46(8): 952–9.

58. Schoen RT, Aversa JM, Rahn DW, et al. Treatment of refractory chronic Lyme arthritis with arthroscopic synovectomy. Arthritis Rheum 1991;34(8):1056–60.

Nervous System Lyme Disease–Facts and Fallacies

John J. Halperin, MD[a,b],*

KEYWORDS

- Lyme disease • *Borrelia burgdorferi* • Neuroborreliosis
- Garin–Bujadoux–Bannwarth syndrome • Nervous system
- Peripheral nervous system • Central nervous system • Intrathecal antibody

KEY POINTS

- The nervous system is involved in 10% to 15% of patients with untreated infection with *B. burgdorferi*, a proportion that is the same with both Eurasian and North American strains of the spirochete.
- Nervous system infection causes either meningitis or multifocal inflammatory changes in the peripheral (frequent) or central (rare) nervous system, evidenced by objective changes on neurologic examination or other objective tests.
- As in many other systemic infectious and inflammatory states, patients may experience cognitive and memory difficulty; these symptoms are neither indicative of CNS infection nor diagnostic of Lyme disease.
- Treatment with standard courses of oral antimicrobials cures approximately 95% of patients with neuroborreliosis. Parenteral treatment may be needed in those rare patients with parenchymal CNS involvement, but some evidence supports the use of oral therapy in these individuals as well.

"It was the best of times, it was the worst of times, it was the age of wisdom, it was the age of foolishness, it was the epoch of belief, it was the epoch of incredulity…" These famous opening words of Dickens' A Tale of Two Cities aptly describe much of what is said today about Lyme disease and its effects on the nervous system. Numerous factors contribute to this[1,2]; probably the single most important is that patients, the public in general and even many physicians struggle with the concept of what does–and does not–constitute nervous system disease. While nervous system function is essential for all behavior, many things affect behavior in the absence of damage to the nervous system–the defining requirement of neurologic disorders. Conditions as diverse as sleep deprivation, sepsis, depression, uremia, psychosis, and learned behaviors can profoundly alter how we function–but none of these necessarily implies the presence of neurologic disease. Since the possibility of neurologic diseases–stroke,

---

[a] Overlook Medical Center, Summit, NJ 07901, USA; [b] Sidney Kimmel Medical College of Thomas Jefferson University
* Department of Neurosciences, Overlook Medical Center, Summit, NJ 07078.
E-mail address: John.halperin@atlantichealth.org

Infect Dis Clin N Am 36 (2022) 579–592
https://doi.org/10.1016/j.idc.2022.02.007
0891-5520/22/© 2022 Elsevier Inc. All rights reserved.

Alzheimer's, Parkinson's, to name a few–is truly terrifying to most of us, it could be argued that these misconceptions about nervous system Lyme disease, or Lyme neuroborreliosis (LNB), contribute substantially to the widespread fear of this tick-borne infection, and some patients' and physicians' willingness to use highly unconventional therapies to try to eradicate what is, in reality, a straightforward infection.

Although the term Lyme disease was coined in the 1970s, with the first reports of nervous system involvement appearing shortly thereafter,[3,4] the first description of neuroborreliosis actually was published in 1922 in a case report[5] that both was brilliant in its insights and foreshadowed how misunderstandings about the specifics of neurologic diagnosis can result in confusion.

Three weeks following the bite of an *Ixodes* tick on his left buttock, a French sheep farmer developed severe pain at the site of the bite and an erythroderm that expanded to cover the entire buttock, much of the thigh, and the lower abdomen. The distribution of the pain expanded–he developed bilateral sciatica and severe and intractable pain in the trunk and right arm. When evaluated his examination was normal except for marked right deltoid atrophy and weakness. He had a neutrophilic cerebrospinal fluid (CSF) pleocytosis with elevated protein and normal glucose. In light of a slightly positive Wasserman test, the authors concluded this was a spirochetosis–but went to great pains to explain why this could not possibly have been syphilis–and treated him with neoarsphenamine (standard of care syphilis treatment in 1922) with rapid resolution of his pain.

While this succinctly captured most of the key elements of neuroborreliosis, the authors' discussion also revealed several logical flaws. In attributing the infection to a spirochetosis, they considered spirochetes to be a type of virus, reflecting limitations of medical knowledge at that time. They equated this patient's problem to tick bite paralysis–a noninfectious disorder that occurs while a tick is still attached, not weeks later and is not associated with a rash, pain, or a CSF pleocytosis. Unfortunately, inappropriate linking of superficially similar disorders continues to this day.

As European clinical experience with this disorder grew, these misunderstandings became unimportant. The disorder became known as Garin–Bujadoux (and subsequently Bannwarth) syndrome and by the 1950s was routinely recognized by European neurologists and treated with penicillin.[6] In the 1970s and '80s the essentially identical neurologic syndrome–described in greater detail in Tyler Crissinger and Kelly Baldwin's article, "Early Disseminated Lyme Disease: Cranial Neuropathy, Meningitis and Polyradiculopathy," in this issue–was described in US patients in association with Lyme disease, and similarly found to be responsive to penicillin.[3]

It would be reasonable to assume that there could be little controversy surrounding an illness that has been well characterized for a century, caused by a known, antibiotic-sensitive microorganism. A quick perusal of the over 2000 Lyme disease-related titles at Amazon.com (fortunately a decreasing fraction of the approximately 15,000 published scientific papers listed in a Medline search on the same day, December 28, 2021) suggests challenges persist.

In summarizing what is well known about neuroborreliosis, the goal of this article will be to address 4 key fallacies (**Box 1**): (1) that nervous system infection with *B burgdorferi* can cause every imaginable neurologic presentation, without any pattern or specificity; (2) that nervous system Lyme disease, like some neurologic disorders, is inexorably progressive and difficult if not impossible to cure; (3) that, in a patient with Lyme disease, nonspecific cognitive symptoms are indicative of nervous system disease; and (4) that such nonspecific symptoms are sufficiently indicative of Lyme disease that treatment is appropriate even in the absence of other evidence supporting the diagnosis. Addressing these fallacies requires one key understanding–that for

---

Box 1
Neuroborreliosis *fallacies*

- Nervous system Lyme disease:
  - Can cause every imaginable neurobehavioral abnormality
  - Is incurable and causes progressive brain deterioration

- Symptoms of fatigue, memory or cognitive disorders, or other neurobehavioral changes
  - In patients with Lyme disease are evidence of nervous system infection
  - Are sufficiently specific for Lyme disease that they support the diagnosis absent any other laboratory or clinical support

---

patients to be diagnosed with nervous system Lyme disease they must have (**Box 2**) both nervous system disease and Lyme disease and there must be a rational basis for believing the 2 are causally linked.

REQUIREMENT #1: NERVOUS SYSTEM DISEASE

An underlying premise of neurology is that neurologic disease is caused by structural damage to the nervous system–at either a macroscopic or microscopic level. The clinical signs and symptoms of nervous system disorders can vary widely, reflecting the specific structures involved and the severity of the damage. One patient with a stroke on MRI imaging may have no demonstrable symptoms, another may be incapacitated with hemiparesis and aphasia. The range of clinical presentations does not reflect a biologic mystery but rather that for any given pathophysiologic process, the size, site, and severity of damage may vary widely. However, if considered within a logical framework, specific patterns are usually evident and can be helpful in inferring an appropriate differential diagnosis, pathophysiology, and therapy.

This framework typically begins with categorization based on either structural or functional neuroanatomy. At its most basic, neuroanatomic localization begins with separating central nervous system (CNS) from peripheral nervous system (PNS) disorders. Primary nervous system disorders usually affect the central or the peripheral nervous system, and only rarely both, frequently with localizing patterns within the affected system. A single localized site of a CNS lesion suggests, in the appropriate context, a stroke, tumor, or other structural abnormality. Localization of a single PNS lesion suggests nerve compression, inflammation, ischemia, or other focal abnormality. Recognition that a disorder involves the meninges will point to an infectious, hemorrhagic, or rarely neoplastic cause. Involvement of function-related populations of neurons can point to specific neurodegenerative processes such as amyotrophic lateral sclerosis (upper and lower motor neurons), Parkinson's (substantia nigra), and so forth.

In contrast to these localizable primary disorders of the nervous system, systemic illnesses often affect the nervous system in a more widespread fashion. Despite being

---

Box 2
Prerequisites to diagnose nervous system Lyme disease

Evidence of:
- Lyme disease
- Nervous system disease
- Causal relation between the 2
  - Syndrome within the clinical/pathophysiologic spectrum linked to Lyme disease *and/or*
  - In CNS disorders evidence of CNS inflammation and intrathecal antibody production

very well protected–mechanically by the skull and vertebral column and physiologically by the blood–brain, blood–CSF, and blood–nerve barriers–the CNS and PNS are occasionally involved in systemic inflammatory or infectious processes. Some infectious agents have developed highly specific mechanisms to invade the nervous system. In some circumstances circulating immune molecules and cells, though normally excluded from the nervous system, enter the CNS and PNS and contribute to damage. Consequently, the absence of a well-defined anatomic pattern usually suggests a disseminated process such as the immune dysregulation of Guillain Barre syndrome, or the widespread involvement of CNS and PNS in vasculitis or diabetic vasculopathy.

In contrast, many systemic illnesses can affect behavior without causing nervous system damage. From psychiatric disease to altered mental status in hypoglycemia, there is a broad range of biochemical, medical, environmental and physiologic alterations that impact behavior but are not neurologic. One of the most frequently seen in medicine is the encephalopathy that accompanies a systemic inflammatory state. A patient with pneumonia, particularly if older, can easily develop delirium. This is not indicative of CNS infection but rather is the effect of fever and circulating cytokines on the nervous system.

REQUIREMENT #2: LYME DISEASE INVOLVING THE NERVOUS SYSTEM

The diagnosis of Lyme disease itself is well addressed in Takaaki Kobayashi and Paul G. Auwaerter's article, "Diagnostic Testing for Lyme Disease," in this issue; the diagnosis of nervous system Lyme disease requires compelling evidence the patient actually has Lyme disease and also has causally related nervous system involvement. European and US neurologists have adopted slightly different diagnostic criteria for neuroborreliosis[7,8] (**Boxes 3** and **4**) but differences relate more to emphasis than substance.

Neuroborreliosis occurs with any of the 3 most common strains of *B burgdorferi* (*B burgdorferi sensu stricto, Borrelia garinii,* and B. *afzelii*). In Europe, neuroborreliosis is more common with *B garinii* than *Borrelia afzelii.*[9] *B burgdorferi sensu stricto* rarely causes neuroborreliosis in Europe, but it is generally an infrequent human pathogen there. In the US, whereby Lyme disease is caused by *B burgdorferi sensu stricto,* neuroborreliosis is said to occur in about 12% of untreated infected patients,[10] essentially the same proportion described in Europe. Much is made of the apparent differences between European and US *B burgdorferi* infection–US patients are, indeed, more likely to have multifocal erythema migrans and arthritis, However, the range and frequency of neurologic manifestations actually seem to be quite similar.

Once the diagnosis of Lyme disease is established, it is helpful to recognize the common neurologic presentations of neuroborreliosis. As described in Tyler

---

Box 3
European Federation of Neurologic Societies (EFNS) criteria for the diagnosis of neuroborreliosis[8]

1. Neurologic disorder within the spectrum of those known to be caused by neuroborreliosis without other apparent cause

2. CSF pleocytosis

3. Intrathecal antibody production

Definite neuroborreliosis if 3/3, possible if 2/3; except in patients with acrodermatitis chronica atrophicans, who may develop a peripheral neuropathy with normal CSF.

Box 4
American Academy of Neurology (AAN) criteria for the diagnosis of neuroborreliosis[7] (update in progress)

1. Possible exposure to *Ixodes* ticks in Lyme-endemic area

2. One or more of the following:
   a. Erythema migrans
   b. Histopathological, microbiologic, or PCR proof of *B. burgdorferi* infection
   c. immunologic evidence of exposure to *B. burgdorferi*

3. Occurrence of a clinical disorder within the realm of those associated with Lyme disease, without other apparent etiology

---

Crissinger and Kelly Baldwin's article, "Early Disseminated Lyme Disease: Cranial Neuropathy, Meningitis and Polyradiculopathy," in this issue, nervous system involvement most commonly occurs early in infection and is acute in nature; as a result most present in warm weather months when ticks are most likely to feed.[10] As symptoms, by definition, require disseminated infection, which takes time to develop, peripheral blood serologic testing is more likely to be positive than at the onset of erythema migrans. In fact, serologies are often markedly elevated, often with a prominent IgM component. Very rarely neurologic symptoms precede the development of a measurable antibody response,[11] so convalescent serologies may be necessary.

Although the neurologic manifestations of neuroborreliosis are often described as protean, this is no more meaningful than it is in any systemic disorder affecting the nervous system. While Lyme disease can affect any nervous system structure, there are meaningful patterns, presumably reflecting the ability of *B burgdorferi*, and the host response to it, to affect specific parts of the nervous system preferentially. Recognition of these patterns is useful in diagnosis.

Involvement can conveniently be considered (**Box 5, Tables 1** and **2**) to affect one or more of 3 separate compartments–the meninges and subarachnoid space, the PNS, and the parenchymal CNS. The classic triad of neuroborreliosis–meningitis, cranial neuritis and radiculoneuritis–involves the meninges and the PNS; parenchymal CNS involvement is quite rare.

Subarachnoid Space

Just as in Garin and Bujadoux's patient, a CSF pleocytosis (the defining characteristic of meningitis) is quite common, found in 5% to 10% of infected, untreated patients. The pleocytosis is typically lymphocyte predominant with modest numbers of white cells/mm^3(50–200), normal CSF glucose, and modest protein elevation. Symptoms vary widely. Some patients with bland CSF have severe headaches, photophobia, and meningismus; others, such as the one described by Garin and Bujadoux, have

---

Box 5
Alterations of nervous system function in Lyme disease

- Focal/multifocal peripheral nervous system inflammation/infection (common)

- Diffuse meningeal inflammation (common)
  ○ Occasionally with intracranial hypertension, mimicking pseudotumor cerebri

- Focal/multifocal central nervous system inflammation/infection (rare)

- Chronic low-grade encephalopathy *in the absence* of nervous system infection or inflammation

Table 1
Peripheral nervous system disorders associated with Lyme disease

Pathophysiology	Clinical Presentation
Mononeuropathy multiplex	Cranial neuropathy (particularly VII)
	Radiculoneuropathy (painful mono- or oligoradiculopathy)
	Brachial or lumbosacral Plexopathy
	Mononeuropathy
	Mononeuropathy multiplex
	Confluent mononeuropathy multiplex (mimicking diffuse axonal polyneuropathy)
	?acute inflammatory demyelinating polyneuropathy (rare if ever)

a significant pleocytosis but no meningitis-like symptoms. As neuroborreliosis typically occurs in warm weather months, the most common concern in endemic areas is whether a given patient's "aseptic" meningitis is due to Lyme disease or an enteroviral infection. Although clinical algorithms[12–14] have been proposed to differentiate between these 2, the most useful component of these is the presence of other elements of the triad–particularly cranial neuropathy or radiculoneuropathy. In endemic areas, the occurrence of either of these in a patient with clinically symptomatic meningitis–not obviously due to other, more pathogenic bacteria–should lead to a preliminary diagnosis of neuroborreliosis.

More specific diagnosis of Lyme meningitis usually depends on indirect diagnostic evidence. Although *B burgdorferi sensu lato* can be cultured, as a practical matter culture of these slowly reproducing organisms is rarely clinically helpful. Even when technically feasible, CSF cultures are only positive in about 10% to 15% of definite cases of Lyme meningitis. Using nucleic acid detection (eg, PCR)-based testing improves sensitivity minimally. Given the technical sensitivity of PCR, the logical inference is that the number of organisms in CSF is so small that they are simply not present in the obtained samples.

The other CSF-space disorder linked to neuroborreliosis, primarily in children, is pseudotumor cerebri. The clinical presentation is typical, with headaches, papilledema, raised intracranial pressure (ICP), and visual obscurations. Visual loss can occur, so accurate, timely diagnosis and treatment are critically important.[15] Virtually

Table 2
Central nervous system disorders associated with Lyme disease

Pathophysiology	Clinical Presentation
Inflammation in subarachnoid space	Meningitis
	Pseudotumor cerebri-like (children), usually with CSF pleocytosis
Parenchymal CNS inflammation & presumably infection	Short segmental spinal cord inflammation in Garin–Bujadoux–Bannwarth syndrome (primarily in European patients)
	Encephalomyelitis (active brain inflammation with focally abnormal neurologic examination & MRI imaging with inflammatory CSF – extremely rare)

all reported patients have had a significant CSF pleocytosis at the time of presentation, suggesting that it would be more accurate to think of these patients as having Lyme meningitis with secondarily raised ICP, rather than true pseudotumor. This distinction is prognostically important, as the elevated ICP of meningitis may be more self-limited than in pseudotumor. Regardless, immediate management needs to address both the causative infection and the elevated pressure.

Peripheral Nervous System

Peripheral and cranial nerves are both frequently involved. Facial nerve (VIIth cranial nerve, controlling facial muscle function) paresis is the most commonly recognized, probably accounting for three-quarters of patients with cranial nerve involvement, and can be bilateral in up to a quarter of these affected individuals.

Facial nerve palsy consists of marked paresis or paralysis of one side of the face, including lip movement, eye closure, and forehead wrinkling. Patients occasionally receive this diagnosis based on a very subtle, often subjective, sense of facial asymmetry, or even facial paresthesias. Neither of these warrants a diagnosis of VIIth nerve palsy. Most patients with facial nerve palsies (of any etiology) describe pain behind the ear ipsilateral to the palsy, often preceding weakness by a day or 2. Hyperacusis on the symptomatic side is common, as is a perceived but often difficult for the patient to characterize alteration in the sense of taste.

Idiopathic facial nerve palsy is very uncommon in young children; bilateral facial palsies are uncommon at any age, occurring primarily in Lyme disease, sarcoid, HIV infection, other less common basal meningitides, and Guillain Barre syndrome. In Lyme-endemic areas in warm weather months, it is reasonable to entertain a preliminary diagnosis of Lyme disease and even begin antibiotic treatment pending test results, in adults with otherwise unexplained bilateral facial palsies or young children with either a unilateral or bilateral facial palsy.

Other cranial neuropathies occur much less frequently and are insufficiently predictive of a diagnosis of Lyme disease to warrant even a preliminary diagnosis. The nerves to the extraocular muscles (III, IV, and VI) can be involved, causing diplopia. Occasionally the trigeminal nerve (V) can be involved causing unilateral facial paresthesias, pain, and/or hypoesthesia. The acousto-vestibular (VIII) nerve is involved occasionally as well, affecting hearing and balance. Involvement of the lower cranial nerves (IX–XII) is quite uncommon. The optic nerve (II, technically a CNS tract and not a peripheral nerve) is involved so rarely that it is questionable whether the anecdotal reports are anything but coincidental.[16,17]

The radiculoneuropathy of Lyme disease is probably the most commonly misdiagnosed form of nervous system involvement. Much as described by Garin and Bujadoux, patients present with severe, often intractable neuropathic pain, typically in a radicular distribution, often involving one but occasionally several contiguous dermatomes. The European literature suggests this often–but not invariably–affects the limb that was the site of the tick bite[18,19]; there are insufficient data in the US to know if that is the case with *B burgdorferi sensu stricto* infection.

Pain is identical in character to that of mechanical radiculopathies–superficial, burning, or shock-like, often with hyperpathia. Typically, there are sensory, motor (eg, deltoid weakness and atrophy in Garin and Bujadoux's patient) and reflex changes appropriate to the involved dermatome. Symptoms can involve the trunk; as in diabetic truncal neuropathies, this may lead to a focus on possible visceral causes of the pain, resulting in prolonged pursuit of other irrelevant diagnoses. As in patients with Lyme disease-associated cranial neuropathies, there is often–but not invariably–an accompanying CSF pleocytosis, which may help in guiding the diagnosis.[20] When a patient in an endemic area in warm weather months develops otherwise unexplained radicular symptoms or symptoms with no relevant changes on spine imaging, the diagnosis of Lyme radiculoneuropathy should be seriously considered.

In approximately the same time frame as the acute radicular symptoms, patients may develop other acute focal PNS symptoms. Brachial and lumbosacral plexopathies occur, as do acute mononeuropathies. Occasionally patients will have clinical evidence of multiple mononeuropathies, a picture usually associated with a vasculopathic process, and rarely (in developed countries) in infectious neuropathies such as leprosy. Detailed neurophysiologic studies in large numbers of patients with PNS neuroborreliosis indicate that all these presentations–cranial neuropathies, radiculopathies, plexopathies, and mononeuropathies–represent varying presentations of a mononeuropathy multiplex.[21] Rare patients have been described with an acute presentation resembling the Guillain Barre syndrome.[22] Only 1 small series[22] from a Lyme endemic area suggested this was in fact an acute demyelinating polyneuropathy. As other studies of PNS neuroborreliosis do not suggest demyelination, the implication of these isolated observations remains unclear.

Early in the development of our understanding of Lyme disease, patients who had been undiagnosed and untreated for several years presented with more indolent neuropathic symptoms–typically stocking-glove numbness, paresthesias, and occasionally weakness and reflex changes.[23] Neurophysiologic testing in such individuals demonstrated a confluent mononeuropathy multiplex–the same pathophysiologic process found in acute Lyme radiculoneuropathy–and changes improved following antimicrobial treatment.[21,24] As it is now quite uncommon to see patients who have had longstanding untreated Lyme disease, this entity is now seen rarely if ever. Importantly, patients presenting with nothing but acral paresthesias, who lack any objective evidence of PNS dysfunction, should not be diagnosed with PNS neuroborreliosis–or neuropathy of any kind.

Parenchymal Central Nervous System Involvement

Patients with European neuroborreliosis-associated radicular symptoms may have findings indicative of spinal cord involvement at the same spinal level as the symptomatic nerve root, suggesting the local spread of the inflammatory process. This has been observed occasionally in the US but systematic data are unavailable. Other than this, parenchymal CNS involvement is extraordinarily unusual. Reports in the 1980s and '90s primarily involved patients with longstanding untreated infection,[25] something that occurs rarely today. Occasional patients with acute to subacute focal encephalitis have been described. Affected individuals have all had focally abnormal brain MRI scans; abnormalities more commonly–but not exclusively–affecting white matter than gray. Clinical neurologic examinations are significantly abnormal, with findings congruous with the MRI abnormalities. Brain PET and SPECT scans have found hypermetabolism in the affected areas.[26] CSF is invariably inflammatory, typically with increased IgG synthesis and often - particularly with European infections oligoclonal bands–findings seen in other chronic CNS infections such as neurosyphilis and subacute sclerosing panencephalitis. As in those disorders, the increased production of antibodies within the CNS in these patients typically specifically targets the causative organism–that is, there is intrathecal synthesis of organism-specific antibody.

Behavioral Change Without Central Nervous System Infection: Lyme Encephalopathy

Patients with serious infections–not directly affecting the CNS–such as pneumonia or sepsis, inflammatory states such as lupus or active rheumatoid arthritis, or even individuals receiving immunomodulatory therapy such as interferons–commonly describe marked fatigue and cognitive difficulty. In most instances, this relates to physiologic effects on the CNS and not anything that would be considered nervous system damage or a neurologic process. The state is generally reversible with elimination (or suppression) of the causative process and has no long-term neurologic implications.

In the 1980's and '90s, when diagnosis and treatment of Lyme disease were still inconsistent, it was not uncommon to see patients with several years of relapsing, primarily rheumatologic symptoms who were then diagnosed with Lyme disease, and improved with antibiotics. Before treatment, many experienced fatigue and cognitive slowing that interfered with their daily functioning.[23,27,28] Detailed investigations found that (1) their perceived difficulties were quantifiable and verifiable with formal neuropsychologic testing, (2) in most instances neurologic examinations, brain MRI and CSF examinations were normal, and (3) the state was reversible with antibiotic therapy. Nothing about the state was considered unique or diagnostic of Lyme disease but rather this was viewed as an opportunity to better understand this commonplace phenomenon–in patients in whom the symptoms were on the one hand both persistent and not particularly time varying–and therefore measurable–and on the other, reversible with treatment. Exhaustive studies found evidence of CNS infection (past or present) in very few but nothing to suggest this in the vast majority. The entity was labeled "Lyme encephalopathy" to distinguish it from "Lyme encephalitis"—the latter term being reserved for individuals with actual brain infection.[29]

Curiously, some took this ubiquitous symptom complex as diagnostic of Lyme disease and began treating such patients–in the absence of anything else to suggest Lyme disease–with ever more aggressive courses of antibiotics. The epidemiology of Lyme disease and of this symptom complex makes the futility of this approach obvious. The annual incidence of CDC confirmed cases of Lyme disease is approximately 0.01% of the US population. Population studies have found that at any given time 2% of the population suffers from these symptoms to a disabling extent[30] suggesting that no more than 1 in 200 such patients might have Lyme disease–indicating that they have no predictive value for the diagnosis of Lyme disease. Even using estimates that the number of US patients treated annually for Lyme disease might be up to 10 times CDC numbers[31] the positive predictive value of such symptoms for Lyme disease remains no more than 5%. Despite this, the notion that patients with this symptom complex have Lyme disease and require prolonged antibiotic (and other) treatment is one of the major drivers of "the Lyme controversy."

Closely related is the construct of "posttreatment Lyme disease symptoms" (PTLDS), a term adopted in the 2006 IDSA Guideline[32] to provide a framework for further studies of this possible entity, but dropped from the 2021 update.[33] Patients with these same symptoms following standard effective antimicrobial therapy have been postulated to have them as residua of prior neurologic damage. Although there remains debate as to whether these symptoms are any more prevalent in these patients than in the general population[34] it seems quite clear they are unrelated to neuroborreliosis. A meta-analysis of residual symptoms in LNB treatment studies found that when patients were stratified using EFNS criteria as definite versus possible LNB, residual fatigue was not reported in any after the treatment of definite LNB. Other PTLDS symptoms were more common in the "possible" than "definite" group–suggesting that posttreatment PTLDS-like symptoms were not related to CNS infection.[35] Even more helpful, studies of the 2067 Danish patients diagnosed with definite LNB (by EFNS/CSF criteria) over 30 years[36] found "no substantial effect on long-term survival, health, or educational/social functioning"[36] or any "increased long-term risk of dementia, Alzheimer's disease, Parkinson's disease, motor neuron diseases, epilepsy or Guillain-

Barre."[37] While a subsequent study found an increased rate of administratively coded psychiatric diagnoses in these patients,[38] prior studies of the broader Danish population found an even greater increase in coded psychiatric diagnoses in patients with any infection or inflammatory disorder.[39,40]

REQUIREMENT #3: CAUSAL RELATIONSHIP BETWEEN LYME DISEASE AND THE NEUROLOGIC PROCESS

The final element in diagnosing a patient with nervous system Lyme disease is the plausibility that their nervous system disease and their Lyme disease are causally related. Laboratory support can be challenging. Serologies, particularly using 2-tier testing, have high sensitivity and specificity, but like any antibody-based measure can remain elevated long after microbiologic cure.

CSF studies can be more helpful–most informative is the measurement of intrathecal antibody production. There are technically several different ways of quantifying this; all rely on finding proportionately more specific anti-*B burgdorferi* antibody in CSF than in serum. All require measuring both specific and total antibody in serum and CSF and determining if there is proportional excess in CSF.

There are several important limitations of this approach. Most importantly if there is no CNS infection, there should be no expectation that CSF will be informative. Specifically, if the patient's Lyme disease does not affect the nervous system, or their neuroborreliosis is limited to the PNS, or if their only "neurologic" symptom is fatigue and cognitive slowing with an otherwise normal neurologic evaluation, CSF will predictably be normal. The technique is useful in patients with demonstrable inflammatory CNS disease; however, in the absence of another "gold standard" diagnostic test for CNS infection, estimates of the sensitivity of this measure in true CNS neuroborreliosis vary from 50% to nearly 100%. As with peripheral blood serologies, patients have been found to have elevated intrathecal antibody production for a decade or more following clearly successful treatment.[41]

These issues notwithstanding, there are several ways this measurement is clearly useful. In a patient with an active CNS inflammatory process (eg, a picture that resembles multiple sclerosis), whose CSF is clearly inflammatory with increased total antibody production, if the process is caused by this infection, it can be reliably assumed that the antibodies present should be specific for *B burgdorferi*. Similarly, and by analogy to neurosyphilis, if the antibodies are being produced in response to an active infection, the more non-specific - evidence of the immune response to the infection (CSF pleocytosis and elevated protein) should slowly normalize following successful treatment, regardless of whether or not clones of B cells and plasma cells continue to produce specific antibody providing a means of determining if the intrathecal antibody production is evidence of current versus prior infection.

Beyond this laboratory support for CNS infection, inferring causality must rely on a logical approach. If the patient's neurologic symptoms are within the range of those described in Lyme disease, and epidemiologic, serologic and other clinical data support the diagnosis, prudence would dictate treatment. If the disorder is outside the realm of disorders known to be causally related, but other data support the diagnosis, careful case-by-case deliberation, including considering biologic plausibility, would be in order.

Treatment

Although treatment is dealt with in detail elsewhere treatment of nervous system infection requires special comment. The use of first high dose parenteral penicillin, then ceftriaxone, was based on the presumption that in some patients the presence of

CNS infection required treatment with regimens known to achieve high levels in the CSF. Numerous European studies have now convincingly demonstrated that oral doxycycline is as effective as parenteral regimens in patients with Lyme meningitis, cranial neuritis, and radiculoneuritis.[42] Although there are no studies of amoxicillin or cefuroxime axetil, the fact that innumerable patients with Lyme disease have been treated with these regimens and none has progressed to develop neuroborreliosis, suggests these are effective as well.

There are no high-level studies addressing the use of oral regimens in those rare individuals who have parenchymal CNS infection. However, there is at least one longitudinal study supporting the role of oral doxycycline in the treatment of these patients as well.[43] As more data accrue in coming years it may well be that oral treatment will be considered appropriate first-line treatment in all but the most severely affected patients with neuroborreliosis.

SUMMARY

The CNS or PNS may be involved in up to 15% of patients with untreated infection with *B burgdorferi*. The efficacy of antimicrobial therapy (which is curative in the overwhelming majority of patients) in reversing the resulting disorders supports the hypothesis that these are caused by direct infection of the nervous system and not by immune or other indirect mechanisms. Neurologic involvement often includes meningitis (inflammation of the meninges) and/or multifocal inflammatory changes in peripheral nerve or rarely, in the brain or spinal cord. PNS involvement most often presents as cranial neuropathy, particularly the facial nerve, or other peripheral mononeuropathies. The latter not infrequently presents as quite painful dysfunction of one or several spinal nerve roots, mimicking mechanical radiculopathy. All but the most severely affected patients with neuroborreliosis respond well to oral antimicrobial therapy.

CLINICS CARE POINTS

- In patients with likely exposure to Lyme disease-carrying ticks, consider this diagnosis in patients with lymphocytic meningitis, facial nerve palsy or other cranial neuropathies, or otherwise unexplained radiculopathy or mononeuropathy.
- 2 tier serology (ELISA confirmed by either Western blot or orthogonal ELISA) is usually positive in Lyme neuroborreliosis.
- CNS. involvement almost always includes a CSF pleocytosis.
- In patients with CNS inflammation, intrathecal synthesis of anti-B. burgdorferi antibody can usually be demonstrated by testing serum and CSF antibody simultaneously.

DISCLOSURE

Expert witness defending physicians in medical malpractice cases in which they have been accused of failure to diagnose or treat Lyme disease; consultant to Pfizer regarding possible development of a Lyme disease vaccine; equity in several pharmaceutical companies none of which is relevant to this topic. Royalties from Up-to-date and "Lyme Disease, an evidence-based approach" 2nd edition published by CABI in 2018.

REFERENCES

1. Halperin JJ, Baker P, Wormser GP. Common misconceptions about lyme disease. Am J Med 2013;126(3):264.e1-7.

2. Halperin JJ. Lyme disease – neurology, neurobiology and behavior. Clin Infect Dis 2014;58(9):1267–72.
3. Steere AC, Pachner AR, Malawista SE. Neurologic abnormalities of Lyme disease: successful treatment with high-dose intravenous penicillin. Ann Intern Med 1983;99:767–72.
4. Reik L, Steere AC, Bartenhagen NH, et al. Neurologic abnormalities of Lyme disease. Medicine 1979;58(4):281–94.
5. Garin C, Bujadoux A. Paralysie par les tiques. J Med Lyon 1922;71:765–7.
6. Hollstrom E. Successful treatment of erythema migrans Afzelius. Acta Derm Venereol 1951;31(2):235–43.
7. Halperin J, Logigian E, Finkel M, et al. Practice parameter for the diagnosis of patients with nervous system Lyme borreliosis (Lyme disease). Neurology 1996;46: 619–27.
8. Mygland A, Ljostad U, Fingerle V, et al. EFNS guidelines on the diagnosis and management of European Lyme neuroborreliosis. Eur J Neurol 2010;17(1): 8–16, e1-4. doi:ENE2862 [pii].
9. Ogrinc K, Lotric-Furlan S, Maraspin V, et al. Suspected early lyme neuroborreliosis in patients with erythema migrans. Clin Infect Dis 2013; 57(4):501–9.
10. Bacon RM, Kugeler KJ, Mead PS. Surveillance for Lyme Disease — United States, 1992–2006. MMWR Morb Mortal Wkly Rep 2008;57(SS10):1–9.
11. Halperin JJ, Golightly M. Lyme borreliosis in Bell's palsy. Long Island Neuroborreliosis Collaborative Study Group. Neurology 1992;42(7):1268–70.
12. Tuerlinckx D, Bodart E, Garrino MG, et al. Clinical data and cerebrospinal fluid findings in Lyme meningitis versus aseptic meningitis. Eur J Pediatr 2003; 162(3):150–3.
13. Shah SS, Zaoutis TE, Turnquist J, et al. Early differentiation of Lyme from enteroviral meningitis. Pediatr Infect Dis J 2005;24(6):542–5.
14. Garro AC, Rutman M, Simonsen K, et al. Prospective validation of a clinical prediction model for Lyme meningitis in children. Pediatrics 2009;123(5): e829–34.
15. Kan L, Sood SK, Maytal J. Pseudotumor cerebri in Lyme disease: a case report and literature review. Pediatr Neurol 1998;18(5):439–41.
16. Sibony P, Halperin J, Coyle P, et al. Reactive Lyme serology in patients with optic neuritis and papilledema. J Neuroophthalmol 2005;25(2):71–82.
17. Blanc F, Ballonzoli L, Marcel C, et al. Lyme optic neuritis. J Neurol Sci 2010;295: 117–9.
18. Ogrinc K, Lusa L, Lotric-Furlan S, et al. Course and outcome of early european lyme neuroborreliosis (bannwarth syndrome): clinical and laboratory findings. Clin Infect Dis 2016;63(3):346–53.
19. Halperin JJ. Editorial Commentary: Neuroborreliosis: What Is It, What Isn't It? Clin Infect Dis 2016;63(3):354–5.
20. Halperin JJ. Facial nerve palsy associated with Lyme disease. Muscle Nerve 2003;28:516–7.
21. Halperin JJ, Luft BJ, Volkman DJ, et al. Lyme neuroborreliosis - peripheral nervous system manifestations. Brain 1990;113:1207–21.
22. Muley SA, Parry GJ. Antibiotic responsive demyelinating neuropathy related to Lyme disease. Neurology 2009;72(20):1786–7.
23. Logigian EL, Kaplan RF, Steere AC. Chronic neurologic manifestations of Lyme disease. N Engl J Med 1990;323(21):1438–44.

24. Halperin JJ, Little BW, Coyle PK, et al. Lyme disease - a treatable cause of periph-eral neuropathy. Neurology 1987;37:1700–6.
25. Ackermann R, Rehse KB, Gollmer E, et al. Chronic neurologic manifestations of erythema migrans borreliosis. Ann N Y Acad Sci 1988;539:16–23.
26. Kalina P, Decker A, Kornel E, et al. Lyme disease of the brainstem. Neuroradi-ology 2005;47(12):903–7.
27. Halperin JJ, Luft BJ, Anand AK, et al. Lyme neuroborreliosis: central nervous sys-tem manifestations. Neurology 1989;39(6):753–9.
28. Kaplan RF, Jones-Woodward L. Lyme encephalopathy: a neuropsychological perspective. Semin Neurol 1997;17(1):31–7.
29. Halperin JJ, Krupp LB, Golightly MG, et al. Lyme borreliosis-associated enceph-alopathy. Neurology 1990;40:1340–3.
30. Luo N, Johnson J, Shaw J, et al. Self-reported health status of the general adult U.S. population as assessed by the EQ-5D and Health Utilities Index. Med Care 2005;43(11):1078–86.
31. Hinckley AF, Connally NP, Meek JI, et al. Lyme disease testing by large commer-cial laboratories in the United States. Clin Infect Dis 2014;59(5):676–81.
32. Wormser GP, Dattwyler RJ, Shapiro ED, et al. The clinical assessment, treatment, and prevention of Lyme disease, human granulocytic anaplasmosis, and babesi-osis: Clinical practice guidelines by the Infectious Diseases Society of America. Clin Infect Dis 2006;43:1089–134.
33. Lantos PM, Rumbaugh J, Bockenstedt LK, et al. Clinical practice guidelines by the infectious diseases society of america (IDSA), american academy of neurology (AAN), and american college of rheumatology (ACR): 2020 guidelines for the prevention, diagnosis and treatment of lyme disease. Clin Infect Dis 2021; 72(1):1–8.
34. Wormser GP, McKenna D, Shaffer KD, et al. Evaluation of selected variables to determine if any had predictive value for, or correlated with, residual symptoms at approximately 12 months after diagnosis and treatment of early lyme disease. Diagn Microbiol Infect Dis 2021;100(3):115348.
35. Dersch R, Sommer H, Rauer S, et al. Prevalence and spectrum of residual symp-toms in Lyme neuroborreliosis after pharmacological treatment: a systematic re-view. J Neurol 2016;263(1):17–24.
36. Obel N, Dessau RB, Krogfelt KA, et al. Long term survival, health, social func-tioning, and education in patients with European Lyme neuroborreliosis: nation-wide population based cohort study. BMJ 2018;361:k1998.
37. Haahr R, Tetens MM, Dessau RB, et al. Risk of neurological disorders in patients with European Lyme neuroborreliosis. A nationwide population-based cohort study. Clin Infect Dis 2019. https://doi.org/10.1093/cid/ciz997.
38. Tetens MM, Haahr R, Dessau RB, et al. Assessment of the risk of psychiatric dis-orders, use of psychiatric hospitals, and receipt of psychiatric medication among patients with lyme neuroborreliosis in denmark. JAMA Psychiatry 2021;78(2): 177–86.
39. Benros ME, Waltoft BL, Nordentoft M, et al. Autoimmune diseases and severe in-fections as risk factors for mood disorders: a nationwide study. JAMA Psychiatry 2013;70(8):812–20. https://doi.org/10.1001/jamapsychiatry.2013.1111.
40. Lund-Sorensen H, Benros ME, Madsen T, et al. A nationwide cohort study of the association between hospitalization with infection and risk of death by suicide. JAMA Psychiatry 2016;73(9):912–9.

41. Hammers Berggren S, Hansen K, Lebech AM, et al. *Borrelia burgdorferi*-specific intrathecal antibody production in neuroborreliosis: a follow-up study. Neurology 1993;43(1):169–75.
42. Halperin JJ, Shapiro ED, Logigian EL, et al. Practice parameter: treatment of nervous system Lyme disease. Neurology 2007;69(1):91–102.
43. Bremell D, Dotevall L. Oral doxycycline for Lyme neuroborreliosis with symptoms of encephalitis, myelitis, vasculitis or intracranial hypertension. Eur J Neurol 2014; 21(9):1162–7.

Lyme Disease in Children

Carol A. McCarthy, MD[a,b,c,]*, Jason A. Helis, MD[b,d,e],
Brian E. Daikh, MD[b,f,g]

KEYWORDS

- Lyme disease • Child • Tick-borne diseases • Intracranial hypertension • Tick bites

KEY POINTS

- Erythema migrans is sometimes diagnosed as other conditions.
- Children with central nervous system Lyme disease can develop intracranial hypertension.
- Lyme arthritis in children can have a presentation similar to septic arthritis.
- Doxycycline is recommended for short-term administration in children.
- Prevention and monitoring for tick bites is important.

INTRODUCTION

The manifestations and management of Lyme disease in children are similar to those in adults with some exceptions. This article presents an overview of Lyme disease in children, highlighting the differences. The discussion focuses on Lyme disease in North America and does not describe the spectrum of Lyme disease that is observed in Europe.

In the United States, Lyme disease is primarily caused by the spirochete, *Borrelia burgdorferi* sensu stricto and rarely, in the upper Midwest, by *Borrelia mayonii*.

EPIDEMIOLOGY

First recognized in 1977 in children evaluated for juvenile rheumatoid arthritis in Connecticut,[1] Lyme disease is now the most commonly reported vector-borne disease in the United States.[2] It is predominately found in New England and the eastern mid-Atlantic states to Virginia. It is also seen in the upper Midwestern states, particularly

[a] Department of Pediatrics, Division of Pediatric Infectious Disease, Barbara Bush Children's Hospital at Maine Medical Center, Portland, ME, USA; [b] Tufts University School of Medicine, Boston, MA, USA; [c] Maine Medical Partners Pediatric Specialty Care, 887 Congress Street, Suite 310, Portland, ME 04102, USA; [d] Department of Pediatrics, Division of Pediatric Neurology, Barbara Bush Children's Hospital at Maine Medical Center, Portland, ME, USA; [e] Maine Medical Partners Neurology, 92 Campus Drive Suite B, Scarborough, ME 04074, USA; [f] Department of Medicine, Maine Medical Center; [g] Rheumatology Associates, 51 Sewall Street, Portland, ME, USA
* Corresponding author. Maine Medical Partners Pediatric Specialty Care, 887 Congress Street, Suite 310, Portland, ME 04102.
E-mail address: Carol.McCarthy@mainehealth.org

Infect Dis Clin N Am 36 (2022) 593–603
https://doi.org/10.1016/j.idc.2022.03.002

Wisconsin and Minnesota, as well as on the west coast, primarily in northern California. B burgdorferi, the predominant bacterial cause of Lyme disease, is transmitted to humans through infected blacklegged ticks, Ixodes scapularis in the northeastern, mid-Atlantic and north central states, and Ixodes pacificus in the Pacific coast. The primary vectors are the nymphal ticks that often go undetected because of their small size. The earlier forms of Lyme disease are most frequently seen when blacklegged ticks are prevalent. The highest incidence occurs in children aged 5 to 9 years with a male predominance.[2] The median incubation period from tick bite to appearance of erythema migrans is 11 days, with an estimated range from 3 to 32 days.[3] In untreated patients, manifestations may occur months after the tick bite. Reinfection is possible. The impact of Lyme disease in pregnancy is not clear. There has not been a defined pathologic sequelae of this organism on the fetus.[4]

CLINICAL MANIFESTATIONS

The clinical presentations of Lyme disease can be conceptualized in 3 stages. The hallmark of early localized disease is erythema migrans. Children may also have fevers, fatigue, headaches, and arthralgias.[5] Manifestations of the next stage, early disseminated disease, include multiple erythema migrans, cranial nerve palsies, meningitis, and carditis. The most common late presentation of Lyme is arthritis. Late neurologic manifestations, which are rare in children, include encephalitis and polyneuropathy. These different presentations are further described.

Dermatologic

The typical rash of Lyme disease, erythema migrans, is the most common manifestation of Lyme disease in children.[5] It often occurs at the site of the tick bite several days to weeks later. It is classically a flat, erythematous, oval, or circular lesion generally noticed when it is 5 cm or larger in size. Early lesions often consist of homogeneous erythema or a central area of erythema with a paler peripheral ring rather than a textbook "bulls-eye" lesion.[6,7] If not treated, the lesion typically expands, forming concentric circles in a target or "bulls-eye" pattern. There may be an initial reaction to the tick bite, which may be mistaken for erythema migrans. However, unlike true erythema migrans, tick bite reactions appear immediately after tick removal or during tick attachment. They are often pruritic, and resolve, rather than expand over the ensuing days. Solitary erythema migrans also may be confused with cellulitis or sunburn from uneven application of sunscreen. The outline of the lesion on the head may be obscured by hair so the circular nature of the rash is not identified.

The skin lesions seen with multiple erythema migrans are usually smaller than single erythema migrans and may be fleeting over days. Children with these lesions tend to have more systemic symptoms. They are commonly misdiagnosed as erythema multiforme or tinea corporis. Continued education of clinicians in endemic areas regarding the spectrum of skin lesions seen with Lyme disease is critical to decrease later complications.

Neurologic

Lyme neuroborreliosis is considered a manifestation of early disseminated disease. The exact pathogenic mechanism for this remains uncertain. Neuroborreliosis generally manifests clinically as cranial neuropathies (most commonly cranial nerve [CN] VII), lymphocytic meningitis, and radiculoneuritis (extremity pain and weakness). Patients may demonstrate clinical overlap among these syndromes. In contrast to Europe, where radiculoneuritis is common in adults, it is thought to be a rare phenomenon in the United States.[8]

Data from the Centers for Disease Control and Prevention show that neurologic manifestations occur in 12.5% of confirmed cases of Lyme disease in the United States (adults and children). Facial nerve palsy is the most common manifestation in children, occurring in 8.4% of cases.[2] In Canada, surveillance data (adults and children) show the prevalence of facial paralysis in Lyme disease at 8.2% and other neurologic manifestations in 14.5% of confirmed cases.[9]

As noted, cranial neuropathy is the most common neurologic manifestation of Lyme neuroborreliosis in the United States, with CN VII the most frequently affected. Rarely, other cranial nerves will be involved.[10] In endemic areas, Lyme disease may be the most common etiology of facial nerve palsy in children.[11] Like other causes of peripheral facial nerve palsy, patients typically have facial weakness affecting the upper and lower parts of the face. Bilateral facial paralysis is not uncommon, with one study documenting the occurrence in 22.8% of cases.[12] The facial palsy may be accompanied by other symptoms, including erythema migrans, malaise, and temporomandibular joint dysfunction. Antibiotic treatment does not affect the course of the facial palsy but is used to prevent late disease.[3] Corticosteroids are not recommended in children for the treatment of facial palsy secondary to Lyme disease.[3] Eye care may include artificial tears as well as nighttime patching. Prognosis for Lyme facial palsy is good, with the vast majority of patients making a complete recovery. Bilateral facial nerve involvement is a risk factor for having minor residual deficits.[12]

Clinical characteristics of Lyme meningitis can be similar to those in aseptic meningitis, making the diagnosis challenging, especially during warmer months when the incidence of enteroviral infections increases. Although patients in either condition have headache as a cardinal feature, there are clinical characteristics that make Lyme neuroborreliosis more likely. Patients with Lyme meningitis tend to have a longer duration of symptoms on presentation (usually longer than 1 week) and lower temperatures.[13] Clinical prediction models to help differentiate between viral and Lyme meningitis have been developed. One model known as the "Rule of 7's" has been validated to show that a child with meningitis who has the following features: cerebrospinal fluid (CSF) with less than or equal to 70% mononuclear cells, absence of CN VII palsy, and headaches less than 7 days, has a low-risk chance of Lyme meningitis.[14] Cranial neuropathy and erythema migrans are often present on evaluation.[13,15] Another common manifestation of Lyme meningitis in children is increased intracranial hypertension.[16] In this condition, the pressure of the CSF surrounding the brain is elevated. This can result in headaches and damage to the optic nerves and, very rarely, loss of vision. Ophthalmologic evaluation is important in these cases. Given the high incidence of increased intracranial pressure in childcare with Lyme meningitis, CSF opening pressure should be obtained when lumbar punctures are performed. Acetazolamide is often used for treatment in children with central nervous system Lyme disease and increased intracranial hypertension. Painful radiculoneuritis is a rare manifestation of Lyme neuroborreliosis in North America, but has been reported. The triad of painful radiculopathy, cranial neuropathy, and CSF lymphocytic pleocytosis is known as Garin–Bujadeux–Bannwarth syndrome. Peripheral nerve involvement likely represents a painful mononeuritis multiplex. Pain can be severe and burning and weakness can occur.[17] Transverse myelitis is a rare condition that has been reported to occur as a manifestation of neuroborreliosis in the United States.[18]

Long-term outcomes in children with Lyme neuroborreliosis are noted to be very favorable, with most patients making a complete recovery. Patients with Lyme neuroborreliosis have a similar cognitive outcome compared with disease-matched and healthy controls.[19]

Serum Lyme antibody measurement is recommended in children with suspected Lyme neuroborreliosis. Routine testing for Lyme disease is not recommended for children with developmental, behavioral, or psychiatric disorders.[20]

Cardiac

Cardiac findings in children with Lyme disease are uncommon and occur early in the course of disease. Children may have palpitations, chest pain, or syncope or no cardiopulmonary symptoms.[21] The most common cardiac findings are atrioventricular heart block ranging from first-degree block to third-degree block. Temporary pacing occasionally may be necessary. Although unusual, myocarditis with decreased myocardial function has been reported.[21] In an analysis comparing children with adults hospitalized with Lyme carditis, most patients of all ages were male without prior cardiac history.[22] Earlier recognition and treatment of suspected Lyme might prevent subsequent cardiac involvement.

Rheumatologic

In North America, Lyme arthritis is the second most common Lyme disease–specific clinical manifestation after erythema migrans and is the most common clinical manifestation of the late, disseminated stage of Lyme disease.[2,23,24] Lyme arthritis typically presents with an inflammatory monoarticular or oligoarticular arthritis with a predilection for large, weight-bearing joints, most commonly the knee.[23,25,26] The mean time interval to the development of arthritis after tick bite is approximately 3.4 months, but with a very broad range[27] and can be the presenting manifestation of Lyme disease. The diagnosis of Lyme arthritis is established by the presence of an inflammatory monoarticular or oligoarticular arthritis and positive blood enzyme-linked immunoassay (ELISA) and confirmatory Western blot or other second-tier test.[20] Synovial fluid polymerase chain reaction (PCR) for *Borrelia* is neither sensitive nor specific and should not be used to make the initial diagnosis of Lyme arthritis.

In children, the clinical presentation of Lyme arthritis is variable. Lyme arthritis may present as a waxing and waning, migratory pattern over months.[23] Compared with adults, children are more likely to present to their health care provider within 2 weeks of the onset of arthritis.[25] Arthritis may be the initial clinical manifestation of Lyme disease.[26] Frequently there is a disparity between clinical examination and symptoms. The child may have a significant degree of swelling and stiffness, but have little pain, often leading to initial evaluation by an orthopedic surgeon for question of suspected trauma or internal derangement of the joint. However, the presentation may be very abrupt. The child may stop ambulating and there may be fever, leukocytosis, and elevated acute phase reactants, all concerning for septic arthritis or toxic synovitis. The diagnosis of Lyme arthritis may be especially challenging when it affects the hip joint. It has been our and others' experience that sometimes children with Lyme arthritis affecting the hip first undergo surgical irrigation and debridement for presumed septic arthritis, only later to be diagnosed with Lyme arthritis.[25]

The major differential diagnoses of Lyme arthritis in children include septic arthritis, toxic synovitis, and juvenile inflammatory arthritis. In several studies of children living in Lyme-endemic areas and presenting with mono-arthritis of the knee or hip joints, Lyme arthritis occurred in 51% to 67% of knees, whereas septic arthritis occurred in only 3.0% to 5.5%.[28,29] The remainder of the cases constituted other forms of inflammatory arthritis. In contrast, when the hip was affected, Lyme arthritis constituted only 13% to 18% of cases. Septic arthritis occurred between 11% and 43% of cases and the remaining cases constituted toxic synovitis or other forms of inflammatory arthritis.[30,31]

Although synovial fluid white blood cell (WBC) counts in Lyme arthritis frequently fall within the range observed in inflammatory arthritis in adults, children with Lyme arthritis may manifest much higher synovial WBC counts suggestive of septic arthritis. In a study comparing Lyme arthritis in children and adults, the mean synovial WBC in children was 49,924 cells/mm^2 compared with 12,396 cells/mm^2 in adults.[25] The highest recorded synovial WBC in a child in that study was 139,700. Thus, there can be considerable overlap of synovial fluid WBC counts between Lyme and septic arthritis, with Lyme arthritis cell counts frequently exceeding 50,000 cells/mm^2.[29,31] Therefore, synovial fluid WBC count alone cannot be relied on to differentiate between septic and Lyme arthritis.

In Lyme-endemic areas, a peripheral blood absolute neutrophil count of $\geq$10,000 and erythrocyte sedimentation rate of $\geq$40 mm/h have been shown to be predictors of septic knee arthritis.[32] Ultimately, synovial fluid cell count, Gram stain, and culture, along with serologic tests for Lyme disease may all be necessary to establish the diagnosis. However, the lack of rapidly available serologic tests for Lyme disease can hamper a timely diagnosis, leading to unnecessary surgical intervention.

The treatment of Lyme arthritis is outlined in **Table 1**. Initial treatment of Lyme arthritis should consist of a 28-day course of oral antibiotics.[3,20] Most children will have resolution of their arthritis after a single course of oral antibiotic.[25,33] Children are more likely to have normal function and joint examination within 4 weeks of starting antibiotic therapy, compared with adults, likely in part because of prior trauma or presence of underlying joint pathology, such as osteoarthritis in adults.[25] In our experience, concomitant use of nonsteroidal anti-inflammatory drugs with antibiotics may hasten clinical improvement. However, up to 10% to 28% of children may experience antibiotic-resistant synovitis.[34–37] Age older than 10, prolonged arthritis before treatment, and poor initial response to antibiotics have been identified as risk factors for antibiotic-refractory Lyme arthritis in children,[37] but not others.[34] Nonadherence with antibiotic therapy always should be considered as a possible explanation for lack of clinical improvement.

If there is incomplete response with a first course of oral antibiotics, a second course of oral antibiotics, followed by a 28-day course of intravenous (IV) antibiotic therapy can be used,[3,38] although there is very little and poor-quality evidence-based data to support these recommendations. The Infectious Disease Society of North America guidelines for the treatment of Lyme arthritis make no recommendations for a second course of oral antibiotics if there is a partial response to an initial course, but do recommend a course of IV antibiotics over a second course of oral antibiotics if there is no clinical improvement after an initial course of oral antibiotics.[20] Previously, additional courses of antibiotic therapy have been recommended if there is a positive PCR result from synovial fluid after antibiotic therapy.[39] However, positive PCR results may not predict active infection,[40] but rather nonviable *Borrelia* spirochetes or their remnants in the joint matrix, perpetuating an ongoing immune response.[41] See Sheila L. Arvikar and Allen C. Steere's article. "Lyme Arthritis," elsewhere in this issue.

Children with persistent joint swelling after a course of IV antibiotics are not likely to improve with prolonged antibiotic therapy. They have synovial inflammation similar to that found in inflammatory arthritis.[38] Formerly labeled as antibiotic-refractory Lyme arthritis, these cases are now referred to as postinfectious Lyme arthritis. These children should be referred to a rheumatologist or other specialist for consideration of

Table 1
Treatment of Lyme disease in children

Clinical Manifestation	Antibiotic
Erythema migrans	Doxycycline 4.4 mg/kg/d by mouth (po) divided every 12 h for 10 d (maximum 200 mg/d) OR Amoxicillin 50 mg/kg/d po divided every 8 h for 14 d (maximum 1.5 g/d) OR Cefuroxime 30 mg/kg/d po divided every 12 h for 14 d (maximum 1 g/d) Second-line agent for those unable to take doxycycline or beta lactams Azithromycin 10 mg/kg/d po once daily for 7 d (maximum 500 mg)
Facial palsy	Doxycycline 4.4 mg/kg/d po divided every 12 h for 14 d (maximum 200 mg/d)
Cardiac	Ceftriaxone 50–75 mg/kg/d for 14–21 d (maximum 2 g daily) in hospitalized children Course can be completed with oral therapy as for early disease when discharged home
Meningitis	Ceftriaxone 50–75 mg/kg/d for 14 d (maximum 2 g daily) in hospitalized children OR Doxycycline 4.4 mg/kg/d po divided every 12 h for 14 d (maximum 200 mg/d) in selected children
Arthritis	
Children <8 y	Amoxicillin 50 mg/kg/d po divided every 8 h for 28 d (maximum 1.5 gm/d) OR Cefuroxime 30 mg/kg/d divided every 12 h for 28 d (maximum 1 g/d)
Children ≥8 y	Doxycycline 4.4 mg/kg/d po divided every 12 h for 28 d (maximum 200 mg/d) OR Treatment as for children <8 y of age
Persistent arthritis	Repeat 28-d course of oral antibiotics OR Ceftriaxone 50–75 mg/kg/d for 14–28 days (maximum 2 g daily) if no response to initial oral therapy

Data from American Academy of Pediatrics. Committee on Infectious Diseases, Kimberlin DW, Barnett ED, Lynfield R, Sawyer MH. Red Book: 2021–2024 Report of the Committee on Infectious Diseases. American Academy of Pediatrics; 2021; and Lantos PM, Rumbaugh J, Bockenstedt LK, et al. Clinical Practice Guidelines by the Infectious Diseases Society of America (IDSA), American Academy of Neurology (AAN), and American College of Rheumatology (ACR): 2020 Guidelines for the Prevention, Diagnosis and Treatment of Lyme Disease. Clin Infect Dis. Jan 23 2021;72(1):1-8. https://doi.org/10.1093/cid/ciab049.

disease-modifying antirheumatic drugs, biologic agents, intra-articular steroids, or arthroscopic synovectomy, although recommendations for these second-line therapies are derived largely from clinical experience and expert opinion and are not supported by randomized clinical trials or other high-quality evidence.[20,38,39] Small retrospective studies do support the use of intra-articular corticosteroid therapy as second-line therapy for refractory Lyme arthritis in children,[36,42] with resultant potentially lower frequency of antibiotic-resistant Lyme arthritis and faster rates of clinical resolution compared with children receiving a second course of oral antibiotics alone.[42] Until more data evaluating the use of intra-articular steroids are available, we recommend only using this treatment after adequate antibiotic therapy and as a bridge to systemic anti-inflammatory treatment. Further prospective data on optimal therapy for postinfectious Lyme arthritis are needed.

DIAGNOSTICS

Testing for Lyme disease is over used and often misinterpreted. It is important to consider the patient's presentation, geographic location, and travel history before testing for Lyme disease. Because a serologic response may take 2 to 4 weeks to develop, testing is not recommended for erythema migrans, the early manifestation of Lyme.[3,20] The recommended testing in patients with compatible clinical syndromes with either residence or travel to Lyme-endemic areas is a 2-step process. The initial screening test is an ELISA or enzyme immunoassay (EIA) or immunofluorescent antibody test. If this testing is equivocal or positive, a Western blot or a Food and Drug Administration–cleared secondary tier EIA is done as a confirmatory test.[43] A positive Western blot result is defined as the presence of at least 2 immunoglobulin (Ig)M bands or the presence of at least 5 IgG bands. The Western blot should not be ordered as a standalone test. In Lyme arthritis, a late-stage presentation, the Western blot IgG should be positive. Testing is not recommended to determine efficacy of treatment. Serologic testing in patients with prior Lyme disease is often difficult to interpret because antibodies may be present for years after initial infection.

PCR testing is sometimes done on joint fluid in patients suspected of having Lyme arthritis. It is not recommended for the initial diagnosis but is used by some clinicians for patients who have persistent joint swelling despite an adequate 1-month course of therapy, or in cases of relapse. However, PCR positivity may persist in the absence of evidence of viable bacterial infection.[40]

In selected patients with neurologic symptoms, a CSF/serum antibody index may be calculated with simultaneously obtained serum and CSF samples.[20]

TREATMENT

The recommended antimicrobials and treatment duration for the different forms of Lyme disease in children are outlined in **Table 1**.[3,20] Although previously not used in children younger than 8 years, doxycycline can be prescribed in children of all ages for shorter periods. Its use is not recommended for more than 2 weeks in children younger than 8 years. Because Lyme arthritis is treated with a 28-day course of antibiotics, these younger children should be treated with an alternative agent. Doxycycline is the recommended oral therapy for facial palsy and peripheral nervous system disease. Families should be counseled to avoid prolonged sun exposure and use of sunscreen while on the doxycycline. Ceftriaxone is used for children hospitalized with carditis and meningitis.

Azithromycin is second-line therapy for erythema migrans in children who are unable to take one of the first-line agents.

PREVENTION

Families should be counseled regarding different strategies that can be used to help prevent tick-borne infection. Long-sleeve shirts and socks pulled over long pants will limit areas of exposed skin. Clothing may be treated with 0.5% permethrin. The repellant that has been used most extensively on skin is N,N-diethyl-meta-toluamide (DEET) at concentrations of 30%, but other repellants approved by the Environmental Protection Agency may be used (see Paul Mead's article, "Epidemiology of Lyme Disease," in this issue). They should be applied sparingly on young children (>2 months of age) and care should be taken that they are not ingested. When hiking, families should try to stay on boardwalks and the center of trails, avoiding long, uncut grass. Playsets can be set back from wooded areas using a gravel buffer. Clothes can be put in the dryer after outdoor activity. It has been demonstrated that ticks are most effectively killed by high heat in a dryer for a minimum of 6 minutes.[44] Finally, routine daily bathing and tick checks are important during the months when ticks and children are active. There should be particular attention paid to exposed areas of skin, especially the head and neck. Ticks can be removed by pulling straight up with fine-tipped tweezers held at the surface of skin. Testing ticks for the presence of *B burgdorferi* is not recommended.[20]

In areas where Lyme is prevalent, doxycycline prophylaxis at a dose of 4.4 mg/kg (maximum 200 mg) is recommended for engorged tick bites (ticks attached for more than 36 hours) within 72 hours of tick removal.

There are no currently licensed vaccines against Lyme disease, but candidate vaccines are being evaluated.[45]

COINFECTIONS

Children with Lyme may become coinfected with another tick-borne disease transmitted by blacklegged ticks. Routine testing for coinfections, however, is not necessary in most children. Notably, the 2 most common infections transmitted by these ticks after Lyme disease, anaplasmosis and babesiosis, uncommonly cause illness in infected children.[46,47] Because PCR panels for anaplasmosis and babesiosis are available, and often included with a serologic screen for Lyme disease, many are done even when the clinical presentation makes these other infections very unlikely. An example is testing for coinfections in the evaluation of possible Lyme arthritis in the winter months. Anaplasmosis should be considered in children with abnormalities on complete blood count or transaminitis. Doxycycline will treat this infection. Babesia should be considered in children with splenic dysfunction, immunocompromised children, and neonates because of potential life-threatening infection. In healthy children, infection with babesia is often asymptomatic.[47]

SUMMARY

Early Lyme disease may go undetected in children because tick bites are not noticed and skin lesions may be attributed to other conditions. Prompt recognition is essential to reduce the risk of neurologic, cardiac, and rheumatologic disease. It is important that families are educated to decrease exposures to ticks and routinely monitor for tick bites.

CLINICS CARE POINTS

- Familiarity with the skin manifestations of Lyme disease is important.
- In Lyme-endemic areas during the appropriate seasons, facial palsy is most likely caused by Lyme disease and the recommended therapy is antibiotics.
- Children with Lyme meningitis should be closely monitored for increased intracranial pressure.
- Children with Lyme carditis may need cardiac pacing, which is usually temporary.
- A careful history may help differentiate Lyme arthritis from septic arthritis, avoiding surgical intervention.
- Education regarding tick exposures is necessary.
- Expanded tick panel testing is often not needed in children.

DISCLOSURE

The authors do not have any commercial or financial conflicts of interest. No funding was received for this article.

REFERENCES

1. Steere AC, Malawista SE, Snydman DR, et al. Lyme arthritis: an epidemic of oligoarticular arthritis in children and adults in three Connecticut communities. Arthritis Rheum 1977;20(1):7–17.
2. Schwartz AM, Hinckley AF, Mead PS, et al. Surveillance for Lyme disease - United States, 2008-2015. MMWR Surveill Summ 2017;66(22):1–12.
3. American Academy of Pediatrics, Committee on infectious diseases, Kimberlin DW, Barnett ED, Lynfield R, et al. Red Book: 2021–2024 Report of the Committee on Infectious Diseases. Am Acad Pediatr 2021;482–9.
4. Waddell LA, Greig J, Lindsay LR, et al. A systematic review on the impact of gestational Lyme disease in humans on the fetus and newborn. PLoS One 2018;13(11):e0207067.
5. Gerber MA, Shapiro ED, Burke GS, et al. Lyme disease in children in southeastern Connecticut. Pediatric Lyme Disease Study Group. N Engl J Med 1996;335(17):1270–4.
6. Nadelman RB, Nowakowski J, Forseter G, et al. The clinical spectrum of early Lyme borreliosis in patients with culture-confirmed erythema migrans. Am J Med 1996;100(5):502–8.
7. Smith RP, Schoen RT, Rahn DW, et al. Clinical characteristics and treatment outcome of early Lyme disease in patients with microbiologically confirmed erythema migrans. Ann Intern Med 2002;136(6):421–8.
8. Halperin JJ. A neurologist's view of Lyme disease and other tick-borne infections. Semin Neurol 2019;39(4):440–7.
9. Gasmi S, Ogden NH, Lindsay LR, et al. Surveillance for Lyme disease in Canada: 2009-2015. Can Commun Dis Rep 2017;43(10):194–9.
10. Belman AL, Iyer M, Coyle PK, et al. Neurologic manifestations in children with North American Lyme disease. Neurology 1993;43(12):2609–14.
11. Cook SP, Macartney KK, Rose CD, et al. Lyme disease and seventh nerve paralysis in children. Comparative study. Am J Otolaryngol 1997;18(5):320–3.
12. Clark JR, Carlson RD, Sasaki CT, et al. Facial paralysis in Lyme disease. Laryngoscope 1985;95(11):1341–5.
13. Eppes SC, Nelson DK, Lewis LL, et al. Characterization of Lyme meningitis and comparison with viral meningitis in children. Pediatrics 1999;103(5 Pt 1):957–60.
14. Cohn KA, Thompson AD, Shah SS, et al. Validation of a clinical prediction rule to distinguish Lyme meningitis from aseptic meningitis. Pediatrics 2012;129(1): e46–53.
15. Shah SS, Zaoutis TE, Turnquist J, et al. Early differentiation of Lyme from enteroviral meningitis. Pediatr Infect Dis J 2005;24(6):542–5.
16. Kan L, Sood SK, Maytal J. Pseudotumor cerebri in Lyme disease: a case report and literature review. Pediatr Neurol 1998;18(5):439–41.
17. Dutta A, Hunter JV, Vallejo JG. Bannwarth syndrome: a rare manifestation of pediatric lyme neuroborreliosis. Pediatr Infect Dis J 2021;40(11):e442–4.
18. Khan S, Singh N, Dow A, et al. Pediatric acute longitudinal extensive transverse myelitis secondary to neuroborreliosis. Case Rep Neurol 2015;7(2):162–6.
19. Adams WV, Rose CD, Eppes SC, et al. Cognitive effects of Lyme disease in children. Pediatrics 1994;94(2 Pt 1):185–9.

20. Lantos PM, Rumbaugh J, Bockenstedt LK, et al. Clinical Practice Guidelines by the Infectious Diseases Society of America (IDSA), American Academy of Neurology (AAN), and American College of Rheumatology (ACR): 2020 guidelines for the prevention, diagnosis and treatment of Lyme disease. Clin Infect Dis 2021;72(1):1–8.

21. Costello JM, Alexander ME, Greco KM, et al. Lyme carditis in children: presentation, predictive factors, and clinical course. Pediatrics 2009;123(5):e835–41.

22. Shen RV, McCarthy CA, Smith RP. Lyme carditis in hospitalized children and adults, a case series. Open Forum Infect Dis 2021;8(7):ofab140.

23. Steere AC, Schoen RT, Taylor E. The clinical evolution of Lyme arthritis. Ann Intern Med 1987;107(5):725–31.

24. Gerber MA, Zemel LS, Shapiro ED. Lyme arthritis in children: clinical epidemiology and long-term outcomes. Pediatrics 1998;102(4 Pt 1):905–8.

25. Daikh BE, Emerson FE, Smith RP, et al. Lyme arthritis: a comparison of presentation, synovial fluid analysis, and treatment course in children and adults. Arthritis Care Res (Hoboken) 2013;65(12):1986–90.

26. Glaude PD, Huber AM, Mailman T, et al. Clinical characteristics, treatment and outcome of children with Lyme arthritis in Nova Scotia. Paediatr Child Health 2015;20(7):377–80.

27. Szer IS, Taylor E, Steere AC. The long-term course of Lyme arthritis in children. N Engl J Med 1991;325(3):159–63.

28. Deanehan JK, Kimia AA, Tan Tanny SP, et al. Distinguishing Lyme from septic knee monoarthritis in Lyme disease-endemic areas. Pediatrics 2013;131(3): e695–701.

29. Deanehan JK, Nigrovic PA, Milewski MD, et al. Synovial fluid findings in children with knee monoarthritis in Lyme disease endemic areas. Pediatr Emerg Care 2014;30(1):16–9.

30. Cruz AI Jr, Aversano FJ, Seeley MA, et al. Pediatric Lyme arthritis of the hip: the great imitator? J Pediatr Orthop 2017;37(5):355–61.

31. Dart AH, Michelson KA, Aronson PL, et al. Hip synovial fluid cell counts in children from a Lyme disease endemic area. Pediatrics 2018;141(5). https://doi.org/10.1542/peds.2017-3810.

32. Grant DS, Neville DN, Levas M, et al. Validation of septic knee monoarthritis prediction rule in a Lyme disease endemic area. Pediatr Emerg Care 2021. https://doi.org/10.1097/PEC.0000000000002455.

33. Steere AC, Levin RE, Molloy PJ, et al. Treatment of Lyme arthritis. Arthritis Rheum 1994;37(6):878–88.

34. Brescia AC, Rose CD, Fawcett PT. Prolonged synovitis in pediatric Lyme arthritis cannot be predicted by clinical or laboratory parameters. Clin Rheumatol 2009; 28(5):591–3.

35. Tory HO, Zurakowski D, Sundel RP. Outcomes of children treated for Lyme arthritis: results of a large pediatric cohort. J Rheumatol 2010;37(5):1049–55.

36. Nimmrich S, Becker I, Horneff G. Intraarticular corticosteroids in refractory childhood Lyme arthritis. Rheumatol Int 2014;34(7):987–94.

37. Horton DB, Taxter AJ, Davidow AL, et al. Pediatric antibiotic-refractory lyme arthritis: a multicenter case-control study. J Rheumatol 2019;46(8):943–51.

38. Steere AC. Treatment of lyme arthritis. J Rheumatol 2019;46(8):871–3.

39. Steere AC, Angelis SM. Therapy for Lyme arthritis: strategies for the treatment of antibiotic-refractory arthritis. Arthritis Rheum 2006;54(10):3079–86.

40. Li X, McHugh GA, Damle N, et al. Burden and viability of *Borrelia burgdorferi* in skin and joints of patients with erythema migrans or Lyme arthritis. Arthritis Rheum 2011;63(8):2238–47.

41. Wormser GP, Nadelman RB, Schwartz I. The amber theory of Lyme arthritis: initial description and clinical implications. Clin Rheumatol 2012;31(6):989–94.

42. Horton DB, Taxter AJ, Davidow AL, et al. Intraarticular glucocorticoid injection as second-line treatment for Lyme arthritis in children. J Rheumatol 2019;46(8): 952–9.

43. Branda JA, Steere AC. Laboratory diagnosis of Lyme borreliosis. Clin Microbiol Rev 2021;17(2):34. https://doi.org/10.1128/CMR.00018-19.

44. Nelson CA, Hayes CM, Markowitz MA, et al. The heat is on: killing blacklegged ticks in residential washers and dryers to prevent tickborne diseases. Ticks tick-borne Dis 2016;7(5):958–63.

45. Gomes-Solecki M, Arnaboldi PM, Backenson PB, et al. Protective immunity and new vaccines for Lyme disease. Clin Infect Dis 2020;70(8):1768–73.

46. Schotthoefer AM, Hall MC, Vittala S, et al. Clinical presentation and outcomes of children with human granulocytic anaplasmosis. J Pediatr Infect Dis Societ 2018; 7(2):e9–15.

47. Vannier E, Krause PJ. Human babesiosis. N Engl J Med 2012;366(25):2397–407.

Diagnostic Testing for Lyme Disease

Takaaki Kobayashi, MD[a],*, Paul G. Auwaerter, MD[b]

KEYWORDS

- Lyme disease • Borrelia burgdorferi • Laboratory diagnosis • Serology testing

KEY POINTS

- Clinicians need to combine knowledge of Lyme disease serologic testing performance and its limitations with potential epidemiologic exposure and clinical presentation to gauge the relative usefulness of the testing results.
- Frequent misuses of serology include testing asymptomatic patients after a tick bite; reliance on testing patients with characteristic erythema migrans (EM); and using IgM immunoblot positivity for symptoms of more than 4 weeks duration.
- A modified 2-tier test strategy (MTTT) approved in 2019 by the Food and Drug Administration that uses 2 different EIAs offers faster results and better sensitivity for detecting early Lyme disease than the standard 2-tier test strategy (STTT, using immunoblots) without compromising specificity.
- In the US, a positive STTT or MTTT in appropriate clinical presentations is sufficient to diagnose most *B. burgdorferi* infections involving the nervous system or causing arthritis with joint effusions without additional fluid or tissue sampling.
- Emerging diagnostic technologies using biomarkers, which examine earlier immune responses instead of humoral immunity, may offer higher sensitivity than STTT or MTTT in early Lyme disease, though the data are still limited.

BACKGROUND

Lyme disease is the most common vector-borne infection in North America and Europe, caused by one of the 3 common pathogenic genospecies of the spirochete *Borrelia*.[1,2] *Borrelia burgdorferi sensu stricto* is transmitted solely in North America by the *Ixodes* genus of hard ticks. In Europe and Asia, Lyme disease is predominantly caused by *Borrelia afzelii* and *Borrelia garinii*. As outlined in the preceding articles,

[a] Division of Infectious Diseases, Department of Internal Medicine, University of Iowa Hospitals & Clinics, 200 Hawkins Drive, Iowa City, IA 52242, USA; [b] Sherrilyn and Ken Fisher Center for Environmental Infectious Diseases, Johns Hopkins University School of Medicine, Baltimore, MD, USA
* Corresponding author.
E-mail address: takaaki-kobayashi@uiowa.edu

Infect Dis Clin N Am 36 (2022) 605–620
https://doi.org/10.1016/j.idc.2022.04.001
0891-5520/22/© 2022 Elsevier Inc. All rights reserved.

B. burgdorferi infection may cause dermatologic, musculoskeletal, neurologic, and/or cardiac illnesses.

Lyme disease can be characterized as presenting within 3 forms: early localized, early disseminated, and late stages. Early localized infection presents as a single erythematous skin lesion called erythema migrans (EM) arising from the tick bite site[3]; see Franc Strle and Gary P. Wormser's article, "Early Lyme Disease (Erythema Migrans) and Its Mimics (STARI and TARI)," in this issue. However, EM may be absent in approximately 20% to 30% of cases.[4,5] If EM is absent or missed and untreated, the spirochete can subsequently disseminate, causing presentations such as multifocal EM rash, nonspecific viral-like illness, polyarthralgia, meningitis, neuropathy, or carditis. For some, late infection may occur after incubating for weeks or months. An oligoarthritis of larger joints, characteristically the knee in adults, is the most common form (see Sheila L. Arvikar and Allen C. Steere's article, "Lyme Arthritis," in this issue).

Serologic testing for Lyme disease is not recommended for asymptomatic patients after a tick bite. Even if *B. burgdorferi* has been introduced, antibody-based testing at this time will not reflect a new infection if present. Furthermore, background seropositivity of up to 5% to 10% in some parts of the US may complicate result interpretation.[6–8] Early localized Lyme disease is clinically diagnosed by the presence of EM since standard 2-tier testing (STTT) is insensitive at this early stage of infection when the humoral response has not been mounted sufficiently. Seropositivity improves as the infection continues, becoming reliable for diagnosing later clinical manifestations, including neurologic manifestations, carditis, and arthritis if an EM history is not solidly established.

Confusion regarding Lyme disease diagnosis has accompanied this infection since its discovery in 1976. Though the causative spirochete was identified in 1981 by Willy Burgdorfer, its fastidiousness and low bacterial burden in human infection meant that neither culture nor molecular techniques were easily performed or frequently positive. Instead, indirect methods reliant on antibody responses have been the dominant method for securing a laboratory diagnosis. A 2-tier approach was recommended in 1995 by CDC[9] to improve the specificity of early generation antibody testing by using immunoblots to confirm the presence of specific restricted antibody responses to *B. burgdorferi* antigens. Although serology is part of the CDC case definition which incorporates the most frequent clinical manifestations of Lyme disease, its inclusion is not intended to restrict diagnosis to seropositive cases. In one survey among practitioners in a Lyme endemic region, a majority did not rely on the CDC case definition for diagnosis.[10] Serologic testing comes with inherent limitations, making it imperative for anyone ordering these tests to sufficiently understand their utility.

Both under- and over-diagnosis of Lyme disease have been well-described.[11–15] The reasons for high misdiagnosis rates in recent years are likely multifactorial. One explanation is that Lyme disease serologic testing reports are prone to misinterpretation, such as reliance on IgM results outside of acute disease or giving undue significance to immunoblot bands not meeting criteria.[16,17] In addition, a variety of non–FDA-approved Lyme tests developed by self-designated Lyme specialty laboratories add to the confusion and often mislead clinicians as these tests are rarely clinically validated.[18] Examples of these laboratory-developed tests that are not recommended include urine antigen, quantitative CD57 lymphocyte assays, in-house criteria for the alternative interpretation of immunoblots, specialized culture techniques, and immunologic stimulation tests.[19] This article reviews the recommended laboratory diagnostics for Lyme disease (focusing on the United States) and potential developments to improve diagnosis.

THE STANDARDIZED 2-TIERED SEROLOGY TEST: STANDARD 2-TIER TESTING

In 1994, the Association of State and Territorial Public Health Laboratory Directors, CDC, FDA, the National Institutes of Health, the Council of State and Territorial Epidemiologists, and the National Committee for Clinical Laboratory Standards convened the Second National Conference on Serologic Diagnosis of Lyme Disease. The recommended methodology uses a quantitative, sensitive enzyme immunoassay (EIA) or immunofluorescence assay (IFA) as a first test. The second-tier Western blot (immunoblot) assays follow if the first tier yields positive or equivocal results based on data showing that the immunoblots improved specificity.[9] Professional society guidelines have endorsed the US Food and Drug Administration (FDA)-approved STTT to support the diagnosis of Lyme disease in patients who have objective manifestations other than acute EM.[20,21]

The schematic summarizing the features of STTT is shown in **Fig. 1**. The first tier of STTT serves as a screening test for antibodies by sensitive EIA or IFA. EIAs examine blood for the existence of IgM and IgG (together or separately) antibodies recognizing *B. burgdorferi* antigens. The initial basis for the first-tier used in FDA-approved tests was a whole-cell sonicate (WCS) of culture-grown *B. burgdorferi*. Though still used, modifications improving the accuracy of the WCS approach have been incorporated including adsorption steps to reduce cross-reacting antibodies, antibody capture techniques, fractionation of the cells, and adding synthetically produced antigens such as surface lipoprotein VlsE (variable major protein-like sequence, expressed) or C6 (invariable region 6 of VlsE) or C10 (the conserved amino-terminal portion of outer surface protein C) peptide.[22,23] Studies have demonstrated that EIAs using the C6 epitope or VlsE protein are more specific than WCS EIAs.[22–25] IFA is now rarely used as it requires skilled technical expertise, whereas automated methodologies make EIA the modern customary choice. Suppose the results of first-tier testing are less than the clinically validated threshold. In that case, the serum is reported as negative for antibodies to *B. burgdorferi* and no further testing is needed. If the result is positive or indeterminate, second-tier testing is performed proceeding to individual IgM and IgG immunoblots.

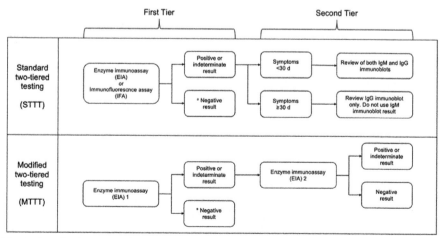

Fig. 1. Standard 2-tier and modified 2-tier tests for Lyme disease. [a] When STTT or MTTT is negative in acute disease, consider obtaining convalescent-phase serum in 4 to 6 weeks if highly suspicious for Lyme disease.

The second tier detects antibodies produced against *B. burgdorferi*, though limited to specific standardized antigens. This process uses proteins derived from *B. burgdorferi* separated in a porous gel by an electrical field. Positions of the proteins are determined by their molecular mass and then transferred to a membrane surface that is probed by serum that may contain antibodies generated to *B. burgdorferi* bacterial antigens. Such antibody–antigen binding results in detecting specific bands in the immunoblot.

The IgM immunoblot is positive if at least 2 of 3 bands (21–24, 39, and 41 kDa) stain greater than with control sera. This finding should only be used if clinical symptoms are 4 weeks or less in duration due to high rates of false positivity in patients who have longer-term symptoms.[9,26] The IgG immunoblot is considered positive if 5 or more of 10 predetermined bands (18, 21–24, 28, 30, 39, 41, 45, 58, 66, and 93 kDa) are found. These blots have been validated for *B. burgdorferi* sensu stricto for Lyme disease in North America but are less reliable for diagnosing other *Borrelia* genospecies in Europe, such as *B. afzelii and B. garinii*.[27]

Early localized Lyme disease is usually diagnosed on clinical grounds alone when a characteristic EM rash (see Franc Strle and Gary P. Wormser's article, "Early Lyme Disease (Erythema Migrans) and Its Mimics (STARI and TARI)," in this issue) is present in a patient who lives in or has recently traveled to areas with a high incidence.[21] Testing for early Lyme disease in the first week of illness may yield rates as low as 20% with STTT as humoral responses take several weeks to fully mount.[25,28,29] If there is clinical suspicion for Lyme disease, but no rash is seen or a skin lesion is atypical, and initial testing in acute illness is negative, repeating serologic testing about 3 to 4 weeks later may be helpful since the immunoblots should be positive. For later stages of Lyme disease, the sensitivity ranges from 70% to 100% with a greater than 95% specificity, including current FDA-approved testing kits[30–33] Late manifestations of Lyme disease, such as arthritis, have nearly universal IgG positive results according to 2-tier criteria, with similar seroreactivity in late neuroborreliosis.[25] Conversely, negative serologic testing among those with long-term symptoms rules out Lyme disease.[34]

THE MODIFIED 2-TIERED SEROLOGY TEST: MODIFIED 2-TIERED TESTING

FDA has recently approved a modified 2-tiered testing (MTTT) algorithm for Lyme disease serology. There is only one MTTT testing (Zeus) commercially available in the U.S as of this writing. A second EIA is used instead of an immunoblot for positive or equivocal samples on the first EIA. This may combine IgM and IgG antibodies or be performed separately. The schematic summarizing the features of MTTT is shown in **Fig. 1**. The CDC now supports MTTT as an alternative to STTT.[35] When these 2 tests are part of MTTT, specificity is greater than that of either test alone and equal to the specificity of traditional STTT.[23,36] Several recent studies comparing STTT and MTTT revealed specificity greater than 98% with MTTT.[24,25,37,38] (**Table 1**). In addition, the MTTT algorithm was more sensitive in early Lyme disease than STTT.[24,25,37,38] Similar results were reported in Canada and central Europe.[38,39] Moreover, MTTT has been shown to be more cost-effective than STTT.[33]

Although there are some features representing an improvement over STTT, limitations of MTTT remain. Similar to STTT, MTTT does not distinguish between active and past infections as antibody responses can persist for months to years. Although better than STTT for detecting early localized Lyme disease, the sensitivity of MTTT is still around 60% to 70% in early Lyme disease, which means that patients who present with EM should still be clinically diagnosed without routine serologic testing. One of

Table 1
Sensitivity and specificity of assays for the diagnosis of Lyme disease

Assay	Specimen Type	Clinical Manifestation	Sensitivity (%)	Selected References	Specificity (%)	Selected References
Standard 2-tiered testing	Serum	Early localized	<40% (acute)	32,33,97	~99%	Branda et al,[36] 2017
			27% (convalescent)	Wormser et al,[33] 2013		
			61% (convalescent)	Molins et al,[32] 2014		
	Serum	Early disseminated	86% (carditis)	Molins et al,[32] 2014	~99%	Waddell et al,[98] 2016
			90%	Waddell et al,[98] 2016		
			42%–87%	99		
	Serum	Neuroborreliosis	90%	Molins et al,[32] 2014	96%–100%	Davis et al,[39] 2020
	Serum	Late disseminated	100% (arthritis)	Molins et al,[32] 2014	99%–100%	Molins et al,[24] 2016, Davis et al,[39] 2020
			97%–100%	99		
Modified 2-tiered testing	Serum	Early localized	53% (acute)	Branda et al,[37] 2011	~99%	Branda et al,[36] 2017
			58% (acute)	Wormser et al,[25] 2013, Wormser et al,[33] 2013	96%–100%	Davis et al,[39] 2020
			89% (convalescent)	Branda et al,[37] 2011		
			67% (convalescent)	Wormser et al,[25] 2013, Wormser et al,[33] 2013		
	Serum	Early disseminated	71%–86% (carditis)	Pegalajar-Jurado et al,[100] 2018	96%–100%	Davis et al,[39] 2020
	Serum	Neuroborreliosis	98%–100%	22,37,100	96%–100%	22,37,39
	Serum	Late disseminated	~100% (arthritis)	Molins et al,[24] 2016, Pegalajar-Jurado et al,[100] 2018	96%–100%	Molins et al,[24] 2016, Davis et al,[39] 2020
Polymerase chain reaction	Serum and/or skin Serum/Plasma	Early localized	64%–81% 62%	Nowakowski et al,[97] 2001 Eshoo et al,[101] 2012	~100%	Nocton et al,[102] 1994 [a], [103,104]
	Serum	Early disseminated	29% (carditis)	Molins et al,[32] 2014		
	CSF	Neuroborreliosis	25%–38% 73%	Nocton et al,[102] 1994 [a][99]		
	Synovial fluid	Late disseminated	85% (arthritis) 83% (arthritis)	Nocton et al,[102] 1994 [a][99]		

(continued on next page)

Table 1
(continued)

Assay	Specimen Type	Clinical Manifestation	Sensitivity (%)	Selected References	Specificity (%)	Selected References
Culture	Skin	Early localized	51%	Nowakowski et al,[97] 2001	N/A	N/A
	Serum		45%	Nowakowski et al,[97] 2001		
	Skin + serum		44%	Molins et al,[32] 2014		
	Skin + serum	Early disseminated	0% (carditis)	Molins et al,[32] 2014		
	Serum	Neuroborreliosis	25%	Molins et al,[32] 2014		
	CSF		10%–30%	Theel et al,[105] 2019		
	Synovial fluid	Late disseminated	N/A	N/A		
CSF: serum antibody index	Serum and CSF	Neuroborreliosis	70% (<6 wk), and ~100% thereafter 82%	Koedel[76] 2015, Ljostad[77] 2007 Djukic et al,[70] 2012	97%	Blanc et al,[106] 2007

Abbreviation: CSF, cerebrospinal fluid; N/A, not applicable.
[a] Article published before 2000.

the advantages of MTTT is a shorter turnaround time, as any clinical laboratory with the capability to perform EIAs can avoid the delay incurred by immunoblot assays which take more time to perform or require a send out to a larger lab. However, for late presentations such as Lyme arthritis, STTT might be favored to distinguish the presence of specific IgG immunoblot responses (see Sheila L. Arvikar and Allen C. Steere's article, "Lyme Arthritis," in this issue).

COMMON ISSUES WITH SEROLOGIC TESTING

Serology has poor positive predictive values in areas with a low incidence of Lyme disease. One study revealed less than 20% of seropositive patients in North Carolina, an area with low incidence, had actual Lyme disease.[40] Therefore, serologic testing for Lyme disease is most useful for patients with at least an intermediate pretest probability. In addition, an EIA can be positive due to other infections or inflammatory processes. For example, both EIA and IgM immunoblots may be falsely positive due to cross-reacting antibodies to other spirochetal diseases, including relapsing fever borreliosis, syphilis, leptospirosis, and viral infections including Epstein–Barr virus, cytomegalovirus and parvovirus B19.[41–46]

Moreover, positive IgM immunoblot alone without positive IgG immunoblot is associated with overdiagnosis of Lyme disease. In a retrospective study from Boston, Lantos and colleagues[16] revealed that 30% of patients with only positive IgM immunoblots were unlikely to have Lyme disease. In the United States, the CDC recommends that a positive IgM response alone should not support Lyme disease diagnosis if symptoms have been present for more than 4 weeks since most patients will have a positive IgG immunoblot.[9] If the patient has an isolated IgM Western blot after 4 to 6 weeks from the onset of the symptoms, the IgM test is likely a false-positive result or, possibly, evidence of past infection.

Lyme disease is not an immunizing condition in early disease, and people can have second or more bouts of EM due to repeated infection.[47] However, serology for the diagnosis of subsequent infection is problematic since antibodies, including IgM and IgG, can remain positive for many years after the initial infection and successful treatment.[48] These persistent positive antibodies often render confusion due to IgM presence that could be interpreted as new or active infection requiring treatment.[48] If a subsequent extracutaneous manifestation of *B. burgdorferi* infection is suspected, it can be helpful to compare quantitative EIA values or see if additional bands are present. In these circumstances, performing acute and convalescent serologic tests would be informative to detect an increase in EIA titers or modification in the seroreactivity pattern by immunoblot.[49] However, serial testing to monitor treatment response is not recommended, although antibody responses generally decline months to years after treatment.[50,51] In addition, it is important to emphasize that immunoblots are only clinically validated for use in serum. Use in other specimens, such as cerebrospinal fluid (CSF) or synovial fluid, is not recommended as a positive result may lead to an inappropriate diagnosis of Lyme disease.[52]

Borrelia miyamotoi is a relapsing fever Borrelia group spirochete transmitted by the same hard-bodied tick species that transmit Lyme disease. *B. miyamotoi* may resemble Lyme disease but uncommonly has a rash, and frequently patients can be found to have identifiable spirochetemia, which is rare for *B. burgdorferi* infection.[53] In a study conducted in New England and New York State, the seroprevalence of *B. miyamotoi* was about one-third of *B. burgdorferi*.[6] Recent studies indicated that the C6 peptide ELISA might be positive in patients infected with *B. miyamotoi,* though do not develop *B. burgdorferi* positive immunoblots.[54] Therefore, careful interpretation is required whereby the first-tier STTT relies solely on C6 peptide in an appropriate patient to include the consideration of *B. miyamotoi* if immunoblot negative.

A newly described spirochete, *Borrelia mayonii,* was identified in patients from Minnesota and Wisconsin with systemic symptoms and rash.[55] Currently, the diagnosis of *B. mayonii* relies on the use of a PCR test, though suspicion may also be garnered by seeing spirochetes in a Giemsa-stained blood smear. While limited studies are available on the utility of *B. burgdorferi* serologic testing on *B. mayonii* infection, available information suggests that patients with *B.mayonii* infection develop antibodies similar to those of patients with *B. burgdorferi*.[55]

CULTURE

While culture remains a standard reference method to confirm microbiological infection, it is not routinely available for diagnosing Lyme disease in most clinical settings. Culture has relatively low sensitivity, long incubation requirements (up to 12 weeks), and is technically demanding, requiring special media. Several methods can be used to confirm growth, including polymerase chain reaction (PCR) and either dark field microscopy or light microscopy using stains such as acridine orange to detect characteristic spirochetes.[56] Due to low organism burden and brief spirochetemia in early infection, culture is relatively insensitive for detecting *B. burgdorferi* in human disease.[57]

Studies have isolated *B. burgdorferi* from skin biopsy specimens, blood, and rarely CSF. Two widely used media are the modified Kelly-Pettenkofer and Barbour-Stoenner-Kelly II. The culture of skin biopsies taken from the leading border of EM has a 40% to 60% sensitivity.[58,59] One report found that blood cultures from untreated patients with EM have a sensitivity of around 45%, increasing to 70% by frequently testing culture aliquots with a sensitive PCR.[56] The sensitivity of blood culture falls to approximately 20% among those with early disseminated disease, including neurologic, cardiac or musculoskeletal manifestations.[60] Spirochetemia is principally found in patients with Lyme disease who have a relatively early infection, and *B. burgdorferi* is seldom cultured from the blood of Lyme disease patients with later disease manifestations.

The culture of CSF is rarely positive and is not recommended. CSF culture is associated with low sensitivity, ranging from 10% to 30%, in European patients with neuroborreliosis, likely lower in the relatively less neurotropic *B. burgdorferi* sensu lato genospecies causing infection in North America.[61,62] *B. burgdorferi* has not been reliably cultivated from synovial fluid, with only isolated reports of successful cultivation.[63] Finally, antibiotic treatment decreases all culture positivity rates, making it useful only in untreated patients.[64]

MOLECULAR TECHNIQUES

Though PCR technology is offered in many laboratories, it is neither an FDA-approved test nor firmly established in clinical practice. It could be pursued using a reliable laboratory backed by the clinical validation of their assay. PCR has been used in many research studies examining skin, blood, synovial fluid, and CSF. While PCR is highly specific, the sensitivity of PCR for borrelial DNA depends on the type of sample. A skin biopsy sample from the leading edge of an EM lesion has a sensitivity of 69% but a specificity of 100%.[64] In patients with Lyme arthritis, PCR of the synovial fluid has a sensitivity ranging from 46% to 96%.[65] However, the sensitivity of PCR of the CSF of patients with neurologic manifestations of Lyme disease is only 20% to 40%.[61,66] PCR of other clinical samples, including blood and urine, is not recommended, as spirochetes are primarily confined to tissues, and very few are present in these body fluids.[64]

In practice, *B. burgdorferi* DNA detection by PCR is most often used to evaluate Lyme arthritis. In patients with suspected Lyme arthritis, synovial fluid analyzed by *B. burgdorferi* PCR is highly specific but less sensitive than serum IgG seroreactivity, which is nearly always positive. Patients with characteristic knee joint effusions may not require arthrocentesis if other explanations (eg, septic arthritis, inflammatory diseases, or microcrystalline disorders) seem unlikely. Lyme arthritis in children is more likely to cause a clinically inflamed joint and fever than in adults; therefore, it can be confused with septic arthritis.[67] The disadvantage of PCR is that a positive result does not always mean active infection. The DNA of nonviable microbes may persist for several months even after successful treatment.[65] When the diagnosis of Lyme arthritis is unclear, such as in patients with a prior history of Lyme disease and existing seropositivity, PCR testing of synovial fluid may help to clarify the likelihood of active infection.

CEREBROSPINAL FLUID ANALYTICS

Common neuroborreliosis manifestations in North America and Europe are cranial neuropathies, lymphocytic meningitis, or radiculitis. Studies have demonstrated that most patients with early Lyme neuroborreliosis are seropositive by conventional 2-tiered testing at initial clinical presentation.[25,68] Lumbar puncture is not routinely required for facial palsy presentations in patients with positive serology.[21] CSF examination in Lyme neuroborreliosis typically shows a pleocytosis of more than 90% lymphocytes (mostly between 30 and 300 cells/mm^3), a slightly raised protein concentration, and a normal glucose concentration[69–71]

If CSF testing is performed in patients with suspected Lyme neuroborreliosis involving the central nervous system, it is recommended to obtain simultaneous samples of CSF and serum for determining the CSF: serum antibody index using the validated methodology in a laboratory with experience in the assay.[21] The index normalizes the level of anti-*Borrelia* antibodies to total IgG and albumin in the CSF. It establishes the antibody index ratio of anti-*Borrelia* antibodies in CSF-to-serum to suggest authentic intrathecal antibody production. Measuring the total antibody concentration only in the CSF can be misleading because a positive result may be caused by the passive transfer of antibodies from the serum. The sensitivity of the CSF: serum antibody index is considered to range from 70% to 90% in those with Lyme neuroborreliosis with less than 6 weeks of symptoms, while it is ~95% in untreated patients with longer symptom durations.[72–77] However, the index may remain elevated for years following successful treatment; therefore, careful interpretation is required.[78]

INVESTIGATIONAL TESTS
CXCL13

The chemokine CXCL13 has been proposed as an early biomarker for detecting Lyme neuroborreliosis.[79] Elevated levels of CSF CXCL13 are known to correlate with intrathecal *B. burgdorferi* antibody response in patients with acute Lyme meningitis.[80–83] However, CSF CXCL13 concentrations may be elevated in numerous conditions, including HIV infection and neoplasia. The role of CSF CXCL13 levels in CNS infection remains unestablished.[84,85]

B. Burgdorferi-Specific Cell-Mediated Responses

T cell-based assays have been the subject of research for decades to improve testing for Lyme disease, especially early infection[86]. Infection with *B. burgdorferi* elicits a T-cell response that exhibits different kinetics than the humoral response.[86,87] These tests include immunosequencing T-cell receptor (TCR) repertoires and detection of

INF-γ secretion.[88–90] Previous studies demonstrated that an active T-cell response is induced during the acute phase of infection, even in the absence of seroconversion, and returns to normal levels after antibiotic treatment and symptom resolution.[91–93] In contrast, humoral responses vary widely, demonstrating attenuated responses and a lack of IgM to IgG seroconversion that can persist for decades.[48,94] One study demonstrated a higher sensitivity with INF-γ at 69% compared with C6 ELISA at 59% and Western blotting at 17% to detect early Lyme disease.[89] In addition, a recent study from NY demonstrated that the level of INF-γ detected by the QuantiFERON ELISA significantly decreased after treatment.[95] These data may suggest that assays examining the -cellular responses may have utility for diagnosing Lyme disease, especially in an early stage, as well as evaluating the response after treatment However, each study included a small number of patients and might have included patients with other or cobacterial and viral infections concerning cross-reactivity. Moreover, controversial results and/or poor methodological quality of studies investigating T-cell response have been reported.[96] More extensive prospective studies are needed to investigate the clinical utility of immunologic cell-mediated responses for Lyme disease diagnosis.

SUMMARY

The 2-tiered serologic strategies, including STTT and MTTT, are currently the mainstays for Lyme disease diagnosis among all patients without EM. PCR of synovial fluid and CSF: serum index can be helpful in selected patients with Lyme disease. However, arthrocentesis or lumbar puncture may not be required in characteristic cases. Clinicians need to be wary of specialty laboratories offering Lyme disease testing using assays whose accuracy and clinical usefulness have not been adequately established. Moreover, clinicians should understand the clinical context of ordering serology to gauge positive and negative predictive values depending on clinical presentation, geography, and symptom duration.

Needed improvements in Lyme disease diagnostics include aiming for accurate direct pathogen-detection methods that are sufficiently sensitive and specific to detect infection by multiple pathogenic Borrelia species. Among indirect methods, serology is hampered by its inherently lagging responses in early infection. Cell-mediated immune changes may narrow the window between acquiring infection and yielding a positive test but need further study. Lastly, a future test for Lyme disease that correlates with microbiologic eradication would help staunch unnecessary antibiotic use in symptomatic people with chronic symptoms that may or may not be due to *B. burgdorferi* infection.

CLINICS CARE POINTS

- In an area with a low incidence of human *Borrelia burgdorferi* infection, positive Lyme disease test results are often false positives.
- In patients with negative serologic testing but high clinical suspicion, consider repeating serology in 3 to 4 weeks.
- MTTT has better sensitivity in early Lyme disease than STTT, with a shorter turnaround time.
- IgM results should be used only for patients with symptoms less than 4 weeks; solely relying on positive IgM responses in patients with symptoms longer than 4 weeks increases the likelihood of overdiagnosis of Lyme disease due to lack of test specificity.

- Clinicians need to be leery of insufficiently validated testing approaches such as alternative immunoblot criteria, immunoblots of CSF or synovial fluid, and testing techniques from self-described Lyme specialty laboratories.
- Synovial or CSF fluid analysis is not always required in the appropriate clinical presentations if diagnostic serum *B. burgdorferi* IgG responses are present.

DISCLOSURE

T. Kobayashi: no disclosure. P.G. Auwaerter: Pfizer (Scientific Consulting), Adaptive Biotechnologies (Scientific Consulting), medical-legal expert consulting.

REFERENCES

1. O'Connell S, Granstrom M, Gray JS, et al. Epidemiology of european lyme borreliosis. Zentralbl Bakteriol 1998;287(3):229–40.
2. Rosenberg R, Lindsey NP, Fischer M, et al. Vital signs: trends in reported vectorborne disease cases - united states and territories, 2004-2016. MMWR Morb Mortal Wkly Rep 2018;67(17):496–501.
3. Sanchez E, Vannier E, Wormser GP, et al. Diagnosis, treatment, and prevention of lyme disease, human granulocytic anaplasmosis, and babesiosis: a review. JAMA 2016;315(16):1767–77.
4. Steere AC, Sikand VK. The presenting manifestations of lyme disease and the outcomes of treatment. N Engl J Med 2003;348(24):2472–4.
5. Esposito S, Leone S, Noviello S. Management of severe bacterial infections. Expert Rev Anti Infect Ther 2005;3(4):593–600.
6. Krause PJ, Narasimhan S, Wormser GP, et al. Borrelia miyamotoi sensu lato seroreactivity and seroprevalence in the northeastern united states. Emerg Infect Dis 2014;20(7):1183–90.
7. Krause PJ, Telford SR 3rd, Spielman A, et al. Concurrent lyme disease and babesiosis. Evidence for increased severity and duration of illness. JAMA 1996;275(21):1657–60.
8. Hilton E, DeVoti J, Benach JL, et al. Seroprevalence and seroconversion for tick-borne diseases in a high-risk population in the northeast united states. Am J Med 1999;106(4):404–9.
9. Centers for Disease C and Prevention. Recommendations for test performance and interpretation from the second national conference on serologic diagnosis of lyme disease. MMWR Morb Mortal Wkly Rep 1995;44(31):590–1.
10. Perea AE, Hinckley AF, Mead PS. Evaluating the potential misuse of the lyme disease surveillance case definition. Public Health Rep 2020;135(1):16–7.
11. Nigrovic LE, Bennett JE, Balamuth F, et al. Accuracy of clinician suspicion of lyme disease in the emergency department. Pediatrics 2017;140(6):e20171975.
12. Nelson CA, Starr JA, Kugeler KJ, et al. Lyme disease in hispanics, united states, 2000-2013. Emerg Infect Dis 2016;22(3):522–5.
13. Schutzer SE, Berger BW, Krueger JG, et al. Atypical erythema migrans in patients with pcr-positive lyme disease. Emerg Infect Dis 2013;19(5):815–7.
14. Kobayashi T, Higgins Y, Samuels R, et al. Misdiagnosis of lyme disease with unnecessary antimicrobial treatment characterizes patients referred to an academic infectious diseases clinic. Open Forum Infect Dis 2019;6(7):ofz299.
15. Kobayashi T, Higgins Y, Melia MT, et al. Mistaken identity: Many diagnoses are frequently misattributed to lyme disease. Am J Med 2022;135(4). 503–511.e5.

16. Lantos PM, Lipsett SC, Nigrovic LE. False positive lyme disease igm immuno-blots in children. J Pediatr 2016;174:267–269 e1.

17. Seriburi V, Ndukwe N, Chang Z, et al. High frequency of false positive igm immunoblots for borrelia burgdorferi in clinical practice. Clin Microbiol Infect 2012;18(12):1236–40.

18. Moore A, Nelson C, Molins C, et al. Current guidelines, common clinical pitfalls, and future directions for laboratory diagnosis of lyme disease, united states. Emerg Infect Dis 2016;22(7):1169–77.

19. Bills H, Snell G, Levvey B, et al. Mycobacterium abscessus and lung transplantation: an international survey. J Heart Lung Transplant 2015;34(4):S304.

20. Wormser GP, Dattwyler RJ, Shapiro ED, et al. The clinical assessment, treatment, and prevention of lyme disease, human granulocytic anaplasmosis, and babesiosis: Clinical practice guidelines by the infectious diseases society of america. Clin Infect Dis 2006;43(9):1089–134.

21. Lantos PM, Rumbaugh J, Bockenstedt LK, et al. Clinical practice guidelines by the infectious diseases society of america (idsa), american academy of neurology (aan), and american college of rheumatology (acr): 2020 guidelines for the prevention, diagnosis and treatment of lyme disease. Clin Infect Dis 2021;72(1):1–8.

22. Branda JA, Body BA, Boyle J, et al. Advances in serodiagnostic testing for lyme disease are at hand. Clin Infect Dis 2018;66(7):1133–9.

23. Theel ES. The past, present, and (possible) future of serologic testing for lyme disease. J Clin Microbiol 2016;54(5):1191–6.

24. Molins CR, Delorey MJ, Sexton C, et al. Lyme borreliosis serology: Performance of several commonly used laboratory diagnostic tests and a large resource panel of well-characterized patient samples. J Clin Microbiol 2016;54(11):2726–34.

25. Wormser GP, Schriefer M, Aguero-Rosenfeld ME, et al. Single-tier testing with the c6 peptide elisa kit compared with two-tier testing for lyme disease. Diagn Microbiol Infect Dis 2013;75(1):9–15.

26. Engstrom SM, Shoop E, Johnson RC. Immunoblot interpretation criteria for serodiagnosis of early lyme disease. J Clin Microbiol 1995;33(2):419–27.

27. Wormser GP, Tang AT, Schimmoeller NR, et al. Utility of serodiagnostics designed for use in the united states for detection of lyme borreliosis acquired in europe and vice versa. Med Microbiol Immunol 2014;203(1):65–71.

28. Steere AC, Malawista SE, Hardin JA, et al. Erythema chronicum migrans and lyme arthritis. The enlarging clinical spectrum. Ann Intern Med 1977;86(6):685–98.

29. Wormser GP, Nowakowski J, Nadelman RB, et al. Impact of clinical variables on borrelia burgdorferi-specific antibody seropositivity in acute-phase sera from patients in north america with culture-confirmed early lyme disease. Clin Vaccin Immunol 2008;15(10):1519–22.

30. Dressler F, Whalen JA, Reinhardt BN, et al. Western blotting in the serodiagnosis of lyme disease. J Infect Dis 1993;167(2):392–400.

31. Johnson BJ, Robbins KE, Bailey RE, et al. Serodiagnosis of lyme disease: accuracy of a two-step approach using a flagella-based elisa and immunoblotting. J Infect Dis 1996;174(2):346–53.

32. Molins CR, Sexton C, Young JW, et al. Collection and characterization of samples for establishment of a serum repository for lyme disease diagnostic test development and evaluation. J Clin Microbiol 2014;52(10):3755–62.

33. Wormser GP, Levin A, Soman S, et al. Comparative cost-effectiveness of two-tiered testing strategies for serodiagnosis of lyme disease with noncutaneous manifestations. J Clin Microbiol 2013;51(12):4045–9.
34. Tugwell P, Dennis DT, Weinstein A, et al. Laboratory evaluation in the diagnosis of lyme disease. Ann Intern Med 1997;127(12):1109–23.
35. Mead P, Petersen J, Hinckley A. Updated cdc recommendation for serologic diagnosis of lyme disease. MMWR Morb Mortal Wkly Rep 2019;68(32):703.
36. Branda JA, Strle K, Nigrovic LE, et al. Evaluation of modified 2-tiered serodiagnostic testing algorithms for early lyme disease. Clin Infect Dis 2017;64(8): 1074–80.
37. Branda JA, Linskey K, Kim YA, et al. Two-tiered antibody testing for lyme disease with use of 2 enzyme immunoassays, a whole-cell sonicate enzyme immunoassay followed by a vlse c6 peptide enzyme immunoassay. Clin Infect Dis 2011;53(6):541–7.
38. Branda JA, Strle F, Strle K, et al. Performance of united states serologic assays in the diagnosis of lyme borreliosis acquired in europe. Clin Infect Dis 2013; 57(3):333–40.
39. Davis IRC, McNeil SA, Allen W, et al. Performance of a modified two-tiered testing enzyme immunoassay algorithm for serologic diagnosis of lyme disease in nova scotia. J Clin Microbiol 2020;58(7):e01841-19.
40. Lantos PM, Branda JA, Boggan JC, et al. Poor positive predictive value of lyme disease serologic testing in an area of low disease incidence. Clin Infect Dis 2015;61(9):1374–80.
41. Magnarelli LA, Anderson JF, Johnson RC. Cross-reactivity in serological tests for lyme disease and other spirochetal infections. J Infect Dis 1987;156(1):183–8.
42. Magnarelli LA, Anderson JF. Enzyme-linked immunosorbent assays for the detection of class-specific immunoglobulins to borrelia burgdorferi. Am J Epidemiol 1988;127(4):818–25.
43. Goossens HA, Nohlmans MK, van den Bogaard AE. Epstein-barr virus and cytomegalovirus infections cause false-positive results in igm two-test protocol for early lyme borreliosis. Infection 1999;27(3):231.
44. Tuuminen T, Hedman K, Soderlund-Venermo M, et al. Acute parvovirus b19 infection causes nonspecificity frequently in borrelia and less often in salmonella and campylobacter serology, posing a problem in diagnosis of infectious arthropathy. Clin Vaccin Immunol 2011;18(1):167–72.
45. Pavletic AJ, Marques AR. Early disseminated lyme disease causing false-positive serology for primary epstein-barr virus infection: Report of 2 cases. Clin Infect Dis 2017;65(2):336–7.
46. Patriquin G, LeBlanc J, Heinstein C, et al. Cross-reactivity between lyme and syphilis screening assays: Lyme disease does not cause false-positive syphilis screens. Diagn Microbiol Infect Dis 2016;84(3):184–6.
47. Nadelman RB, Wormser GP. Reinfection in patients with lyme disease. Clin Infect Dis 2007;45(8):1032–8.
48. Kalish RA, McHugh G, Granquist J, et al. Persistence of immunoglobulin m or immunoglobulin g antibody responses to borrelia burgdorferi 10-20 years after active lyme disease. Clin Infect Dis 2001;33(6):780–5.
49. Pfister HW, Neubert U, Wilske B, et al. Reinfection with borrelia burgdorferi. Lancet 1986;2(8513):984–5.
50. Philipp MT, Wormser GP, Marques AR, et al. A decline in c6 antibody titer occurs in successfully treated patients with culture-confirmed early localized or early disseminated lyme borreliosis. Clin Diagn Lab Immunol 2005;12(9):1069–74.

51. Marangoni A, Sambri V, Accardo S, et al. A decrease in the immunoglobulin g antibody response against the vlse protein of borrelia burgdorferi sensu lato correlates with the resolution of clinical signs in antibiotic-treated patients with early lyme disease. Clin Vaccin Immunol 2006;13(4):525–9.

52. Barclay SS, Melia MT, Auwaerter PG. Misdiagnosis of late-onset lyme arthritis by inappropriate use of borrelia burgdorferi immunoblot testing with synovial fluid. Clin Vaccin Immunol 2012;19(11):1806–9.

53. Pritt BS, Mead PS, Johnson DKH, et al. Identification of a novel pathogenic borrelia species causing lyme borreliosis with unusually high spirochaetaemia: A descriptive study. Lancet Infect Dis 2016;16(5):556–64.

54. Koetsveld J, Platonov AE, Kuleshov K, et al. Borrelia miyamotoi infection leads to cross-reactive antibodies to the c6 peptide in mice and men. Clin Microbiol Infect 2020;26(4):513 e1–13 e6.

55. What you need to know about borrelia mayonii. Centers for disease control and preventions. Available at: https://www.cdc.gov/lyme/mayonii/index.html. Accessed March 24.

56. Liveris D, Schwartz I, Bittker S, et al. Improving the yield of blood cultures from patients with early lyme disease. J Clin Microbiol 2011;49(6):2166–8.

57. Coulter P, Lema C, Flayhart D, et al. Two-year evaluation of borrelia burgdorferi culture and supplemental tests for definitive diagnosis of lyme disease. J Clin Microbiol 2005;43(10):5080–4.

58. Picken MM, Picken RN, Han D, et al. A two year prospective study to compare culture and polymerase chain reaction amplification for the detection and diagnosis of lyme borreliosis. Mol Pathol 1997;50(4):186–93.

59. Liveris D, Wang G, Girao G, et al. Quantitative detection of borrelia burgdorferi in 2-millimeter skin samples of erythema migrans lesions: Correlation of results with clinical and laboratory findings. J Clin Microbiol 2002;40(4):1249–53.

60. Nowakowski J, McKenna D, Nadelman RB, et al. Blood cultures for patients with extracutaneous manifestations of lyme disease in the united states. Clin Infect Dis 2009;49(11):1733–5.

61. Cerar T, Ogrinc K, Cimperman J, et al. Validation of cultivation and pcr methods for diagnosis of lyme neuroborreliosis. J Clin Microbiol 2008;46(10):3375–9.

62. Mygland A, Ljostad U, Fingerle V, et al. Efns guidelines on the diagnosis and management of european lyme neuroborreliosis. Eur J Neurol 2010;17(1):8–16, e1-4.

63. Snydman DR, Schenkein DP, Berardi VP, et al. Borrelia burgdorferi in joint fluid in chronic lyme arthritis. Ann Intern Med 1986;104(6):798–800.

64. Aguero-Rosenfeld ME, Wang G, Schwartz I, et al. Diagnosis of lyme borreliosis. Clin Microbiol Rev 2005;18(3):484–509.

65. Li X, McHugh GA, Damle N, et al. Burden and viability of borrelia burgdorferi in skin and joints of patients with erythema migrans or lyme arthritis. Arthritis Rheum 2011;63(8):2238–47.

66. Nocton JJ, Bloom BJ, Rutledge BJ, et al. Detection of borrelia burgdorferi DNA by polymerase chain reaction in cerebrospinal fluid in lyme neuroborreliosis. J Infect Dis 1996;174(3):623–7.

67. Deanehan JK, Kimia AA, Tan Tanny SP, et al. Distinguishing lyme from septic knee monoarthritis in lyme disease-endemic areas. Pediatrics 2013;131(3):e695–701.

68. Steere AC, McHugh G, Damle N, et al. Prospective study of serologic tests for lyme disease. Clin Infect Dis 2008;47(2):188–95.

69. Stanek G, Wormser GP, Gray J, et al. Lyme borreliosis. Lancet 2012;379(9814): 461–73.
70. Djukic M, Schmidt-Samoa C, Lange P, et al. Cerebrospinal fluid findings in adults with acute lyme neuroborreliosis. J Neurol 2012;259(4):630–6.
71. Lakos A. Csf findings in lyme meningitis. J Infect 1992;25(2):155–61.
72. Halperin JJ, Volkman DJ, Wu P. Central nervous system abnormalities in lyme neuroborreliosis. Neurology 1991;41(10):1571–82.
73. Tumani H, Nolker G, Reiber H. Relevance of cerebrospinal fluid variables for early diagnosis of neuroborreliosis. Neurology 1995;45(9):1663–70.
74. Cerar T, Ogrinc K, Strle F, et al. Humoral immune responses in patients with lyme neuroborreliosis. Clin Vaccin Immunol 2010;17(4):645–50.
75. Steere AC, Berardi VP, Weeks KE, et al. Evaluation of the intrathecal antibody response to borrelia burgdorferi as a diagnostic test for lyme neuroborreliosis. J Infect Dis 1990;161(6):1203–9.
76. Koedel U, Fingerle V, Pfister HW. Lyme neuroborreliosis-epidemiology, diagnosis and management. Nat Rev Neurol 2015;11(8):446–56.
77. Ljostad U, Skarpaas T, Mygland A. Clinical usefulness of intrathecal antibody testing in acute lyme neuroborreliosis. Eur J Neurol 2007;14(8):873–6.
78. Clark JR, Carlson RD, Sasaki CT, et al. Facial paralysis in lyme disease. Laryngoscope 1985;95(11):1341–5.
79. Yang J, Han X, Liu A, et al. Chemokine cxc ligand 13 in cerebrospinal fluid can be used as an early diagnostic biomarker for lyme neuroborreliosis: A meta-analysis. J Interferon Cytokine Res 2017;37(10):433–9.
80. Eckman EA, Pacheco-Quinto J, Herdt AR, et al. Neuroimmunomodulators in neuroborreliosis and lyme encephalopathy. Clin Infect Dis 2018;67(1):80–8.
81. Wutte N, Berghold A, Loffler S, et al. Cxcl13 chemokine in pediatric and adult neuroborreliosis. Acta Neurol Scand 2011;124(5):321–8.
82. Hytonen J, Kortela E, Waris M, et al. Cxcl13 and neopterin concentrations in cerebrospinal fluid of patients with lyme neuroborreliosis and other diseases that cause neuroinflammation. J Neuroinflammation 2014;11:103.
83. Cerar T, Ogrinc K, Lotric-Furlan S, et al. Diagnostic value of cytokines and chemokines in lyme neuroborreliosis. Clin Vaccin Immunol 2013;20(10):1578–84.
84. Schmidt C, Plate A, Angele B, et al. A prospective study on the role of cxcl13 in lyme neuroborreliosis. Neurology 2011;76(12):1051–8.
85. Bremell D, Mattsson N, Edsbagge M, et al. Cerebrospinal fluid cxcl13 in lyme neuroborreliosis and asymptomatic hiv infection. BMC Neurol 2013;13(2). https://doi.org/10.1186/1471-2377-13-2.
86. Dressler F, Yoshinari NH, Steere AC. The t-cell proliferative assay in the diagnosis of lyme disease. Ann Intern Med 1991;115(7):533–9.
87. Vaz A, Glickstein L, Field JA, et al. Cellular and humoral immune responses to borrelia burgdorferi antigens in patients with culture-positive early lyme disease. Infect Immun 2001;69(12):7437–44.
88. Auwaerter PG, Aucott J, Dumler JS. Lyme borreliosis (lyme disease): Molecular and cellular pathobiology and prospects for prevention, diagnosis and treatment. Expert Rev Mol Med 2004;6(2):1–22.
89. Callister SM, Jobe DA, Stuparic-Stancic A, et al. Detection of ifn-gamma secretion by t cells collected before and after successful treatment of early lyme disease. Clin Infect Dis 2016;62(10):1235–41.
90. Greissl J, Pesesky M, Dalai SC, et al. Immunosequencing of the t-cell receptor repertoire reveals signatures specific for diagnosis and characterization of early lyme disease. medRxiv 2021. https://doi.org/10.1101/2021.07.30.21261353.

91. Soloski MJ, Crowder LA, Lahey LJ, et al. Serum inflammatory mediators as markers of human lyme disease activity. PLoS One 2014;9(4):e93243.

92. Jin C, Roen DR, Lehmann PV, et al. An enhanced elispot assay for sensitive detection of antigen-specific t cell responses to borrelia burgdorferi. Cells 2013;2(3):607–20.

93. Forsberg P, Ernerudh J, Ekerfelt C, et al. The outer surface proteins of lyme disease borrelia spirochetes stimulate t cells to secrete interferon-gamma (ifn-gamma): Diagnostic and pathogenic implications. Clin Exp Immunol 1995; 101(3):453–60.

94. Rebman AW, Crowder LA, Kirkpatrick A, et al. Characteristics of seroconversion and implications for diagnosis of post-treatment lyme disease syndrome: Acute and convalescent serology among a prospective cohort of early lyme disease patients. Clin Rheumatol 2015;34(3):585–9.

95. Arnaboldi PM, D'Arco C, Hefter Y, et al. Detection of ifn-gamma secretion in blood samples collected before and after treatment of varying stages of lyme disease. Clin Infect Dis 2021;73(8):1484–91.

96. Raffetin A, Saunier A, Bouiller K, et al. Unconventional diagnostic tests for lyme borreliosis: a systematic review. Clin Microbiol Infect 2020;26(1):51–9.

97. Nowakowski J, Schwartz I, Liveris D, et al. Laboratory diagnostic techniques for patients with early lyme disease associated with erythema migrans: A comparison of different techniques. Clin Infect Dis 2001;33(12):2023–7.

98. Waddell LA, Greig J, Mascarenhas M, et al. The accuracy of diagnostic tests for lyme disease in humans, a systematic review and meta-analysis of north american research. PLoS One 2016;11(12):e0168613.

99. Centers for disease control and prevention. Hhs federal research updates on lyme disease diagnostics. Available at: https://www.cdc.gov/lyme/diagnosistesting/HHS-research-updates.html. Accessed January 15, 2022.

100. Pegalajar-Jurado A, Schriefer ME, Welch RJ, et al. Evaluation of modified two-tiered testing algorithms for lyme disease laboratory diagnosis using well-characterized serum samples. J Clin Microbiol 2018;56(8):e01943-17.

101. Eshoo MW, Crowder CC, Rebman AW, et al. Direct molecular detection and genotyping of borrelia burgdorferi from whole blood of patients with early lyme disease. PLoS One 2012;7(5):e36825.

102. Nocton JJ, Dressler F, Rutledge BJ, et al. Detection of borrelia burgdorferi DNA by polymerase chain reaction in synovial fluid from patients with lyme arthritis. N Engl J Med 1994;330(4):229–34.

103. Nigrovic LE, Lewander DP, Balamuth F, et al. The lyme disease polymerase chain reaction test has low sensitivity. Vector Borne Zoonotic Dis 2020;20(4): 310–3.

104. Ruzic-Sabljic E, Cerar T. Progress in the molecular diagnosis of lyme disease. Expert Rev Mol Diagn 2017;17(1):19–30.

105. Theel ES, Aguero-Rosenfeld ME, Pritt B, et al. Limitations and confusing aspects of diagnostic testing for neurologic lyme disease in the united states. J Clin Microbiol 2019;57(1):e01406-18.

106. Blanc F, Jaulhac B, Fleury M, et al. Relevance of the antibody index to diagnose lyme neuroborreliosis among seropositive patients. Neurology 2007;69(10): 953–8.

Persistent Symptoms After Treatment of Lyme Disease

Adriana Marques, MD

KEYWORDS

- Lyme disease • Posttreatment Lyme disease syndrome • Chronic Lyme disease
- Long-term symptoms • Misdiagnosis

KEY POINTS

- Lyme disease is treated successfully with recommended antibiotics in most of the cases; however, some patients have persisting nonspecific symptoms after treatment, referred to as posttreatment Lyme disease symptoms (PTLDs) or syndrome (PTLDS).
- Chronic Lyme disease (CLD) is a controversial term, with no defined diagnostic criteria, used to describe different patient populations. Patients with PTLDs represent a small portion of patients with CLD.
- Most patients with CLD suffer from other conditions or are patients with medically unexplained physical symptoms and are diagnosed with CLD based on unvalidated tests and criteria.
- There is a critical need for more research to elucidate the mechanisms underlying PTLDs, together with research into patients diagnosed with CLD .

"Confusion worse confounded." John Milton, Paradise Lost. Book ii.

CHRONIC LYME DISEASE AND POSTTREATMENT LYME DISEASE

Lyme disease, caused by infection with *Borreliella (Borrelia) burgdorferi* and transmitted by the bite of the ticks of the *Ixodes ricinus* complex, is the most common vector-borne disease in the United States and Europe.[1] Antibiotic treatment is effective for most patients, but some patients report persisting or relapsing nonspecific symptoms after treatment.[2] These symptoms are referred to as posttreatment Lyme disease symptoms (PTLDs) or syndrome (PTLDS), depending on their severity and functional impact.[3]

Patients with PTLDs are a small subset of what is called "chronic Lyme disease" (CLD) (**Fig. 1**), a term avoided by academic literature and mainstream medical providers, as there are no clear criteria or agreement as to what constitutes "chronic Lyme disease" and the term can refer to very different groups of patients. For example,

---

Laboratory of Clinical Immunology and Microbiology, National Institute of Allergy and Infectious Diseases, National Institutes of Health, BG 10 RM 12C118 MSC 1888 10 Center, Bethesda, MD 20892-1888, USA
E-mail address: amarques@niaid.nih.gov

Infect Dis Clin N Am 36 (2022) 621–638
https://doi.org/10.1016/j.idc.2022.04.004
0891-5520/22/Published by Elsevier Inc.

id.theclinics.com

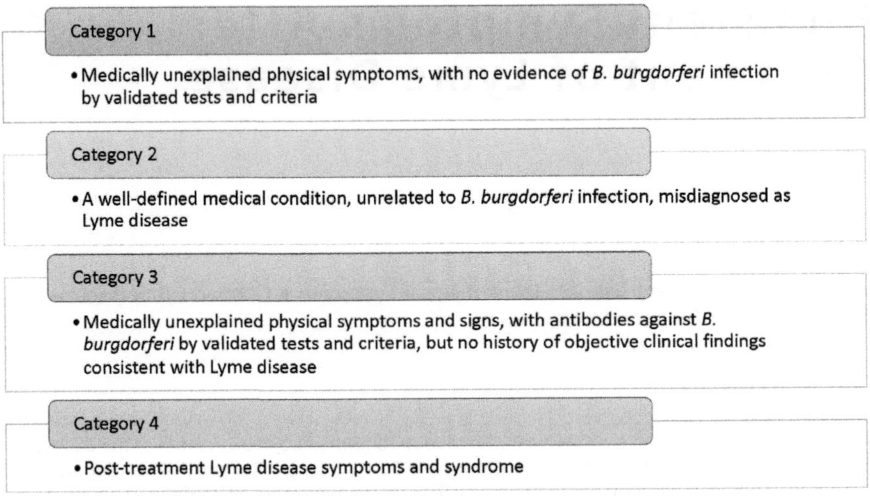

Category 1

- Medically unexplained physical symptoms, with no evidence of *B. burgdorferi* infection by validated tests and criteria

Category 2

- A well-defined medical condition, unrelated to *B. burgdorferi* infection, misdiagnosed as Lyme disease

Category 3

- Medically unexplained physical symptoms and signs, with antibodies against *B. burgdorferi* by validated tests and criteria, but no history of objective clinical findings consistent with Lyme disease

Category 4

- Post-treatment Lyme disease symptoms and syndrome

Fig. 1. Categories of "Chronic Lyme Disease." (*Data from* Feder HM, Jr., Johnson BJ, O'Connell S, et al. A critical appraisal of "chronic Lyme disease." N Engl J Med. Oct 42,007;357(14):1422–30. https://doi.org/10.1056/NEJMra072023).

CLD is defined by one society as a "multisystem illness with a wide range of symptoms and/or signs that are either continuously or intermittently present for a minimum of 6 months." CLD has evolved into a "multiple chronic infectious disease syndrome" and patients are diagnosed with multiple infections (*Babesia, Ehrlichia, Anaplasma, Rickettsia, Bartonella*, Powassan virus, *Mycoplasma, Chlamydia,* multiple herpesviruses*)* and poorly defined conditions ("immune dysfunction, inflammation, toxin damage by heavy metals and mold, food and environmental allergies, nutritional and metabolic abnormalities, hormonal imbalances, mitochondrial dysfunction, free radical/oxidative stress, and autonomic system dysfunction." These diagnoses are based on clinical judgment, together with unvalidated tests and interpretation criteria. A study found that 57.5% of healthy controls could be interpreted as positive using the in-house criteria of a Lyme specialty laboratory.[4] Culture assays claiming high positivity have raised serious concerns[5,6] and could not be replicated.[7] A urine antigen assay had false-positive results and the same sample varied from negative to highly positive when testing 5 fractions from each of 10 negative control samples.[8] Natural killer cells measurements are unhelpful.[9] Practitioners treating CLD often market themselves as integrative, functional, naturopathic, and Lyme-literate. Patients are charged high fees and spend a significant amount of money on multiple unproven tests and unvalidated treatments that range from innocuous to highly dangerous.[10–16] Once a patient has received the diagnosis of "chronic Lyme disease," the inclination is to assign any signs and symptoms to it, leading to missed or delayed diagnosis of other medical conditions.[17,18] Patients diagnosed with "chronic Lyme disease" can be reluctant to accept the diagnosis of other diseases, even when this can have dire consequences.[14,18] These patients frequently disagree with the different diagnosis provided, seeking further evaluation and receiving additional antibiotic therapy for Lyme disease.[19]

Most of the patients diagnosed with CLD have conditions whose symptoms are misdiagnosed or are patients with medically unexplained physical symptoms (MUPS) who receive the diagnosis based on unproven and/or nonvalidated laboratory tests and clinical criteria (**Fig. 2**). Studies have shown that 47% to 80% of the patients seeking further evaluation for Lyme disease had no evidence of *B. burgdorferi* infection.[19–26]

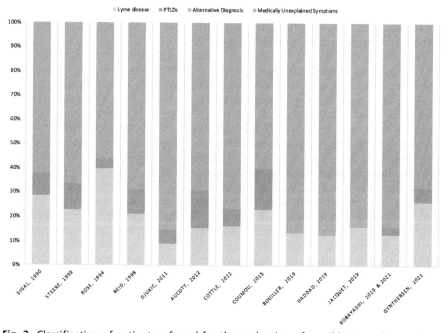

Fig. 2. Classification of patients referred for the evaluation of possible Lyme disease. Posttreatment Lyme disease symptoms (PTLDs).

An alternative diagnosis was made in 15% to 55% (median 34%) of the cases, while MUPS accounted for 19% to 54% (median 32%). Patients with PTLDs accounted for 3% to 15% (median 9%) of the cases.

Patients with MUPS, or persistent physical symptoms, are common across general medicine.[27–29] MUPS encompasses a range of conditions, including fibromyalgia and myalgic encephalomyelitis/chronic fatigue syndrome (ME/CFS); with the substantial overlap of symptoms between patients.[30] These symptoms are caused and maintained by complex interactions between biological, psychological, and social mechanisms.[31] A possible mechanism is central sensitization, whereby maladaptive changes lead to alterations in how pain and other sensory stimuli are processed with the development of chronic symptoms.[31] Interestingly, patients with "alternatively diagnosed chronic Lyme syndrome" (another name for CLD) were similar to patients with ME/CFS when compared with controls, with no differences in gene expression, B-cell/T-cell receptor profiles, and potential viral infections. The CLD diagnosis was due to false-positive results from alternative laboratory tests.[32,33]

POSTTREATMENT LYME DISEASE SYMPTOMS AND SYNDROME

The remainder of this article will focus on research addressing PTLDs. To fulfill the criteria for PTLDs,[34] patients must have a documented episode of Lyme disease, have received a recommended course of antibiotic therapy, with resolution or stabilization of the objective manifestation(s) of Lyme disease, have nonspecific symptoms (persistent or relapsing) that started within 6 months of the Lyme disease diagnosis and lasted for at least 6 months after the completion of antibiotic therapy and have no other condition that explains the symptoms. Symptoms need to cause a substantial reduction in previous levels of activity to be classified as PTLD syndrome. A standardized approach is very important as it would allow for systematical quantification of the severity level of symptoms in patients with PTLDs and allow for comparison between studies of outcomes and other data.[3,35,36]

Most patients who present with defined manifestations of Lyme disease will have a good outcome after antibiotic treatment with recommended regimens,[2] returning to their previous level of health. Patients with later manifestations may have a delayed response to therapy, and recovery can take weeks or months.[37] Incomplete resolution due to nonreversible damage can occur, as seen in patients with facial palsy and residual facial weakness.[38] Some patients with Lyme arthritis have persistent synovitis after antibiotic therapy, known as postinfectious Lyme arthritis.[39] Treatment failure with current antibiotic regimens (whereby patients have objective signs of disease after treatment) can occur, but it is very uncommon.

Persisting or relapsing subjective nonspecific complaints, mostly of mild to moderate intensity, occurred in between 0% and 26% of patients with erythema migrans evaluated 6 to 12 months after the completion of treatment (**Fig. 3**).[36,40–62] Risk factors for PTLDs include antibiotic treatment delay, symptom severity at the time of treatment, presentation with multiple erythema migrans or with nonerythema migrans manifestations of Lyme disease, and presence of tingling or an abnormal skin sensation at the initial visit.[42,49,63–65] Other risk factors include a history of stressful events,[61,65] the presence of comorbidities unrelated to Lyme disease,[66] older age, and female sex.[42,61] Children are less likely to develop PTLDs.[45,51,52,56,62]

Possible Causes of Posttreatment Lyme Disease Symptoms

The mechanisms underlying PTLDs are not known and are likely to be multifactorial. The pathogenesis of the nonspecific symptoms is likely to differ among individuals (**Box 1**).[67] Possible explanations include both related and unrelated causes.

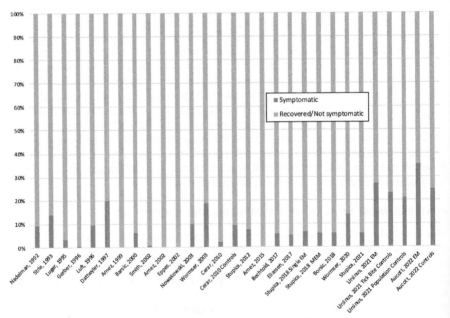

Fig. 3. Symptoms after antibiotic therapy in patients with erythema migrans. Erythema migrans (EM). Multiple erythema migrans (MEM).

> **Box 1**
> **Possible causes of posttreatment Lyme disease symptoms**
>
> Part of the expected resolution of symptoms after treatment
>
> New and preexisting conditions unrelated to Lyme disease
>
> Postinfective fatigue syndrome
>
> Other tick-borne infections
>
> Microbiome changes
>
> Metabolome changes
>
> Dysregulated immune response/autoimmunity
>
> Persistence of *B. burgdorferi* remnants
>
> Persistent infection with *B. burgdorferi*

Natural Course of Response to Treatment

For many individuals, these nonspecific symptoms are part of the natural course of the response to the treatment of the infection, and they will continue to improve after completing antibiotic treatment. Studies of patients with erythema migrans show that the proportion of patients reporting symptoms after antibiotic treatment decreases over time (**Fig. 4**).[36,40,46–48,68] A prospective study of patients with Lyme disease showed that, regardless of disease stage or severity at diagnosis, their quality-of-life scores increased to just above the United States national average after 3 years of follow-up time. Comorbidities unrelated to Lyme disease were the only

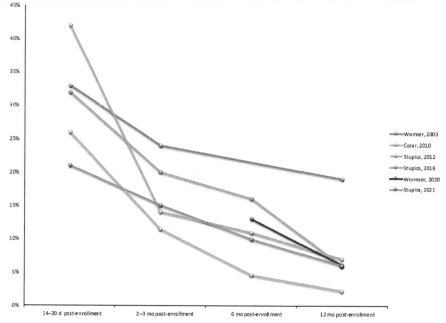

Fig. 4. The number of patients reporting symptoms after antibiotic treatment decreases over time.

factors significantly associated with long-term symptoms or lower quality of life scores.[66] Similar results were seen in a study of patients with culture-confirmed erythema migrans evaluated 11 to 20 years after diagnosis.[69]

Postinfective fatigue syndrome
Prolonged fatigue after infections is relatively common, can be disabling and persistent, and is associated with the severity of the acute illness.[70–74] The mechanisms triggered during the acute illness that sustain the persistent symptoms are currently unknown. However, prolonged fatigue in patients with early Lyme disease after treatment is not common, with only 3% of patients with erythema migrans having persistent fatigue possibly due to Lyme disease when evaluated 11 to 20 years after treatment.[75]

Misattribution and other conditions, including background prevalence of nonspecific symptoms and coinfections
Symptoms and signs due to other conditions can be wrongly attributed to Lyme disease, and these patients would be expected to have a less favorable response to specific antiborrelial therapy. This was shown in a study of patients with disseminated Lyme disease, whereby 90% of the patients with definite diagnosis had excellent or good outcomes, comparing with only 47% of possible cases.[76] Similarly, patients with definite Lyme neuroborreliosis had better long-term outcomes than those with possible Lyme neuroborreliosis.[37,77,78]

Nonspecific symptoms such as fatigue, chronic pain, and sleep disorders are common in the general population, often reported together and associated with anxiety and depression.[79] Studies whereby patients with Lyme disease and matched controls were followed prospectively showed similar prevalence of symptoms at follow-up,[36,41,46,47,68,80,81] while 2 studies showed a higher prevalence of persistent symptoms in a small subset of patients with Lyme disease.[60,61] All these studies demonstrate substantial (some more than 20%) background prevalence of nonspecific symptoms in the general population.

Coinfection with other tick-borne pathogens is rare in patients with PTLDs.[82–84] Patients with concurrent Lyme disease and untreated Babesia infection had increased symptoms in one study[85] but another study showed no difference in symptoms between patients with and without Babesia coinfection.[86]

Microbiome changes
A study compared patients with PTLDS with healthy controls and intensive care unit patients.[87] As expected, intensive care unit controls were distinct from both PTLDS and healthy controls. There was a relative abundance of Blautia sp and Enterobacteriaceae over 10% in patients with PTLDS when compared with healthy controls but patients with PTLDS had received extensive antibiotic therapy (median of 56 days) and the effect of antibiotics on the gut microbiome can be prolonged.[88] A prospective study of patients with Lyme disease before and at intervals after antibiotic therapy will be necessary to assess the validity and relevance of these findings.

Metabolic changes
The metabolic response was studied in 23 non-PTLDs and 24 patients with PTLDs (11 symptoms and 13 syndrome).[89] Metabolite classes including glycerophospholipid, bile acid, and acylcarnitine metabolism were altered between the groups. Interestingly, patients with PTLDs' metabolic patterns looked similar at posttreatment and 1-year follow-up, while there were greater differences for the patients with non-

PTLDs, particularly at the posttreatment timepoint, suggesting the end of treatment as the most informative metabolic biosignature.

Immune Dysregulation or Maladaptive Host Responses

Immune dysregulation or maladaptive host responses has been best studied in patients with postinfectious Lyme arthritis,[39] which is associated with both host genetic factors and *B. burgdorferi* factors that together contribute to dysregulated and excessive inflammatory immune responses, increased T-helper 1 and T-helper 17 immune responses, and autoreactive T and B cells. PTLDs differ substantially from postinfectious Lyme arthritis. However, it is possible that immune dysregulation and/or infection-induced autoimmune mechanisms could contribute to symptoms. A few studies considered this question, but no reproducible marker has been identified. An important issue is that, in prospective studies, the number of patients with early Lyme disease who will develop PTLDs is small. Because many variables are being examined with a small number of patients, there is a risk of a type I error. Other reasons include differences in methods and technologies used, and differences in the patient groups studied.

Patients with PTLDS had higher levels of antibodies against neural proteins than recovered patients or healthy controls[90,91] and higher antibody reactivity frequencies against certain *B. burgdorferi* antigens.[91–93] PTLDS cases had higher levels of antilysoganglioside GM1 antibody than controls, but not other antineuronal antibodies.[94] Antibodies against endothelial cell growth factor were found more frequently in patients with persistent symptoms in one study,[95] but not in another study.[96]

Differences in the host response and their association with persistent symptoms have been investigated in the Study of Lyme disease Immunology and Clinical Events (SLICE) cohort.[97] One study measured 58 cytokines and chemokines, and 6 acute-phase markers, on 76 patients with erythema migrans (36 recovered, 29 patients with symptoms-only and 11 PTLDS), and 26 healthy controls. C-C motif chemokine ligand 19 (CCL19), ferritin, fibrinogen, C-X-C motif chemokine ligand (CXCL) 10, CXCL9, C-reactive protein, and serum amyloid A were differentially regulated between Lyme disease and healthy controls at the pretreatment visit. Generalized logistical regressions were used to predict Lyme disease clinical outcome group using these 7 markers. An increase in CCL19 of 0.5 standard deviation for the Lyme disease group at posttreatment visits was associated with PTLDS, and the hypothesis was that elevated CCL19 levels could reflect an ongoing reaction at distal sites to the secondary lymphoid tissue. For comparison, a European study measured 23 cytokines in the serum of 45 patients with erythema migrans with at least 1 posttreatment Lyme symptom, compared with 41 recovered patients. In this study, interleukin (IL)-23 levels were higher before therapy and stayed higher up to 12-month follow-up in patients with persistent symptoms,[95] a finding not seen in the previous study.[97] CCL19 was not found to be significantly different between the groups. A study evaluating serum samples from 19 patients with a history of Lyme disease and objective memory impairment showed increased serum interferon-alpha activity in patients when compared with recovered (n = 11) and healthy controls (n = 20). There were no changes with prolonged antibiotic therapy.[91]

Blum et al.[98] showed that blood plasmablasts were increased in 32 patients with untreated Lyme (7 PTLDS and 25 recovered patients, also part of the SLICE study) and returned to baseline levels by 6 months following antibiotic treatment. As expected, patients with disseminated erythema migrans (10 recovered and 1 PTLDS) had higher plasmablasts numbers compared with those with single erythema migrans (15 recovered and 6 PTLDS). Patients with PTLDS had significantly lower blood plasmablasts than patients who returned to health at the pretreatment timepoint, and less seroreactivity to surface proteins and peptides from *B. burgdorferi*. This finding contrast with the studies showing patients with PTLDS have higher levels of autoantibodies and certain *B. burgdorferi* antigens.[90–96]

The longitudinal transcriptomic response in blood was studied in 29 individuals with Lyme disease (15 who returned to health, 9 with symptoms only, and 4 PTLDS) and 13 matched controls, part of the SLICE study.[99] There were no genes significantly differentially expressed at any single time point between the 15 patients who returned to health and the 13 patients with persistent symptoms. Four differentially expressed genes were identified when all timepoints were combined, and GPR15 was found differentially expressed when comparing patients with resolved Lyme disease with PTLDS at the time of diagnosis visit. A recent publication (also using data from the SLICE study) claims that, based on the projection of the RNA-seq data, cases are separated from controls and stay separate over time, but could not distinguish the patients that would go on to develop posttreatment persistent symptoms.[100] Further corroboration of the results will need to wait until the actual dataset for this study is made available to the scientific community.

Persistence of B. burgdorferi Remnants

It is possible that leftover *B. burgdorferi* products may stay trapped and preserved in tissue after infection, playing a role in posttreatment symptoms.[101] Deposits of antigens were shown to persist near the cartilage and within joint entheses after antibiotic treatment in mice, and this material was capable of stimulating an inflammatory and immune response in uninfected mice.[102] Recently *B. burgdorferi* peptidoglycan was detected in synovial fluid samples from patients with Lyme arthritis, including patients with postinfectious Lyme arthritis after antibiotic therapy, and its systemic administration elicited acute arthritis in mice.[103] Although these observations do not exclude the possibility that these antigens could be produced by residual live bacteria, treatment of patients with postinfectious Lyme arthritis with potent immunosuppressive agents have not led to the reemergence of infection.

Persistent Infection with B. burgdorferi

The possibility that a persistent infection could be driving PTLDs has been a major concern. Arguments against this hypothesis include studies showing that symptomatic patients were not more likely to be seropositive than recovered patients and that patients did not develop objective manifestations of late Lyme disease.[49,104] Also, no direct evidence of *B. burgdorferi* infection was found in these patients (however, *B. burgdorferi* culture and PCR have low sensitivity in most body fluids from patients with Lyme disease).[105]

In animal studies, *B. burgdorferi* DNA and RNA can be detected in tissues for months after antibiotic treatment but are not found by culture in antibiotic-treated animals, while untreated control mice are culture positive, and have significantly higher DNA and RNA copy numbers.[106–108] One hypothesis is that some of the spirochetes could become "persisters." Persistence is a survival mechanism that allows organisms to endure diverse adverse environmental conditions by entering a physiologically dormant state.[109] This mechanism is nongenetic and nonheritable (as opposed to the acquisition of antibiotic resistance, which does not appear to occur with *B. burgdorferi*). Resuscitation (exiting the persistent state) is a hallmark of the persistence phenotype, and persister cells will restart proliferating when the adverse condition is removed.[110] For *B. burgdorferi*, persister bacteria have been identified *in vitro*, whereby, as expected, *B. burgdorferi* persisters are able to grow back after removal of the adverse condition.[111] The inability to culture bacteria from animals, particularly mice, months after antibiotic therapy is difficult to explain if persisters remained in the tissues of treated animals. One possibility would be that the bacteria are in a viable, but nonculturable (VBNC) state. It is unclear if VBNC actually occurs, or that persisters that do not resuscitate are dead cells.[112] There is no convincing data that *B. burgdorferi* forms true biofilms.[113]

B. burgdorferi DNA was detected by xenodiagnosis after antibiotic treatment in mice and nonhuman primate studies, while cultures of tick contents were almost always negative. A clinical study showed that xenodiagnosis using pathogen-free *I. scapularis* larval ticks was safe; and the procedure, while quite cumbersome, was well tolerated.[114] Xenodiagnosis was positive for *B. burgdorferi* DNA in one of the 10 patients with PTLDS tested. The discussion has been the significance of the detection of borrelial DNA by xenodiagnosis in relation to the presence (or not) of viable spirochetes, when it was not possible to demonstrate the recovery of live spirochetes by culture.[115] On the other side, the question is how *B. burgdorferi* DNA reached the xenodiagnostic ticks if the spirochetes were not alive. The possibility that very sensitive PCR tests could be detecting rare DNA fragments leftover in the skin is unlikely, as all 39 skin biopsy specimens collected 6 months posttherapy from the area of erythema migrans lesions were negative using the same assay as the clinical study.[116] Another interesting question is how to interpret a negative result in a nonreservoir competent host for *B. burgdorferi* and what these findings can teach us about borrelial infection in humans. A larger study to assess whether a positive xenodiagnosis correlates with the persistence of symptoms is ongoing.

The Results From the Antibiotic Treatment Trials

An important question is if patients with PTLDs benefit from additional treatment. To answer this question, 5 randomized, placebo-controlled, double-blind clinical trials have been conducted.[82,83,117,118] These studies have shown that prolonged antibiotic treatment offered no sustained benefit, while having potential serious risks.

The first 2 studies, one for patients who were IgG seropositive for *B. burgdorferi* at enrollment, and the other for seronegative patients, were published together.[82] Participants were randomized to either ceftriaxone 2 g intravenous daily for 30 days, followed by oral doxycycline, 200 mg daily for 60 days (n = 64), or matching intravenous and oral placebos (n = 65). The studies were stopped early when a planned interim analysis showed it was highly unlikely that a significant difference in treatment efficacy between the groups would be observed. There were no significant differences in quality-of-life scores between the treatment groups at 30, 90, and 180 days in the studies, with about a third of the patients improving, a third worsening, and a third unchanged. There were 2 severe adverse events related to treatment.

The next study was the STOP-LD (Study and Treatment of Post-Lyme Disease) and enrolled 55 patients with PTLDS with persistent significant fatigue.[117] Patients were randomized to 28 days of intravenous ceftriaxone 2 g or placebo. There was improvement in fatigue with ceftriaxone therapy at 6 months but no improvement in mental speed or other neurocognitive measures. Exploratory analysis showed that patients who had positive immunoblot, had not received previous intravenous antibiotic therapy, and had less pain were more likely to improve. Three patients in each group discontinued therapy due to side effects, and 4 had to be hospitalized.

The fourth study enrolled patients with PTLDS treated with at least 3 weeks of intravenous antibiotic therapy, seropositive by IgG Western blot, and had objective memory impairment.[83] Patients were randomized 2:1 to receive 10 weeks of intravenous ceftriaxone (23 patients) or placebo (14 patients), with 20 patients in the ceftriaxone group and 12 patients in the placebo group completing follow-up. Using a model with an aggregate of the 6 domains of neurocognitive performance measured in the study (chosen by a data-driven selection process, which complicated the interpretation of the results),[119] the authors reported a borderline significant small improvement at 12 weeks in the ceftriaxone group. However, both placebo and ceftriaxone groups had similar improvements from baseline when analyzed at 24 weeks. Nine patients discontinued therapy due to side effects. These included 3 allergic reactions, 2 thrombus, one staphylococcal infection, and 2 due to pain. One patient on ceftriaxone underwent cholecystectomy at week 16.

The fifth study is the Persistent Lyme Empiric Antibiotic Study Europe (PLEASE).[118] This study, performed in the Netherlands, enrolled 280 participants with persistent symptoms attributed to Lyme disease. About 90% of the patients had received anti-biotic treatment, and the median duration of symptoms was more than 2 years. After an initial 2-week treatment with open-label intravenous ceftriaxone, participants were randomized to receive 12 weeks of oral doxycycline with a placebo twice a day, clar-ithromycin with hydroxychloroquine twice a day, or 2 placebos twice a day. All groups improved when compared with their initial scores but there were no differences be-tween groups at any time point during follow-up.[120] Because all participants received ceftriaxone therapy, it is unknown if the initial improvement was due to the therapy or a placebo effect. The improvement in fatigue was similar to the improvement seen in the intravenous placebo arm of 2 other studies.[121] Regarding safety, 9 patients had a serious adverse event, and 19 patients had an adverse event that led to the discontin-uation of the study drug.

An interesting analysis, derived from the PLEASE study, examined predictors of symptom improvement.[122] Pretreatment functioning, higher pretreatment expectancy to improve, and thinking that one had received antibiotics at the end of therapy were positively associated with physical and mental improvement at both end-of-treatment and at follow-up. This highlights the important role of patients' positive or negative ex-pectancies on symptom course and treatment outcome. This is a well-known issue within the area of placebo (and nocebo) research, and it is important to consider the patient's expectations of therapeutic benefit as a confounding aspect in clinical trials. Similarly, these considerations apply when evaluating personal reports of the success of alternative therapies and practices. In these contexts, the many variables shown to increase the placebo effect are being combined. These include costly doctor's visits and tests, perceived expertise, complex (and expensive) treatment regimens, priming, social influence, and emotional investment, to cite a few.[123] How to integrate these multiple variables into therapeutic research is an interesting and challenging topic.

SUMMARY

The controversy regarding the underlying mechanisms of PTLDs and the increasingly bitter debate over CLD, continues unabated over the past years. If anything, it has become more contentious. For health care providers, it is important that patients be offered the best advice based on current, evidence-based information. Patients treated for Lyme disease can be reassured that most will fully recover after recom-mended antibiotic therapy,[2] and that nonspecific symptoms will improve over time. Evaluation of patients with PTLDs and CLD can be quite challenging. Practitioners should carefully review the evidence for the diagnosis of Lyme disease, and not lose sight of that symptoms may be due to unrelated conditions. Most importantly is a collaborative approach to the treatment process with the patient, with warmth, empathy, and positive communication. More research on the pathogenesis of PTLDs, particularly biomarkers that would allow for differentiation accordingly to the underlying process, is urgently needed. Such markers could give insights into pathways and lead to valuable treatments. Current evidence shows that prolonged antibiotic therapy, as tested in the randomized placebo-controlled clinical trials, does not offer substantive benefits for patients with PTLDs. These studies also showed a significant placebo effect and variability of the intensity of subjective symptoms over time. Therefore, interventional studies in this population must have a double-blind, randomized controlled design. There is a critical need for high-quality research to better understand "chronic Lyme disease," and how to best help this large and heterogenous group of patients.

CLINICS CARE POINTS

- Patients treated for Lyme disease can be reassured that most will fully recover after recommended antibiotic therapy and that nonspecific symptoms will improve over time.

- Evaluating patients with symptoms after Lyme disease or with the diagnosis of chronic Lyme disease can be challenging. Different factors are likely to play a role in an individual case.

- Symptoms and signs due to other conditions can be wrongly attributed to Lyme disease. Practitioners should carefully review the evidence for the diagnosis of Lyme disease, and not lose sight that symptoms may be due to unrelated conditions.

- Current evidence shows that prolonged antibiotic therapy for PTLDs provides little benefit and carries significant risk.

DISCLOSURES

A. Marques has a patent US 8,926,989 issued; and is an unpaid Scientific Advisor to the Global Lyme Alliance and to the American Lyme Disease Foundation.

ACKNOWLEDGMENTS

Funding for this study was provided by the Division of Intramural Research, National Institute of Allergy and Infectious Diseases, National Institutes of Health. The content of this publication does not necessarily reflect the views or policies of the Department of Health and Human Services, nor does mention of trade names, commercial products, or organizations imply endorsement by the US Government.

REFERENCES

1. Marques AR, Strle F, Wormser GP. Comparison of lyme disease in the United States and Europe. Emerg Infect Dis 2021;27(8):2017–24.
2. Lantos PM, Rumbaugh J, Bockenstedt LK, et al. Clinical Practice Guidelines by the Infectious Diseases Society of America (IDSA), American Academy of Neurology (AAN), and American College of Rheumatology (ACR): 2020 Guidelines for the Prevention, Diagnosis and Treatment of Lyme Disease. Clin Infect Dis 2021;72(1):1–8.
3. Turk SP, Lumbard K, Liepshutz K, et al. Post-treatment Lyme disease symptoms score: developing a new tool for research. PLoS One 2019;14(11):e0225012.
4. Fallon BA, Pavlicova M, Coffino SW, et al. A comparison of lyme disease serologic test results from 4 laboratories in patients with persistent symptoms after antibiotic treatment. Clin Infect Dis 2014;59(12):1705–10.

5. Johnson BJ, Pilgard MA, Russell TM. Assessment of new culture method for detection of Borrelia species from serum of lyme disease patients. research support, U.S. Gov't, P.H.S. J Clin Microbiol 2014;52(3):721–4.

6. Wormser GP, Shapiro ED, Strle F. Studies that report unexpected positive blood cultures for Lyme borrelia - are they valid? Diagn Microbiol Infect Dis 2017;89(3): 178–81.

7. Marques AR, Stock F, Gill V. Evaluation of a new culture medium for Borrelia burgdorferi. J Clin Microbiol 2000;38(11):4239–41.

8. Klempner MS, Schmid CH, Hu L, et al. Intralaboratory reliability of serologic and urine testing for Lyme disease. Am J Med 2001;110(3):217–9.

9. Marques A, Brown MR, Fleisher TA. Natural killer cell counts are not different between patients with post-Lyme disease syndrome and controls. Clin Vaccin Immunol 2009;16(8):1249–50.

10. Frankl S, Hadar PN, Yakhkind A, et al. Devastating Neurological Injury as a Result of Treatment of "Chronic Lyme Disease. Mayo Clin Proc 2021;96(7): 2005–7.

11. Auwaerter PG, Bakken JS, Dattwyler RJ, et al. Antiscience and ethical concerns associated with advocacy of Lyme disease. Lancet Infect Dis 2011;11(9):713–9.

12. Lantos PM, Shapiro ED, Auwaerter PG, et al. Unorthodox alternative therapies marketed to treat Lyme disease. Clin Infect Dis 2015;60(12):1776–82.

13. Marzec NS, Nelson C, Waldron PR, et al. Serious bacterial infections acquired during treatment of patients given a diagnosis of chronic lyme disease - United States. MMWR Morb Mortal Wkly Rep 2017;66(23):607–9.

14. Shelton A, Giurgea L, Moshgriz M, et al. A case of Mycobacterium goodii infection related to an indwelling catheter placed for the treatment of chronic symptoms attributed to Lyme disease. Infect Dis Rep 2019;11(2):8108.

15. Goodlet KJ, Fairman KA. Adverse events associated with antibiotics and intravenous therapies for post-lyme disease syndrome in a commercially insured sample. Clin Infect Dis 2018;67(10):1568–74.

16. Ettestad PJ, Campbell GL, Welbel SF, et al. Biliary complications in the treatment of unsubstantiated Lyme disease. J Infect Dis 1995;171(2):356–61.

17. Nelson C, Elmendorf S, Mead P. Neoplasms misdiagnosed as "chronic lyme disease. JAMA Intern Med 2015;175(1):132–3.

18. Strizova Z, Patek O, Vitova L, et al. Internet-based self-diagnosis of Lyme disease caused death in a young woman with systemic lupus erythematosus. Joint Bone Spine 2019;86(5):650–1.

19. Reid MC, Schoen RT, Evans J, et al. The consequences of overdiagnosis and overtreatment of Lyme disease: an observational study. Ann Intern Med 1998; 128(5):354–62.

20. Sigal LH. Summary of the first 100 patients seen at a Lyme disease referral center. Am J Med 1990;88(6):577–81.

21. Steere AC, Taylor E, McHugh GL, et al. The overdiagnosis of Lyme disease. JAMA 1993;269(14):1812–6.

22. Rose CD, Fawcett PT, Gibney KM, et al. The overdiagnosis of Lyme disease in children residing in an endemic area. Clin Pediatr 1994;33(11):663–8.

23. Aucott JN, Seifter A, Rebman AW. Probable late lyme disease: a variant manifestation of untreated *Borrelia burgdorferi* infection. BMC Infect Dis 2012; 12:173.

24. Kobayashi T, Higgins Y, Samuels R, et al. Misdiagnosis of lyme disease with unnecessary antimicrobial treatment characterizes patients referred to an

academic infectious diseases clinic. Open Forum Infect Dis 2019;6(7). https://doi.org/10.1093/ofid/ofz299.

25. Gynthersen RMM, Tetens MM, Orbaek M, et al. Classification of patients referred under suspicion of tick-borne diseases, Copenhagen, Denmark. Ticks Tick-borne Dis 2021;12(1):101591.

26. Kortela E, Kanerva M, Kurkela S, et al. Suspicion of Lyme borreliosis in patients referred to an infectious diseases clinic: what did the patients really have? Clin Microbiol Infect 2021;27(7):1022–8.

27. van Westrienen PE, Pisters MF, Veenhof C, et al. Identification of patients with moderate medically unexplained physical symptoms in primary care with a five years follow-up. BMC Fam Pract 2019;20(1):66.

28. Kop WJ, Toussaint A, Mols F, et al. Somatic symptom disorder in the general population: Associations with medical status and health care utilization using the SSD-12. Gen Hosp Psychiatry 2019;56:36–41.

29. Dahli MP, Saltyte-Benth J, Haavet OR, et al. Somatic symptoms and associations with common psychological diagnoses: a retrospective cohort study from Norwegian urban general practice. Fam Pract 2021;38(6):766–72.

30. Chalder T, Willis C. "Lumping" and "splitting" medically unexplained symptoms: is there a role for a transdiagnostic approach? J Ment Health 2017;26(3): 187–91.

31. den Boer C, Dries L, Terluin B, et al. Central sensitization in chronic pain and medically unexplained symptom research: A systematic review of definitions, operationalizations and measurement instruments. J Psychosom Res 2019; 117:32–40.

32. Patrick DM, Miller RR, Gardy JL, et al. Lyme disease diagnosed by alternative methods: a phenotype similar to that of chronic fatigue syndrome. Clin Infect Dis 2015;61(7):1084–91.

33. Bouquet J, Gardy JL, Brown S, et al. RNA-Seq analysis of gene expression, viral pathogen, and B-Cell/T-cell receptor signatures in complex chronic disease. Clin Infect Dis 2017;64(4):476–81.

34. Wormser GP, Dattwyler RJ, Shapiro ED, et al. The clinical assessment, treatment, and prevention of lyme disease, human granulocytic anaplasmosis, and babesiosis: clinical practice guidelines by the Infectious Diseases Society of America. Clin Infect Dis 2006;43(9):1089 134.

35. Aucott JN, Crowder LA, Kortte KB. Development of a foundation for a case definition of post-treatment Lyme disease syndrome. Int J Infect Dis 2013;17(6): e443–9.

36. Wormser GP, McKenna D, Karmen CL, et al. Prospective evaluation of the frequency and severity of symptoms in lyme disease patients with erythema migrans compared with matched controls at baseline, 6 months, and 12 months. Clin Infect Dis 2020;71(12):3118–24.

37. Stupica D, Bajrovic FF, Blagus R, et al. Clinical manifestations and long-term outcome of early Lyme neuroborreliosis according to the European Federation of Neurological Societies diagnostic criteria (definite versus possible) in central Europe. A retrospective cohort study. Eur J Neurol 2021;28(9):3155–66.

38. Marques A, Okpali G, Liepshutz K, et al. Characteristics and outcome of facial nerve palsy from Lyme neuroborreliosis in the United States. Ann Clin Transl Neurol 2022;9(1):41–9.

39. Lochhead RB, Strle K, Arvikar SL, et al. Lyme arthritis: linking infection, inflammation and autoimmunity. Nat Rev Rheumatol 2021;17(8):449–61.

40. Stupica D, Bajrovic FF, Blagus R, et al. Association between statin use and clinical course, microbiologic characteristics, and long-term outcome of early Lyme borreliosis. A post hoc analysis of prospective clinical trials of adult patients with erythema migrans. PLoS One 2021;16(12):e0261194.

41. Stupica D, Maraspin V, Bogovic P, et al. Comparison of clinical course and treatment outcome for patients with early disseminated or early localized lyme borreliosis. JAMA Dermatol 2018;154(9):1050–6.

42. Borsic K, Blagus R, Cerar T, et al. Clinical course, serologic response, and long-term outcome in elderly patients with early lyme borreliosis. J Clin Med 2018; 7(12). https://doi.org/10.3390/jcm7120506.

43. Eliassen KE, Hjetland R, Reiso H, et al. Symptom load and general function among patients with erythema migrans: a prospective study with a 1-year follow-up after antibiotic treatment in Norwegian general practice. Scand J Prim Health Care 2017;35(1):75–83.

44. Bechtold KT, Rebman AW, Crowder LA, et al. Standardized symptom measurement of individuals with early lyme disease over time. Arch Clin Neuropsychol 2017;32(2):129–41.

45. Arnez M, Ruzic-Sabljic E. Azithromycin is equally effective as amoxicillin in children with solitary erythema migrans. Pediatr Infect Dis J 2015;34(10):1045–8.

46. Stupica D, Lusa L, Ruzic-Sabljic E, et al. Treatment of erythema migrans with doxycycline for 10 days versus 15 days. Clin Infect Dis 2012;55(3):343–50.

47. Cerar D, Cerar T, Ruzic-Sabljic E, et al. Subjective symptoms after treatment of early Lyme disease. Am J Med 2010;123(1):79–86.

48. Wormser GP, Ramanathan R, Nowakowski J, et al. Duration of antibiotic therapy for early Lyme disease. a randomized, double-blind, placebo-controlled trial. Ann Intern Med 2003;138(9):697–704.

49. Nowakowski J, Nadelman RB, Sell R, et al. Long-term follow-up of patients with culture-confirmed Lyme disease. Am J Med 2003;115(2):91–6.

50. Smith RP, Schoen RT, Rahn DW, et al. Clinical characteristics and treatment outcome of early Lyme disease in patients with microbiologically confirmed erythema migrans. Ann Intern Med 2002;136(6):421–8.

51. Eppes SC, Childs JA. Comparative study of cefuroxime axetil versus amoxicillin in children with early Lyme disease. Pediatrics 2002;109(6):1173–7.

52. Arnez M, Pleterski-Rigler D, Luznik-Bufon T, et al. Solitary erythema migrans in children: comparison of treatment with azithromycin and phenoxymethylpenicillin. Wien Klin Wochenschr 2002;114(13–14):498–504.

53. Barsic B, Maretic T, Majerus L, et al. Comparison of azithromycin and doxycycline in the treatment of erythema migrans. Infection 2000;28(3):153–6.

54. Dattwyler RJ, Luft BJ, Kunkel MJ, et al. Ceftriaxone compared with doxycycline for the treatment of acute disseminated Lyme disease. N Engl J Med 1997; 337(5):289–94.

55. Luft BJ, Dattwyler RJ, Johnson RC, et al. Azithromycin compared with amoxicillin in the treatment of erythema migrans. A double-blind, randomized, controlled trial. Ann Intern Med 1996;124(9):785–91.

56. Gerber MA, Shapiro ED, Burke GS, et al. Lyme disease in children in southeastern connecticut. pediatric lyme disease study group. N Engl J Med 1996; 335(17):1270–4.

57. Luger SW, Paparone P, Wormser GP, et al. Comparison of cefuroxime axetil and doxycycline in treatment of patients with early Lyme disease associated with erythema migrans. Antimicrob Agents Chemother 1995;39(3):661–7.

58. Strle F, Preac-Mursic V, Cimperman J, et al. Azithromycin versus doxycycline for treatment of erythema migrans: clinical and microbiological findings. Infection 1993;21(2):83–8.

59. Nadelman RB, Luger SW, Frank E, et al. Comparison of cefuroxime axetil and doxycycline in the treatment of early Lyme disease. Ann Intern Med 1992; 117(4):273–80.

60. Ursinus J, Vrijmoeth HD, Harms MG, et al. Prevalence of persistent symptoms after treatment for lyme borreliosis: a prospective observational cohort study. Lancet Reg Health Eur 2021;6:100142.

61. Aucott JN, Yang T, Yoon I, et al. Risk of post-treatment Lyme disease in patients with ideally-treated early Lyme disease: a prospective cohort study. Int J Infect Dis 2022;116:230–7.

62. Arnez M, Radsel-Medvescek A, Pleterski-Rigler D, et al. Comparison of cefuroxime axetil and phenoxymethyl penicillin for the treatment of children with solitary erythema migrans. Wien Klin Wochenschr 1999;111(22–23):916–22.

63. Weitzner E, McKenna D, Nowakowski J, et al. Long-term assessment of post-treatment symptoms in patients with culture-confirmed early lyme disease. Clin Infect Dis 2015;61(12):1800–6.

64. Hirsch AG, Poulsen MN, Nordberg C, et al. Risk factors and outcomes of treatment delays in lyme disease: a population-based retrospective cohort study. Front Med (Lausanne) 2020;7:560018.

65. Wormser GP, McKenna D, Shaffer KD, et al. Evaluation of selected variables to determine if any had predictive value for, or correlated with, residual symptoms at approximately 12 months after diagnosis and treatment of early Lyme disease. Diagn Microbiol Infect Dis 2021;100(3):115348.

66. Wills AB, Spaulding AB, Adjemian J, et al. Long-term follow-up of patients with lyme disease: longitudinal analysis of clinical and quality-of-life measures. Clin Infect Dis 2016;62(12):1546–51.

67. Feder HM Jr, Johnson BJ, O'Connell S, et al. A critical appraisal of "chronic Lyme disease. N Engl J Med 2007;357(14):1422–30.

68. Stupica D, Veluscek M, Blagus R, et al. Oral doxycycline versus intravenous ceftriaxone for treatment of multiple erythema migrans: an open-label alternate-treatment observational trial. J Antimicrob Chemother 2018;73(5):1352–8.

69. Wormser GP, Weitzner E, McKenna D, et al. Long-term assessment of health-related quality of life in patients with culture-confirmed early Lyme disease. Clin Infect Dis 2015;61(2):244–7.

70. Hickie I, Davenport T, Wakefield D, et al. Post-infective and chronic fatigue syndromes precipitated by viral and non-viral pathogens: prospective cohort study. BMJ 2006;333(7568):575.

71. Carter BL, Stiff RE, Elwin K, et al. Health sequelae of human cryptosporidiosis-a 12-month prospective follow-up study. Eur J Clin Microbiol Infect Dis 2019;38(9): 1709–17.

72. Furberg M, Anticona C, Schumann B. Post-infectious fatigue following Puumala virus infection. Infect Dis (Lond) 2019;51(7):519–26.

73. Morch K, Hanevik K, Rivenes AC, et al. Chronic fatigue syndrome 5 years after giardiasis: differential diagnoses, characteristics and natural course. BMC Gastroenterol 2013;13:28.

74. Blomberg B, Mohn KG, Brokstad KA, et al. Long COVID in a prospective cohort of home-isolated patients. Nat Med 2021;27(9):1607–13.

75. Wormser GP, Weitzner E, McKenna D, et al. Long-term assessment of fatigue in patients with culture-confirmed Lyme disease. Am J Med 2015;128(2):181–4.

76. Oksi J, Nikoskelainen J, Hiekkanen H, et al. Duration of antibiotic treatment in disseminated Lyme borreliosis: a double-blind, randomized, placebo-controlled, multicenter clinical study. Eur J Clin Microbiol Infect Di 2007;26(8):571–81.

77. Dersch R, Sommer H, Rauer S, et al. Prevalence and spectrum of residual symptoms in Lyme neuroborreliosis after pharmacological treatment: a systematic review. J Neurol 2016;263(1):17–24.

78. Kortela E, Kanerva MJ, Puustinen J, et al. Oral Doxycycline Compared to Intravenous Ceftriaxone in the Treatment of Lyme Neuroborreliosis: A Multicenter, Equivalence, Randomized, Open-label Trial. Clin Infect Dis 2021;72(8):1323–31.

79. Rohrbeck J, Jordan K, Croft P. The frequency and characteristics of chronic widespread pain in general practice: a case-control study. Br J Gen Pract 2007;57(535):109–15.

80. Skogman BH, Croner S, Nordwall M, et al. Lyme neuroborreliosis in children: a prospective study of clinical features, prognosis, and outcome. Pediatr Infect Dis J 2008;27(12):1089–94.

81. Markowicz M, Kundi M, Stanek G, et al. Nonspecific symptoms following infection with Borrelia burgdorferi sensu lato: A retrospective cohort study. Ticks Tick-Borne Dis 2022;13(1):101851.

82. Klempner MS, Hu LT, Evans J, et al. Two controlled trials of antibiotic treatment in patients with persistent symptoms and a history of Lyme disease. N Engl J Med 2001;345(2):85–92.

83. Fallon BA, Keilp JG, Corbera KM, et al. A randomized, placebo-controlled trial of repeated IV antibiotic therapy for Lyme encephalopathy. Neurology 2008;70(13):992–1003.

84. Lantos PM, Wormser GP. Chronic coinfections in patients diagnosed with chronic lyme disease: a systematic review. Am J Med 2014;127(11):1105–10.

85. Krause PJ, Telford SR 3rd, Spielman A, et al. Concurrent Lyme disease and babesiosis. evidence for increased severity and duration of illness. JAMA 1996;275(21):1657–60.

86. Wang TJ, Liang MH, Sangha O, et al. Coexposure to Borrelia burgdorferi and Babesia microti does not worsen the long-term outcome of lyme disease. Clin Infect Dis 2000;31(5):1149–54.

87. Morrissette M, Pitt N, Gonzalez A, et al. A distinct microbiome signature in post-treatment lyme disease patients. mBio 2020;29(5):11.

88. Zimmermann P, Curtis N. Factors Influencing the Intestinal Microbiome During the First Year of Life. Pediatr Infect Dis J 2018;37(12):e315–35.

89. Fitzgerald BL, Graham B, Delorey MJ, et al. Metabolic Response in Patients With Post-treatment Lyme Disease Symptoms/Syndrome. Clin Infect Dis 2021;73(7):e2342–9.

90. Chandra A, Wormser GP, Klempner MS, et al. Anti-neural antibody reactivity in patients with a history of Lyme borreliosis and persistent symptoms. Brain Behav Immun 2010;24(6):1018–24.

91. Jacek E, Fallon BA, Chandra A, et al. Increased IFNalpha activity and differential antibody response in patients with a history of Lyme disease and persistent cognitive deficits. J Neuroimmunol 2013;255(1–2):85–91.

92. Chandra A, Wormser GP, Marques AR, et al. Anti-Borrelia burgdorferi antibody profile in post-Lyme disease syndrome. Clin Vaccin Immunol 2011;18(5):767–71.

93. Chandra A, Latov N, Wormser GP, et al. Epitope mapping of antibodies to VlsE protein of *Borrelia burgdorferi* in post-Lyme disease syndrome. Clin Immunol 2011;141(1):103–10.
94. Fallon BA, Strobino B, Reim S, et al. Anti-lysoganglioside and other anti-neuronal autoantibodies in post-treatment Lyme Disease and Erythema Migrans after repeat infection. Brain Behav Immun Health 2020;2:100015.
95. Strle K, Stupica D, Drouin EE, et al. Elevated levels of IL-23 in a subset of patients with post-lyme disease symptoms following erythema migrans. Clin Infect Dis 2014;58(3):372–80.
96. Tang KS, Klempner MS, Wormser GP, et al. Association of immune response to endothelial cell growth factor with early disseminated and late manifestations of Lyme disease but not posttreatment Lyme disease syndrome. Clin Infect Dis 2015;61(11):1703–6.
97. Aucott JN, Soloski MJ, Rebman AW, et al. CCL19 as a chemokine risk factor for posttreatment lyme disease syndrome: a prospective clinical cohort study. Clin Vaccin Immunol 2016;23(9):757–66.
98. Blum LK, Adamska JZ, Martin DS, et al. Robust B cell responses predict rapid resolution of lyme disease. Front Immunol 2018;9:1634.
99. Bouquet J, Soloski MJ, Swei A, et al. Longitudinal transcriptome analysis reveals a sustained differential gene expression signature in patients treated for acute lyme disease. mBio 2016;7(1):e00100–16.
100. Clarke DJB, Rebman AW, Bailey A, et al. Predicting lyme disease from patients' peripheral blood mononuclear cells profiled with RNA-sequencing. Front Immunol 2021;12:636289.
101. Wormser GP, Nadelman RB, Schwartz I. The amber theory of Lyme arthritis: initial description and clinical implications. Clin Rheumatol 2012;31(6):989–94.
102. Bockenstedt LK, Gonzalez DG, Haberman AM, et al. Spirochete antigens persist near cartilage after murine Lyme borreliosis therapy. J Clin Invest 2012;122(7):2652–60.
103. Jutras BL, Lochhead RB, Kloos ZA, et al. *Borrelia burgdorferi* peptidoglycan is a persistent antigen in patients with Lyme arthritis. Proc Natl Acad Sci U S A 2019; 116(27):13498–507.
104. Kalish RA, Kaplan RF, Taylor E, et al. Evaluation of study patients with Lyme disease, 10-20-year follow-up. J Infect Dis 2001;183(3):453–60.
105. Schutzer SE, Body BA, Boyle J, et al. Direct diagnostic tests for lyme disease. Clin Infect Dis 2019;68(6):1052–7.
106. Hodzic E, Imai D, Feng S, et al. Resurgence of persisting non-cultivable Borrelia burgdorferi following antibiotic treatment in mice. research support, N.I.H., extramural support, 2014 research support, Non-U.S. Gov't. PLoS One 2014; 9(1):e86907.
107. Embers ME, Hasenkampf NR, Jacobs MB, et al. Variable manifestations, diverse seroreactivity and post-treatment persistence in non-human primates exposed to Borrelia burgdorferi by tick feeding. PLoS One 2017;12(12): e0189071.
108. Hodzic E, Imai DM, Escobar E. Generality of Post-Antimicrobial Treatment Persistence of Borrelia burgdorferi Strains N40 and B31 in Genetically Susceptible and Resistant Mouse Strains. Infect Immun 2019;87(10).
109. Song S, Wood TK. Are we really studying persister cells? Environ Microbiol Rep 2021;13(1):3–7.
110. Harms A, Maisonneuve E, Gerdes K. Mechanisms of bacterial persistence during stress and antibiotic exposure. Science 2016;354:6318.

111. Wilmaerts D, Windels EM, Verstraeten N, et al. General mechanisms leading to persister formation and awakening. Trends Genet 2019;35(6):401–11.
112. Kim JS, Chowdhury N, Yamasaki R, et al. Viable but non-culturable and persistence describe the same bacterial stress state. Environ Microbiol 2018;20(6): 2038–48.
113. Marques A, Lemieux J, Hu L. The widening gyre: controversies in lyme disease. In: JD R, DS S, editors. *Lyme Disease and relapsing Fever spirochetes: Genomics, Molecular Biology, host Interactions and disease pathogenesis* Caister. Academic Press; 2021. p. 685–702, chap 23.
114. Marques A, Telford SR 3rd, Turk SP, et al. Xenodiagnosis to detect *Borrelia burgdorferi* infection: a first-in-human study. Clin Infect Dis 2014;58(7):937–45.
115. Bockenstedt LK, Radolf JD. Xenodiagnosis for posttreatment Lyme disease syndrome: resolving the conundrum or adding to it? comment editorial research support, N.I.H., extramural research support, Non-U.S. Gov't. Clin Infect Dis 2014;58(7):946–8.
116. Mosel MR, Rebman AW, Carolan HE, et al. Molecular microbiological and immune characterization of a cohort of patients diagnosed with early lyme disease. J Clin Microbiol 2020;59(1). https://doi.org/10.1128/JCM.00615-20.
117. Krupp LB, Hyman LG, Grimson R, et al. Study and treatment of post Lyme disease (STOP-LD): a randomized double masked clinical trial. Neurology 2003; 60(12):1923–30.
118. Berende A, ter Hofstede HJ, Vos FJ, et al. Randomized trial of longer-term therapy for symptoms attributed to lyme disease. N Engl J Med 2016;374(13): 1209–20.
119. Marques A, Shaw P, Schmid CH, et al. Re: A randomized, placebo-controlled trial of repeated IV antibiotic therapy for Lyme encephalopathy. Prolonged Lyme disease treatment: enough is enough. Neurology 2009;72(4):383–4, author reply 384.
120. Berende A, Ter Hofstede HJM, Vos FJ, et al. Effect of prolonged antibiotic treatment on cognition in patients with Lyme borreliosis. Neurology 2019;92(13): e1447–55.
121. Wormser GP. Longer-term therapy for symptoms attributed to lyme disease. N Engl J Med 2016;375(10):997.
122. van Middendorp H, Berende A, Vos FJ, et al. Expectancies as predictors of symptom improvement after antimicrobial therapy for persistent symptoms attributed to Lyme disease. Clin Rheumatol 2021;40(10):4295–308.
123. Ashar YK, Chang LJ, Wager TD. Brain mechanisms of the placebo effect: an affective appraisal account. Annu Rev Clin Psychol 2017;13:73–98.

Human Granulocytic Anaplasmosis

Douglas MacQueen, MD, MS[a,b],*, Felipe Centellas, MD[a]

KEYWORDS

- Anaplasmosis • *Ixodes* • Deer tick • Tick-borne • Leukopenia • Thrombocytopenia
- Doxycycline

KEY POINTS

- Anaplasmosis is transmitted by the bite of *Ixodes ricinus* complex ticks, which includes the black-legged or deer tick (*Ixodes scapularis)* in north central and eastern North America, and the western black-legged tick (*Ixodes pacificus*) in western North America.
- Symptoms of anaplasmosis include fever, headache, malaise, loss of appetite, and aches.
- Illness can be mild and self-limited or progress to severe illness and death, particularly in older individuals and those with comorbid conditions.
- Laboratory findings may include leukopenia, thrombocytopenia, and elevated hepatic transaminases.
- The probability of anaplasmosis increases with a history of *Ixodes* tick/habitat exposure and the presence of typical symptoms and can be confirmed with polymerase chain reaction testing.
- A patient with compatible illness and epidemiologic exposures should be treated with doxycycline. Continue treatment if they improve while on doxycycline, regardless of confirmatory test results.

INTRODUCTION

Human granulocytic anaplasmosis (HGA) is a vector-borne bacterial infection caused by *Anaplasma phagocytophilum*. It has one of the most rapidly increasing incidences of tick-borne infections in the United States.[1] It is transmitted to humans when infected nymphal or adult *Ixodes ricinus* complex (black-legged or deer) ticks take a blood meal.[2] These ticks are found in north central and eastern North America and the West coast of North America. Related *I ricinus* complex ticks transmit HGA in much of Eurasia and eastern Asia. In the United States, HGA was first described in 1994 in the upper Midwest[3,4] and then in multiple areas of the Northeast.[5,6] The illness was initially known as human granulocytic ehrlichiosis because the pathogen was named *Ehrlichia phagocytophilum* at the time. Subsequent work involving 16s rRNA

[a] Cayuga Medical Center, 101 Dates Drive, Ithaca, NY 14850, USA; [b] Weill Cornell Medicine
* Corresponding author.
E-mail address: dmac92077@gmail.com

Infect Dis Clin N Am 36 (2022) 639–654
https://doi.org/10.1016/j.idc.2022.02.008
0891-5520/22/© 2022 Elsevier Inc. All rights reserved.

id.theclinics.com

gene sequences led to realignment of families in the order *Rickettsiales* and renaming of the bacteria as *Anaplasma phagocytophilum*.[7] Members of the genera *Anaplasma* cause infections in humans and animals. In addition to HGA, *A phagocytophilum* causes canine and equine granulocytic anaplasmosis, and tick-borne fever in cattle and sheep.[8,9]

BACKGROUND

A phagocytophilum is an obligate intracellular gram-negative bacterium in the order Rickettsiales, family Anaplasmataceae.[10] It multiplies in vacuoles called morulae in the cytoplasm of mammalian host neutrophils. In tick vectors, the organism initially lives in cells of the midgut and then migrates to salivary glands where it develops.[11–13] *A phagocytophilum* has been found in the salivary glands of infected ticks that have yet to begin a blood meal,[11] suggesting the possibility of faster transmission than occurs with other organisms, such as *Borrelia burgdorferi*.[14]

A phagocytophilum is able to interfere with molecular pathways in both tick and host cells to evade the immune response in each. This allows the organism to infect tick midgut cells, evade mammalian host cell defenses, and cause infection.[15]

There are distinct genetic variants of *A phagocytophilum* that have specificity for the host in which they are maintained, and for the type of host in which they cause infection. In North America, genetic variant Ap-ha, which causes HGA in humans, is maintained in a white-footed mouse (*Peromyscus leucopus*) and Eastern chipmunk (*Tamias striatus*) reservoir.[16] Ap-V1, which is found in white-tailed deer (*Odocoileus virginianus*), is not pathogenic to humans. An abundance of Ap-ha–infected host-seeking ticks in the environment is predictive of human anaplasmosis case distribution and incidence based on data from New York State (Melissa Prusinksi, personal communication, January 5, 2022) and other parts of eastern North America.[17]

VECTOR-BORNE TRANSMISSION

A phagocytophilum is transmitted primarily by the bite of *I ricinus* complex ticks.[2] It is important to be familiar with the range of these ticks in order to assess a patient's risk for acquiring HGA. In the eastern and Midwest United States and south central and south eastern Canada, the vector is *Ixodes scapularis*, commonly called the black-legged (deer) tick.[18–20] In the western United States and Canada, it is *Ixodes pacificus*.[21] Throughout much of the United Kingdom and Eurasia, *I ricinus* is the vector.[22–24] *I persulcatus* is the vector in Japan, Korea, and eastern portions of Russia and China.[25]

I ricinus complex ticks are not infected as larvae by transovarial transmission.[26] Instead, larval and nymph forms of these ticks may acquire *A phagocytophilum* when they take a blood meal from an infected host. These ticks feed and acquire a blood meal over the course of several days during the same "bite."

Mammalian models suggest that 24 hours or more of tick attachment is needed to transmit enough *A phagocytophilum* to cause an infection in hosts. *I ricinus* complex ticks required at least 2 days of feeding to cause symptomatic tick-borne fever owing to *A phagocytophilum* in sheep.[27] Infected *I ricinus* ticks that fed on dogs began transmission of *A phagocytophilum* within hours, but more than 48 hours of feeding was needed to transmit a sufficient inoculum of the organism to cause infection.[28] Depending on the study, nymphal *I scapularis* ticks that fed on mice typically required 24 to 48 hours to transmit *A phagocytophilum* to the mouse.[29–32] Some models showed the presence of *A phagocytophilum* DNA in hosts after feeding by infected ticks in less than 24 hours, but those hosts did not develop antibodies against *A phagocytophilum*. This suggests that insufficient inoculum had been transmitted to cause infection during more brief feeding periods.

BLOOD TRANSFUSION AND ORGAN TRANSPLANT–RELATED TRANSMISSION

HGA can be transmitted by both red blood cell and platelet transfusion as well as organ transplantation. Several transfusion-related cases have been reported, including some that were fatal.[33–35] A review of the cases that occurred between 1997 and 2020 identified 10 transfusion-related cases of HGA and 7 solid organ transplant–related cases.[36] The blood supply is not screened for HGA.[37] Leukoreduced blood units may reduce, but not eliminate, the risk of transfusion-related HGA.

EPIDEMIOLOGY

HGA is an emerging disease in parts of North America, East Asia, and Eurasia.[38–40] The geographic range of HGA and overall incidence are increasing.[41–44] The rate of increase is higher than has been seen with other tick-borne infections, and it is estimated that the actual number of cases may be 11 times higher than is reported by public health departments.[45] Seroprevalence of antibodies against *A phagocytophilum* in asymptomatic humans varies by region and exposure type. They were found in 36% of forest workers in Poland,[46] 14.9% of northwestern Wisconsin residents with no known preceding tick bite,[47] and 23% of potential organ donors in Manitoba, where the presence of *I scapularis* had only recently been described.[48]

This increase in HGA cases is multifactorial. Elias and colleagues[40,41] postulated that case recognition and testing for HGA in individuals with compatible illnesses have increased because of better public and clinician awareness of HGA as well as widespread availability of accurate molecular testing. Other factors include the increased population density and range of *I ricinus* complex ticks,[49] and new areas in that range that questing ticks carry *A phagocytophilum*.[17,50] For example, in New York State, the percentage of adult *I scapularis* (black-legged or deer) ticks that were positive for *A phagocytophilum* increased from 4.0% to 9.2% (*P*<.01%) between 2010 and 2018. In eastern New York State, adjacent to HGA endemic areas of New England, the proportion of ticks carrying *A phagocytophilum* increased fourfold during that time.[51] *I scapularis* has been present in many of those areas for years but did not previously transmit *A phagocytophilum*. A similar lag was seen between the time when *I scapularis* populations were established on coastal Maine islands and when *B burgdorferi* was detected in those ticks.[52]

There is a temporal pattern of infection related to timing of tick exposure.[53,54] Infection is most common in ticks[55] and subsequently in humans in late spring and early summer when nymphal *I scapularis* and *I pacificus* ticks are most active (**Fig. 1**). Most reported cases in New York State that occurred between 2010 and 2018 were reported in May, June, and July.[51] This coincides with peak abundance and activity of *I scapularis* nymphs, which cause most human infection. However, HGA should be considered whenever *I ricinus* complex ticks are active. Adults may be present in early spring and fall and during the winter if there is not heavy snow cover and temperatures climb above freezing. Cases of HGA that present outside of peak tick season may be more likely to have a delay in diagnosis.[56]

Older white men are at highest risk of infection, possibly because of behavioral factors that increase risk of exposure. More problematic symptoms are common in older age, and infection may be unrecognized in young and otherwise healthy individuals. Russell and colleagues[51] reported that 63% of reported cases in New York State were in those over age 50 years.

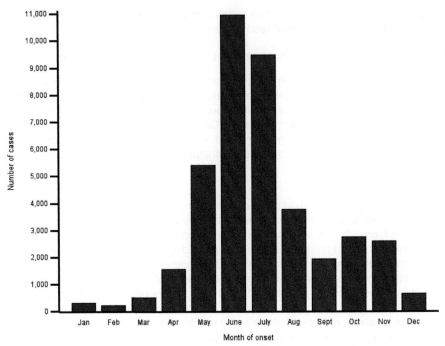

Fig. 1. Number of reported cases of anaplasmosis, by month of onset—United States, 2000 to 2019. (*From* U.S. Centers for Disease Control and Prevention: Anaplasmosis Epidemiology and Statistics. Available at https://www.cdc.gov/anaplasmosis/stats/index.html).

More severe cases have been associated with age over 75 years, higher neutrophil count, lower lymphocyte count, anemia, detection of morulae in neutrophils, immuno-suppression, chronic inflammatory illnesses, and underlying malignancy.[57–59]

HUMAN INFECTION

The incubation period of HGA is 5 to 14 days after a tick bite.[1] HGA symptoms range from minimally symptomatic to fulminant, including sepsis and death.[60] The illness is often mild and self-limited,[1] which makes it difficult to know the true prevalence of infection. Most case series included a preponderance of cases that were severe enough to require hospitalization, so the available data may represent symptoms and complications seen in more severe cases.

SYMPTOMS

The symptoms and presentation of HGA are nonspecific and may not differentiate it from other infections. Symptoms include fever (92%–100%), malaise (97%), myalgia (77%), headache (82%), and anorexia[61] (**Table 1**). The headache can be severe enough to lead to lumbar puncture, but cerebrospinal fluid is normal. In patients unable to give a history, caregivers may report malaise or loss of interest in usual activities and decreased appetite.

One series reported that 76% of patients in a mix of inpatients and outpatients with HGA also had respiratory or gastrointestinal symptoms.[62] When focal symptoms are prominent in HGA, the correct diagnosis may be delayed. For example, several cases

Table 1
Relative frequency of symptoms reported in human granulocytic anaplasmosis

Symptom	Relative Frequency
Fever	+++++
Malaise	++++
Rigors	+++
Myalgia	+++
Headache	+++
Anorexia	++
Nausea	++
Vomiting	++
Diarrhea	++
Cough	++
Arthralgia	++
Nuchal rigidity	+
Confusion	+
Abdominal pain	+

Data from Refs.[57,58,60]

of HGA with respiratory symptoms, hypoxia, and imaging findings of interstitial pneumonitis have been reported.[63,64] A case in France presented as acute respiratory distress syndrome.[65] Others have presented with prominent abdominal pain.[66] If gastrointestinal symptoms are prominent, the initial diagnostic focus may be on an underlying abdominal disorder. As an example, a patient with abdominal pain, transaminitis, and fever underwent cholecystectomy for presumed acute cholecystitis before HGA was diagnosed (Robert Smith, personal communication, January 1, 2022).

Most reported cases of HGA in the literature have been in adults. Children are commonly infected as well, but case reports are few. Pediatric infection may be asymptomatic or cause a mild, self-limited illness in younger people. Symptoms in children are similar to those in adults but may be more likely to include abdominal pain.[67]

PHYSICAL EXAMINATION

There are no physical examination findings that help make the diagnosis of HGA. Fever and muscle or joint tenderness without synovitis may be present. Rash is uncommon, present in 6% of patients who were diagnosed by polymerase chain reaction (PCR).[62] A description of the rashes seen in HGA are not readily available. However, a 14-year-old patient in Slovenia with HGA had a maculopapular rash on the trunk and neck.[68] Rash may be an epiphenomenon related to systemic infection and inflammation.

EVALUATION

When evaluating a patient for HGA, it is important to ask about outdoor exposure or contact with outdoor companion animals to gauge their probability for tick exposure. The lack of a known tick bite does not rule out HGA, as the bite often goes unnoticed. In one case series, less than two-thirds recalled a bite.[62] In nonendemic areas, consider HGA in people who become ill after traveling to an area where it is endemic or emerging.[69]

Complete blood count may reveal leukopenia and thrombocytopenia with occasional anemia. Depending on the case series, leukopenia was present in 47% to 71% of cases, thrombocytopenia in 61% to 91%, and anemia in 6% to 44%.[8] Metabolic panels may show elevated hepatic transaminases in 63% to 98% of cases. These abnormalities may not be present at the same time and not always at the time of initial evaluation. Bakken and colleagues[70] described a fluctuating course of leukopenia, anemia, and thrombocytopenia that varied during the course of illness and resolved with effective antibiotic treatment. They observed that leukocytosis or thrombocytosis in a patient with symptoms for less than a week was unlikely to have HGA. Blood cell and platelet level changes in HGA are due to increases in specific proinflammatory cytokine levels that impact hematopoiesis.[71] Elevated C-reactive protein is typically seen during this and many febrile illnesses.

These blood findings are nonspecific and occur in many viral and bacterial processes. They support the possibility of HGA in a patient with a compatible illness and epidemiologic exposure. They may also resolve spontaneously during the course of illness so if they are absent and symptoms are present for more than a week, HGA remains on the differential diagnosis.

Children with HGA are less likely to have telltale laboratory findings. In children with confirmed or probable HGA, 33% had elevated hepatic transaminases, 24% had leukopenia, and 17% had thrombocytopenia.[72]

Confirmatory blood testing is best accomplished with PCR for the presence of *A phagocytophilum* nucleic acid. PCR was found to have 74% sensitivity and 100% specificity, whereas antibody seroconversion had a sensitivity of 32% and specificity of 97% in a series in France.[73] PCR may have a delayed turnaround time in locations where it is a send-out test.

Empiric coverage of HGA is appropriate in ill patients whereby the diagnosis is suggested while awaiting confirmatory results. A rapid symptomatic response is expected and can be a helpful clue to the cause of illness even before a PCR result has returned.

A Wright-Giemsa–stained blood smear can also be used to detect morulae in neutrophils. Reports in severely ill patients showed diagnostic blood smears in only 25% to 60% of cases, so it is not useful in ruling out HGA.[6,70] It is also labor intensive and requires expertise in staining and smear preparation.[74] A group of pathologists determined that one would need to review 200 granulocytes to detect morulae in their series of 14 hospitalized patients with confirmed HGA.[75]

Acute and convalescent titers that show a fourfold increase are also confirmatory if PCR is not available. Serology may miss some mild cases and overdiagnose others because of cross-reactivity of antibodies.[45] Immunoglobulin G antibodies will persist for years after HGA infection, so they are not helpful to recheck after treatment as proof of cure.[76]

Turbett and colleagues[77] used a complete blood count–based strategy to rule out HGA without PCR testing during acute illness. When they combined a white blood cell count greater than 11,000 and a platelet count greater than 300,000, they rejected performing PCR testing for 25% of true negative (by PCR) HGA cases and 3 (5%) of true positive cases. In the true positive group of 3 patients, 1 patient had a history of splenectomy and another patient had chronic lymphocytic leukemia with a baseline leukocytosis. They implemented a testing stewardship criterion to reject PCR testing for HGA if the white blood cell count was greater than 11,000, the platelet count was greater than 300,000, and the patient was not critically ill or immunocompromised. In the outpatient setting, consider obtaining a complete blood count before proceeding to PCR testing. This would be particularly safe if empiric treatment of HGA was used concomitantly.

In those with HGA, it is worth considering coinfection with Lyme or babesiosis. Black-legged ticks transmit *B burgdorferi*, which causes Lyme infection, and *Babesia microti*, which causes babesiosis. In a group of patients in New York State who presented with erythema migrans rash owing to *B burgdorferi* infection, between 2.3% and 10% also met diagnostic criteria for HGA, depending on the criteria used.[78]

OUTCOMES

Early literature suggests that 36% of HGA infections required hospitalization,[59] and 17% of admitted patients needed critical care.[57] Deaths occurred in less than 1% of patients.[59,79] In patients with HGA in the United States reported to the Centers for Disease Control and Prevention between 2008 and 2012, the fatality rate was 0.3% and the hospitalization rate was 31%.[80]

More recently, a series of 33 patients diagnosed by PCR in Massachusetts showed that 42% were hospitalized, one required critical care, and none died.[62] In this series, the average age of admitted patients was 64 years, whereas the mean age for those who did not need admission was 53 years ($P = .04$). The severity of thrombocytopenia was associated with need for admission, whereas the degree of leukopenia was not. Thirty-five percent of patients in a series of all HGA cases reported in New York State between 2010 and 2018 were hospitalized, and 0.5% died.[51] Delay in diagnosis is correlated with increased length of stay in hospitalized patients with HGA.[56]

In a small case series of pediatric cases with probable or confirmed HGA, 7% of patients required hospital admission, and there were no fatalities.[72] Data in pregnancies complicated by HGA infection also suggest excellent outcomes. There was only 1 case of perinatal transmission in a case series of 6 pregnant women who were diagnosed by PCR and treated with doxycycline or rifampin. There were no adverse outcomes for the pregnancies or for those women and their children in the following 21 months.[81]

There are no reports of relapse or longstanding infection after HGA treatment.

COMPLICATIONS

Evidence of end-organ damage may be present in severe cases, including acute kidney injury, rhabdomyolysis, and multiorgan failure.[82,83] There are 2 reports of nontraumatic splenic rupture in patients with HGA.[84,85] There are reports of pancreatitis[86] and secondary hemophagocytic lymphohistiocytosis that complicate the infection.[87]

Focal neurologic manifestations are rare and should lead to consideration of another diagnosis or coinfection. There is 1 report of meningoencephalitis (and a facial nerve diplegia) putatively owing to *A phagocytophilum*.[88] This is in contrast to human monocytic ehrlichiosis owing to *Ehrlichia chaffeensis*, which more commonly causes central nervous system infection.[89] There are cases of HGA that presented with stroke symptoms that did not have evidence of CNS infection or imaging suggestive of stroke.[56] One patient with stroke symptoms and HGA had brain imaging that showed basal ganglia infarct (but no evidence of CNS infection)[90] and one with bilateral subarachnoid hemorrhage but no evidence of CNS infection.[91] Other neurologic manifestations are reported rarely, including postinfectious brachial plexopathy.[92] In severe cases involving the elderly or compromised hosts, transient encephalopathy from HGA is common.

TREATMENT

Doxycycline is the treatment of choice for HGA in all patients (**Table 2**). Empiric treatment for seriously ill patients with suspected HGA should be initiated while pending confirmatory testing. Doxycycline is also appropriate for treatment of HGA in children. The 2021 Report of the Committee on Infectious Diseases of the American Academy of Pediatrics (Red Book) now recommends doxycycline for the treatment of children of all ages with HGA.[93] Tetracycline has been associated with discoloration of teeth and enamel hypoplasia in children under 8 years of age, but this is not seen with short courses of doxycycline.[94] Doxycycline is taken at a dose of 2.2 mg/kg every 12 hours by mouth. The maximum dose is 100 mg every 12 hours, as in adults. There is a liquid formulation of doxycycline available for those who cannot swallow pills.

As with treatment in children, doxycycline is the treatment of choice during pregnancy. This has evolved with more safety data in young children, recognition of potential severe outcomes with suboptimal treatment of HGA in pregnancy, and a systemic review that did not show adverse effects with doxycycline use during pregnancy.[95] High-dose tetracycline therapy had been associated with acute fatty liver in pregnancy,[96] but this has not been reported with doxycycline treatment.[1]

In children, treatment is continued for a minimum of 72 hours after resolution of fever, although the standard course in children is 5 to 7 days and in adults is 7 to 10 days.[1]

If there is a strong suspicion for HGA, based on potential *I ricinus* complex tick exposure *and* a compatible illness that improves with doxycycline, and no alternative diagnosis made, a full course of doxycycline should be completed per CDC recommendations.[1]

In those who have allergic reaction or severe intolerance to doxycycline, rifampin is the treatment for HGA. Krause and colleagues[97] reported successful treatment of HGA in children with rifampin for 5 to 7 days. Dhand and colleagues[81] reported success in using rifampin to treat pregnant women with HGA. In children, rifampin is taken at a dose of 10 mg/kg every 12 hours up to a maximum of 300 mg per dose. This is the adult dose as well. Like doxycycline, it is taken by mouth. Intravenous formulations are available if medications cannot be taken by mouth or absorbed via the gastrointestinal tract.

In vitro data show favorable minimal inhibitory concentrations attained against *A phagocytophilum* for doxycycline and rifampin but not ampicillin, ceftriaxone, azithromycin, or trimethoprim-sulfamethoxazole.[98–100] In vitro susceptibility to levofloxacin and ciprofloxacin has been demonstrated. However, there are reports of relapse

Table 2
Treatment regimens for human granulocytic anaplasmosis

	Indication	Drug	Age Group	Dose	Duration
First line	Drug of choice	Doxycycline	Adults	100 mg twice a day	7–10 d
		Doxycycline	Pregnant	100 mg twice a day	7 d
		Doxycycline	Children	2.2 mg/kg every 12 h (maximum 100 mg/dose)	5–7 d
Second line	Severe allergy or intolerance	Rifampin	Adults	300 mg twice a day	7–10 d
		Rifampin	Pregnant	300 mg twice a day	7 d
		Rifampin	Children	10 mg/kg every 12 h (maximum 300 mg/dose)	5–7 d

Data from Refs.[1,81,93,97]

and possible inducible resistance when levofloxacin was used to treat HGA.[101] Fluoroquinolones are not recommended treatment options for HGA.

If rifampin or courses of doxycycline are limited to less than 7 days, closer symptom monitoring during and after treatment should be undertaken. Rifampin is not active against *B burgdorferi*. If it is used for HGA and coinfection with Lyme is suspected, a second agent should be added to treat Lyme.

Doxycycline can cause side effects, including profound anorexia and nausea, which is not an allergic reaction but can lead to poor compliance. These symptoms can be mitigated by eating a small meal before taking each dose of the medication. Doubly positive cations, such as calcium and magnesium, decrease its absorption. Separate its use by 2 hours from dairy products and vitamins that contain them. Doxycycline can also cause severe photosensitivity reactions, including a blistering rash, and therefore, direct sunlight should be avoided and sunscreen used along with sun-protective clothing to prevent this reaction. Rifampin has several drug-drug interactions that should be checked before it is used.

PREVENTION

There has not been a study of antibiotics after tick bite to demonstrate efficacy to prevent HGA. There is not a vaccine to prevent HGA in humans. Given an expected 24 hours' time from bite to transmission, development of an "anti-tick" vaccine could theoretically become a tool to prevent HGA.[102]

Preventing tick attachment and removing attached ticks after spending time in black-legged tick habitat are key to preventing tick-borne infections. This includes brief exposure to wooded or brushy areas with leaf litter on the ground and can include yards in urban and suburban settings. Prevention of attachment can be accomplished by tick repellents such as DEET or permethrin,[103] use of long sleeves and long pants while outdoors, and modification of habitat around high-use areas.

As previously discussed, *A phagocytophilum* transmission occurs more rapidly from tick vector to host than *B burgdorferi* transmission. However, daily tick check and removal after outdoor exposure are probably sufficient. The bigger issue is remembering to do the tick check, particularly when outdoor exposure has been minimal. An equally challenging issue is finding minuscule immature ticks during a tick check. Carefully explore the whole anatomy and consider using a magnifying glass. Tick removal is best carried out with either a twisting device or a tweezer at the base of the tick where it attaches to the skin and applying slow gentle pressure over 1 to 2 minutes until the tick releases.[104]

Testing black-legged ticks removed from patients for human pathogens could yield misleading results and is not recommended. Nonhuman disease-causing genetic variants of *A phagocytophilum* have been identified in *I ricinus* complex ticks removed from humans[105] and could return a false positive result. The presence of pathogenic bacterial genetic material in a tick does not mean the organism was transmitted to the human host from which it was removed. In addition, a negative test may lead people to stop monitoring for symptoms of infection after exposure. A more prudent approach is to monitor for symptoms of tick-borne infection in the weeks after exposure to tick habitat.

SUMMARY

HGA is a bacterial infection caused by *A phagocytophilum*. It is transmitted by the bite of the *I ricinus* complex (black-legged) ticks, which include *I scapularis* and *I pacificus*. These ticks are present on the west coast of North America, north central and eastern

North America (where they are known as deer ticks), Eurasia, and eastern Asia. The incidence of HGA is increasing steadily throughout an expanding geographic range. *A phagocytophilum* can be transmitted to humans after 24 hours, and more often after 48 hours, of tick attachment. The incubation period is 5 to 14 days after a tick bite. Many people will not be aware of their tick bite, so ask about exposure to black-legged (deer) tick habitat to assess their risk for HGA. Symptoms vary in severity and include fever, chills, headache, and body aches. HGA is often self-limited in younger and healthy people. Complications of infection include shock, organ dysfunction, and death. Mortality is less than 1%. Blood test findings include leukopenia, thrombocytopenia, and elevated hepatic transaminases. PCR is the confirmatory test of choice. Doxycycline is first-line treatment for all patients, regardless of age. Start it empirically in patients with a compatible illness who have spent time in black-legged tick habitat.[1] Complete a 7- to 10-day course if symptoms resolve with treatment, regardless of confirmatory test results. The keys to preventing HGA are preventing tick bites with repellants and checking for ticks frequently while in tick habitat.

CLINICS CARE POINTS

- To assess for risk of human granulocytic anaplasmosis, inquire as to time spent in black-legged (deer) tick habitat as opposed to presence of recent tick bites.
- Blood test findings may include leukopenia, thrombocytopenia, and elevated hepatic transaminases, sometimes alone or in combination.
- Polymerase chain reaction testing for *A phagocytophilum* is the most sensitive and specific test to confirm human granulocytic anaplasmosis.
- Doxycycline for 7 days in children and 7 to 10 days in adults is the treatment of choice for human granulocytic anaplasmosis.
- Human granulocytic anaplasmosis is a life-threatening infection. If it is deemed a possible cause of a patient's symptoms, start doxycycline while awaiting confirmatory test results.
- Complete a 7- to 10-day course if symptoms resolve with treatment, regardless of confirmatory test results.

DISCLOSURE

Neither author has any commercial or financial conflict of interest. There are no funding sources for either author.

REFERENCES

1. Biggs HM, Behravesh CB, Bradley KK, et al. Diagnosis and management of tickborne rickettsial diseases: Rocky Mountain spotted fever and other spotted fever group rickettsioses, ehrlichioses, and anaplasmosis - United States. MMWR Recomm Rep 2016;65(2):1–44.
2. Gray JS, Kahl O, Lane RS, et al. Diapause in ticks of the medically important Ixodes ricinus species complex. Ticks Tick Borne Dis 2016;7(5):992–1003.
3. Bakken JS, Dumler JS, Chen SM, et al. Human granulocytic ehrlichiosis in the upper Midwest United States. A new species emerging? JAMA 1994;272(3):212–8.

4. Chen SM, Dumler JS, Bakken JS, et al. Identification of a granulocytotropic Ehrlichia species as the etiologic agent of human disease. J Clin Microbiol 1994; 32(3):589–95.

5. Telford SR, Lepore TJ, Snow P, et al. Human granulocytic ehrlichiosis in Massachusetts. Ann Intern Med 1995;123(4):277–9.

6. Aguero-Rosenfeld ME, Horowitz HW, Wormser GP, et al. Human granulocytic ehrlichiosis: a case series from a medical center in New York State. Ann Intern Med 1996;125(11):904–8.

7. Dumler JS, Barbet AF, Bekker CP, et al. Reorganization of genera in the families Rickettsiaceae and Anaplasmataceae in the order Rickettsiales: unification of some species of Ehrlichia with Anaplasma, Cowdria with Ehrlichia and Ehrlichia with Neorickettsia, descriptions of six new species combinations and designation of Ehrlichia equi and 'HGE agent' as subjective synonyms of Ehrlichia phagocytophila. Int J Syst Evol Microbiol 2001;51(Pt 6):2145–65.

8. Bakken JS, Dumler JS. Human granulocytic anaplasmosis. Infect Dis Clin North Am 2015;29(2):341–55.

9. Atif FA. Anaplasma marginale and Anaplasma phagocytophilum: rickettsiales pathogens of veterinary and public health significance. Parasitol Res 2015; 114(11):3941–57.

10. Rikihisa Y. Mechanisms of obligatory intracellular infection with Anaplasma phagocytophilum. Clin Microbiol Rev 2011;24(3):469–89.

11. Telford SR, Dawson JE, Katavolos P, et al. Perpetuation of the agent of human granulocytic ehrlichiosis in a deer tick-rodent cycle. Proc Natl Acad Sci U S A 1996;93(12):6209–14.

12. Foley J, Nieto N. Anaplasma phagocytophilum subverts tick salivary gland proteins. Trends Parasitol 2007;23(1):3–5.

13. Kocan KM, de la Fuente J, Cabezas-Cruz A. The genus Anaplasma: new challenges after reclassification. Rev Sci Tech 2015;34(2):577–86.

14. Piesman J, Mather TN, Sinsky RJ, et al. Duration of tick attachment and Borrelia burgdorferi transmission. J Clin Microbiol 1987;25(3):557–8.

15. de la Fuente J, Estrada-Peña A, Cabezas-Cruz A, et al. Anaplasma phagocytophilum uses common strategies for infection of ticks and vertebrate hosts. Trends Microbiol 2016;24(3):173–80.

16. Massung RF, Mather TN, Priestley RA, et al. Transmission efficiency of the AP-variant 1 strain of Anaplasma phagocytophila. Ann N Y Acad Sci 2003;990:75–9.

17. Werden L, Lindsay LR, Barker IK, et al. Prevalence of anaplasma phagocytophilum and Babesia microti in Ixodes scapularis from a newly established Lyme disease endemic area, the Thousand Islands region of Ontario, Canada. Vector Borne Zoonotic Dis 2015;15(10):627–9.

18. Rich S, Caporale DA, Telford S, et al. Distribution of the Ixodes ricinus-like ticks of eastern North America. Proc Natl Acad Sci 1995;92(14):6284–8.

19. Schwartz I, Fish D, Daniels TJ. Prevalence of the rickettsial agent of human granulocytic ehrlichiosis in ticks from a hyperendemic focus of Lyme disease. N Engl J Med 1997;337(1):49–50.

20. Des Vignes F, Fish D. Transmission of the agent of human granulocytic ehrlichiosis by host-seeking Ixodus scapularis (Acari:Ixodidae) in southern New York state. J Med Entomol 1997;34(4):379–82.

21. Richter PJ, Kimsey RB, Madigan JE, et al. Ixodes pacificus (Acari: Ixodidae) as a vector of Ehrlichia equi (Rickettsiales: Ehrlichieae). J Med Entomol 1996; 33(1):1–5.

22. Rizzoli A, Rosà R, Mantelli B, et al. [Ixodes ricinus, transmitted diseases and reservoirs]. Parassitologia 2004;46(1–2):119–22.

23. Sprong H, Azagi T, Hoornstra D, et al. Control of Lyme borreliosis and other Ixodes ricinus-borne diseases. Parasit Vectors 2018;11(1):145.

24. Hvidsten D, Frafjord K, Gray JS, et al. The distribution limit of the common tick, Ixodes ricinus, and some associated pathogens in north-western Europe. Ticks Tick Borne Dis 2020;11(4):101388.

25. Jaarsma RI, Sprong H, Takumi K, et al. Anaplasma phagocytophilum evolves in geographical and biotic niches of vertebrates and ticks. Parasit Vectors 2019; 12(1):328.

26. Stuen S, Granquist EG, Silaghi C. Anaplasma phagocytophilum–a widespread multi-host pathogen with highly adaptive strategies. Front Cell Infect Microbiol 2013;3:31.

27. Macleod J. Studies on tick-borne fever of sheep. II. Experiment on transmission and distribution of the disease. Parasitology 1936;(28):320–9.

28. Fourie JJ, Evans A, Labuschagne M, et al. Transmission of Anaplasma phagocytophilum (Foggie, 1949) by Ixodes ricinus (Linnaeus, 1758) ticks feeding on dogs and artificial membranes. Parasit Vectors 2019;12(1):136.

29. Katavolos P, Armstrong PM, Dawson JE, et al. Duration of tick attachment required for transmission of granulocytic ehrlichiosis. J Infect Dis 1998;177(5): 1422–5.

30. Hodzic E, Fish D, Maretzki CM, et al. Acquisition and transmission of the agent of human granulocytic ehrlichiosis by Ixodes scapularis ticks. J Clin Microbiol 1998;36(12):3574–8.

31. des Vignes F, Piesman J, Heffernan R, et al. Effect of tick removal on transmission of Borrelia burgdorferi and Ehrlichia phagocytophila by Ixodes scapularis nymphs. J Infect Dis 2001;183(5):773–8.

32. Levin ML, Troughton DR, Loftis AD. Duration of tick attachment necessary for transmission of Anaplasma phagocytophilum by Ixodes scapularis (Acari: Ixodidae) nymphs. Ticks Tick Borne Dis 2021;12(6):101819.

33. Alhumaidan H, Westley B, Esteva C, et al. Transfusion-transmitted anaplasmosis from leukoreduced red blood cells. Transfusion 2013;53(1):181–6.

34. Fine AB, Sweeney JD, Nixon CP, et al. Transfusion-transmitted anaplasmosis from a leukoreduced platelet pool. Transfusion 2016;56(3):699–704.

35. Goel R, Westblade LF, Kessler DA, et al. Death from transfusion-transmitted anaplasmosis, New York, USA, 2017. Emerg Infect Dis 2018;24(8):1548–50.

36. Mowla SJ, Drexler NA, Cherry CC, et al. Ehrlichiosis and anaplasmosis among transfusion and transplant recipients in the United States. Emerg Infect Dis 2021;27(11):2768–75.

37. Prevention CfDCa. Anaplasmosis for healthcare providers: transmission and epidemiology. 2021. Available at: https://www.cdc.gov/anaplasmosis/healthcare-providers/transmission-epidemiology.html.

38. Tsai KH, Chung LH, Chien CH, et al. Human granulocytic anaplasmosis in Kinmen, an offshore island of Taiwan. PLoS Negl Trop Dis 2019;13(9):e0007728.

39. Nelder MP, Russell CB, Lindsay LR, et al. Recent Emergence of Anaplasma phagocytophilum in Ontario, Canada: Early Serological and Entomological Indicators. Am J Trop Med Hyg 2019;101(6):1249–58.

40. Edouard S, Koebel C, Goehringer F, et al. Emergence of human granulocytic anaplasmosis in France. Ticks Tick Borne Dis 2012;3(5–6):403–5.

41. Elias SP, Bonthius J, Robinson S, et al. Surge in anaplasmosis cases in Maine, USA, 2013-2017. Emerg Infect Dis 2020;26(2):327–31.

42. Baker A, Wang HH, Mogg M, et al. Increasing incidence of anaplasmosis in the United States, 2012 through 2016. Vector Borne Zoonotic Dis 2020;20(11): 855–9.

43. Rau A, Munoz-Zanzi C, Schotthoefer AM, et al. Spatio-temporal dynamics of tick-borne diseases in North-Central Wisconsin from 2000-2016. Int J Environ Res Public Health 2020;17(14):5105.

44. O'Connor C, Prusinski MA, Jiang S, et al. A comparative spatial and climate analysis of human granulocytic anaplasmosis and human babesiosis in New York State (2013-2018). J Med Entomol 2021;58(6):2453–66.

45. Services USDoHaH. Ehrlichiosis and Anaplasmosis Subcommittee Report to the Tick-Borne Disease Working Group. 2022. Available at: https://www.hhs.gov/ ash/advisory-committees/tickbornedisease/reports/ehrlichiosis-and- anaplasmosis-subcommittee-report-2020/index.html.   Accessed   January 29,2022.

46. Matei IA, Estrada-Peña A, Cutler SJ, et al. A review on the eco-epidemiology and clinical management of human granulocytic anaplasmosis and its agent in Europe. Parasit Vectors 2019;12(1):599.

47. Bakken JS, Goellner P, Van Etten M, et al. Seroprevalence of human granulo- cytic ehrlichiosis among permanent residents of northwestern Wisconsin. Clin Infect Dis 1998;27(6):1491–6.

48. Kadkhoda K, Gretchen A. Retrospective study investigating the seroprevalence of. Open Forum Infect Dis 2016;3(4):ofw199.

49. Lee X, Hardy K, Johnson DH, et al. Hunter-killed deer surveillance to assess changes in the prevalence and distribution of Ixodes scapularis (Acari: Ixodi- dae) in Wisconsin. J Med Entomol 2013;50(3):632–9.

50. Murphy DS, Lee X, Larson SR, et al. Prevalence and distribution of human and tick infections with the Ehrlichia muris-like agent and anaplasma phagocytophi- lum in Wisconsin, 2009-2015. Vector Borne Zoonotic Dis 2017;17(4):229–36.

51. Russell A, Prusinski M, Sommer J, et al. Epidemiology and spatial emergence of anaplasmosis, New York, USA, 2010–2018. Emerg Infect Dis 2021;27(8): 2154–62.

52. MacQueen DD, Lubelczyk C, Elias SP, et al. Genotypic diversity of an emergent population of Borrelia burgdorferi at a coastal Maine island recently colonized by Ixodes scapularis. Vector Borne Zoonotic Dis 2012;12(6):456–61.

53. Heo DH, Hwang JH, Choi SH, et al. Recent increase of human granulocytic anaplasmosis and co-infection with scrub typhus or Korean hemorrhagic fever with renal syndrome in Korea. J Korean Med Sci 2019;34(11):e87.

54. Prevention CfDCa. Anaplasmosis Stats. 2021. Available at: https://www.cdc. gov/anaplasmosis/stats/index.html.

55. Mysterud A, Easterday WR, Qviller L, et al. Spatial and seasonal variation in the prevalence of Anaplasma phagocytophilum and Borrelia burgdorferi sensu lato in questing Ixodes ricinus ticks in Norway. Parasit Vectors 2013;6:187.

56. Eldaour Y, Hariri R, Yassin M. Severe anaplasmosis presenting as possible CVA: case report and 3-year Anaplasma infection diagnosis data is based on PCR testing and serology. IDCases 2021;24:e01073.

57. Bakken JS. Clinical and laboratory characteristics of human granulocytic ehr- lichiosis. JAMA 1996;275(3):199.

58. Dumler JS, Choi K-S, Garcia-Garcia JC, et al. Human granulocytic anaplas- mosis and anaplasma phagocytophilum. Emerg Infect Dis 2005;11(12): 1828–34.

59. Dahlgren FS, Mandel EJ, Krebs JW, et al. Increasing incidence of Ehrlichia chaffeensis and Anaplasma phagocytophilum in the United States, 2000–2007. Am J Trop Med Hyg 2011;85(1):124–31.

60. Bakken JS, Dumler JS. Clinical diagnosis and treatment of human granulocytotropic anaplasmosis. Ann N Y Acad Sci 2006;1078:236–47.

61. Dumler J, DH W. Ehrlichia chaffeensis (human monocytotropic ehrlichiosis), Anaplasma phagocytophilum (human granulocytotropic anaplasmosis), and other anaplasmataceae Mandell, Douglas, and Bennett's principles and practice of infectious diseases. 2015:2227–33:chap 194.

62. Weil AA, Baron EL, Brown CM, et al. Clinical findings and diagnosis in human granulocytic anaplasmosis: a case series from Massachusetts. Mayo Clin Proc 2012;87(3):233–9.

63. Rivera JE, Young K, Kwon TS, et al. Anaplasmosis presenting with respiratory symptoms and pneumonitis. Open Forum Infect Dis 2020;7(8):ofaa265.

64. Stice MJ, Bruen CA, Grall KJH. Anchoring on COVID-19: a case report of human granulocytic anaplasmosis masquerading as COVID-19. Clin Pract Cases Emerg Med 2021;5(3):328–31.

65. Remy V, Hansmann Y, De Martino S, et al. Human anaplasmosis presenting as atypical pneumonitis in France. Clin Infect Dis 2003;37(6):846–8.

66. Ladzinski AT, Baker M, Dunning K, et al. Human granulocytic anaplasmosis presenting as subacute abdominal pain and hyponatremia. IDCases 2021;25: e01183.

67. Sigurjonsdottir VK, Feder HM, Wormser GP. Anaplasmosis in pediatric patients: case report and review. Diagn Microbiol Infect Dis 2017;89(3):230–4.

68. Pokorn M, Županc TA, Strle F. Pediatric human granulocytic anaplasmosis is rare in Europe. Pediatr Infect Dis J 2016;35(3):358–9.

69. Camprubí-Ferrer D, Portillo A, Santibáñez S, et al. Incidence of human granulocytic anaplasmosis in returning travellers with fever. J Travel Med 2021;28(4): taab056.

70. Bakken JS, Aguero-Rosenfeld ME, Tilden RL, et al. Serial measurements of hematologic counts during the active phase of human granulocytic ehrlichiosis. Clin Infect Dis 2001;32(6):862–70.

71. Schotthoefer AM, Schrodi SJ, Meece JK, et al. Pro-inflammatory immune responses are associated with clinical signs and symptoms of human anaplasmosis. PLoS One 2017;12(6):e0179655.

72. Schotthoefer AM, Hall MC, Vittala S, et al. Clinical presentation and outcomes of children with human granulocytic anaplasmosis. J Pediatr Infect Dis Soc 2018; 7(2):e9–15.

73. Hansmann Y, Jaulhac B, Kieffer P, et al. Value of PCR, serology, and blood smears for human granulocytic anaplasmosis diagnosis, France. Emerg Infect Dis 2019;25(5):996–8.

74. ME R, JS D. Manual of clinical microbiology. 11th ed. 1135-1149:chap Ehrlichia, Anaplasma , and related intracellular bacteria , chapter 65.

75. Rand JV, Tarasen AJ, Kumar J, et al. Intracytoplasmic granulocytic morulae counts on confirmed cases of ehrlichiosis/anaplasmosis in the Northeast. Am J Clin Pathol 2014;141(5):683–6.

76. Bakken JS, Haller I, Riddell D, et al. The serological response of patients infected with the agent of human granulocytic ehrlichiosis. Clin Infect Dis 2002; 34(1):22–7.

77. Turbett SE, Anahtar MN, Pattanayak V, et al. Use of routine complete blood count results to rule out anaplasmosis without the need for specific diagnostic testing. Clin Infect Dis 2020;70(6):1215–21.

78. Horowitz HW, Aguero-Rosenfeld ME, Holmgren D, et al. Lyme disease and human granulocytic anaplasmosis coinfection: impact of case definition on coinfection rates and illness severity. Clin Infect Dis 2013;56(1):93–9.

79. Dumler JS, Madigan JE, Pusterla N, et al. Ehrlichioses in humans: epidemiology, clinical presentation, diagnosis, and treatment. Clin Infect Dis 2007;45(Suppl 1): S45–51.

80. Dahlgren FS, Heitman KN, Behravesh CB, et al. Human granulocytic anaplasmosis in the United States from 2008 to 2012: a summary of national surveillance data. Am J Trop Med Hyg 2015;93(1):66–72.

81. Dhand A, Nadelman RB, Aguero-Rosenfeld M, et al. Human granulocytic anaplasmosis during pregnancy: case series and literature review. Clin Infect Dis 2007;45(5):589–93.

82. Uminski K, Kadkhoda K, Houston BL, et al. Anaplasmosis: an emerging tick-borne disease of importance in Canada. IDCases 2018;14:e00472.

83. Cho JM, Chang J, Kim DM, et al. Human granulocytic anaplasmosis combined with rhabdomyolysis: a case report. BMC Infect Dis 2021;21(1):1184.

84. Khan R, Ali A. Non-traumatic splenic rupture in a patient with human granulocytic anaplasmosis and focused review of the literature. Ticks Tick Borne Dis 2018;9(3):735–7.

85. Hsia K, Johnson J, Rice D. Splenomegaly, non-traumatic splenic rupture, and pancytopenia in patient with human granulocytic anaplasmosis. R Med J (2013) 2021;104(2):60–2.

86. Rocco JM, Mallarino-Haeger C, McCurry D, et al. Severe anaplasmosis represents a treatable cause of secondary hemophagocytic lymphohistiocytosis: two cases and review of literature. Ticks Tick Borne Dis 2020;11(5):101468.

87. Johnson TL, Graham CB, Maes SE, et al. Prevalence and distribution of seven human pathogens in host-seeking Ixodes scapularis (Acari: Ixodidae) nymphs in Minnesota, USA. Ticks Tick Borne Dis 2018;9(6):1499–507.

88. Lee FS, Chu FK, Tackley M, et al. Human granulocytic ehrlichiosis presenting as facial diplegia in a 42-year-old woman. Clin Infect Dis 2000;31(5):1288–91.

89. Ratnasamy N, Everett ED, Roland WE, et al. Central nervous system manifestations of human ehrlichiosis. Clin Infect Dis 1996;23(2):314–9.

90. Kim SW, Kim CM, Kim DM, et al. Manifestation of anaplasmosis as cerebral infarction: a case report. BMC Infect Dis 2018;18(1):409.

91. Mullholand JB, Tolman N, De Obaldia A, et al. Central nervous system involvement of anaplasmosis. BMJ Case Rep 2021;14(12). https://doi.org/10.1136/bcr-2021-243665.

92. Horowitz HW, Marks SJ, Weintraub M, et al. Brachial plexopathy associated with human granulocytic ehrlichiosis. Neurology 1996;46(4):1026–9.

93. Kimberlin DW, Barnett ED, Lynfield R, et al. Ehrlichia, Anaplasma, and related infections (human Ehrlichiosis, anaplasmosis, and related infections attributable to bacteria in the family Anaplasmataceae). Red Book: Report of the Committee on Infectious Diseases; 2021.

94. Todd SR, Dahlgren FS, Traeger MS, et al. No visible dental staining in children treated with doxycycline for suspected Rocky Mountain spotted fever. J Pediatr 2015;166(5):1246–51.

95. Cross R, Ling C, Day NP, et al. Revisiting doxycycline in pregnancy and early childhood–time to rebuild its reputation? Expert Opin Drug Saf 2016;15(3): 367–82.

96. Schultz JC, Adamson JS, Workman WW, et al. Fatal liver disease after intravenous administration of tetracycline in high dosage. N Engl J Med 1963;269: 999–1004.

97. Krause PJ, Corrow CL, Bakken JS. Successful treatment of human granulocytic ehrlichiosis in children using rifampin. Pediatrics 2003;112(3 Pt 1):e252–3.

98. Klein MB, Nelson CM, Goodman JL. Antibiotic susceptibility of the newly cultivated agent of human granulocytic ehrlichiosis: promising activity of quinolones and rifamycins. Antimicrob Agents Chemother 1997;41(1):76–9.

99. Maurin M, Bakken JS, Dumler JS. Antibiotic susceptibilities of Anaplasma (Ehrlichia) phagocytophilum strains from various geographic areas in the United States. Antimicrob Agents Chemother 2003;47(1):413–5.

100. Branger S, Rolain JM, Raoult D. Evaluation of antibiotic susceptibilities of Ehrlichia canis, Ehrlichia chaffeensis, and Anaplasma phagocytophilum by real-time PCR. Antimicrob Agents Chemother 2004;48(12):4822–8.

101. Wormser GP, Filozov A, Telford SR, et al. Dissociation between inhibition and killing by levofloxacin in human granulocytic anaplasmosis. Vector Borne Zoonotic Dis 2006;6(4):388–94.

102. de la Fuente J, Contreras M. Tick vaccines: current status and future directions. Expert Rev Vaccin 2015;14(10):1367–76.

103. Prose R, Breuner NE, Johnson TL, et al. Contact irritancy and toxicity of permethrin-treated clothing for ixodes scapularis, amblyomma americanum, and dermacentor variabilis ticks (Acari: Ixodidae). J Med Entomol 2018;55(5): 1217–24.

104. Needham GR. Evaluation of five popular methods for tick removal. Pediatrics 1985;75(6):997–1002.

105. Rejmanek D, Freycon P, Bradburd G, et al. Unique strains of Anaplasma phagocytophilum segregate among diverse questing and non-questing Ixodes tick species in the western United States. Ticks Tick Borne Dis 2013;4(6):482–7.

Human Babesiosis

Rami Waked, MD[a,*], Peter J. Krause, MD[b]

KEYWORDS

- Babesiosis • *Babesia microti* • Tick • Apicomplexa • Erythrocyte • Protozoan
- Transfusion

KEY POINTS

- Human babesiosis is an emerging tick-borne zoonosis caused by hemoprotozoan parasites that are transmitted primarily by ticks, infrequently through blood transfusion, and rarely through transplacental transmission or organ transplantation.
- *Babesia microti*, the predominant cause for human babesiosis, is endemic in the Northeast and upper Midwest of the United States.
- Babesia infections can range in severity from asymptomatic to fatal, with risk for severe disease highest in the elderly and immunocompromised individuals.
- Diagnosis is confirmed by identification of Babesia parasites on blood smear, amplification, and detection of Babesia DNA by polymerase chain reaction, or a fourfold increase in babesia antibody titers in acute and convalescent sera.
- Treatment of choice for *B microti* infection is the combination of atovaquone plus azithromycin, which is better tolerated than the alternative clindamycin plus quinine combination. Red blood cell exchange transfusion is an additional intervention used in some patients with life-threatening disease.

INTRODUCTION

Babesiosis is an infection caused by intraerythrocytic protozoa of the genus *Babesia*. Different species of *Babesia* infect different vertebrate hosts, but human disease has been documented as a result of infection by only 6 species worldwide.[1–4] In North America, *Babesia microti*, a parasite of white-footed mice and other small rodents, accounts for nearly all human cases. It is transmitted by *Ixodes scapularis* (black-legged tick or deer tick), but infection can also be acquired through contaminated blood products, organ transplantation, or congenitally.[5] Endemic geographic areas and incidence of reported cases have grown rapidly over the past several decades, and the number and range of black-legged ticks have increased.[6] Only a small number of human babesiosis cases in North America are due to infection by other species (*Babesia duncani* and *Babesia divergens*–like species).[7,8] There is increasing recognition of

[a] Division of Infectious Diseases, Maine Medical Center, 22 Bramhall Street, Portland, ME 04102, USA; [b] Division of Epidemiology of Microbial Diseases, Yale School of Public Health and Yale School of Medicine, 60 College Street, New Haven, CT 06520, USA
* Corresponding author.
E-mail address: rami.waked@mainehealth.org

Infect Dis Clin N Am 36 (2022) 655–670
https://doi.org/10.1016/j.idc.2022.02.009
0891-5520/22/© 2022 Elsevier Inc. All rights reserved.

id.theclinics.com

Babesia infection in Europe and Asia owing to *Babesia crassa*–like species, *B divergens*, *B microti*, *Babesia motasi*, and *Babesia venatorum*.

PATHOGENS

Babesia species are grouped in the phylum Apicomplexa, which includes several genera of protozoan human pathogens, that is, Plasmodium, Toxoplasma, and Cryptosporidium. *Babesia* use particular organelles that facilitate their invasion into host red blood cells (RBC) and their ability to persist in ticks.[9] Although at least 4 clades of *Babesia* species are recognized as human pathogens, phylogenetic analysis suggests the *B microti* group is distinct and might be classified in a separate genus in the Apicomplexa phylum. Diverse strains or clades of *B microti* occur worldwide, but human disease focuses on North America, where Northeastern and Midwest lineages of *B microti* have been identified.[10,11]

TRANSMISSION

Babesiosis is a zoonotic disease, primarily transmitted between *Ixodes* ticks and vertebrate animal reservoirs. Humans are incidental hosts.[12] *I scapularis* is the only documented North American tick vector for *B microti*, and the white-footed mouse, *Peromyscus leucopus*, is the primary vertebrate host, although other small rodents can also serve as reservoir hosts. White-footed mice maintain infection for prolonged periods with low parasitemia.[13] Recent work reveals that infected mice may transmit *Babesia* to their progeny.[14] Deer are hosts for all stages of black-legged ticks (larva, nymph, and adult) but do not become infected with *B microti*. Deer are infected by a different babesia species (*Babesia odocoilei*), not known to be a human pathogen.[15] Female ticks do not transmit infection to the eggs.[16]

In the United States, *B microti* is one of the most prevalent transfusion-transmitted pathogens, leading to recent recommendations to screen blood from donors in endemic states. Screening has recently been initiated and has been effective in largely preventing transfusion-transmitted *B microti* infection.[17,18] Blood transfusion–transmitted cases may occur in nonendemic areas owing to national distribution of donated blood and by asymptomatically infected donors traveling from an endemic area and donating contaminated blood in a nonendemic area.[19] A small number of cases of babesiosis have occurred following organ transplantation, as well as transplacental transmission in the newborn.[17,18,20–22]

EPIDEMIOLOGY

B microti infection has been reported from the Americas, Europe, Africa, Asia, and Australia.[23–27] The incidence of *B microti* infections has been increasing in the United Stated over the past decade, as with other tick-borne illnesses transmitted by *I scapularis*.[6,28,29] *B microti* is endemic in the northeastern United States (from Maine to Maryland) and the northern Midwest.[16] Babesiosis and Lyme disease are expanding in these regions in concert with expansion of the range of black-legged ticks. Not all areas endemic for Lyme disease are also endemic for babesiosis, in part because of more limited host species for *B microti*, and in part because of lower efficiency of transmission by ticks. Coinfection of a tick with *Borrelia burgdorferi* may facilitate transmission of *B microti*.[30] Two other *Babesia* species have been found to cause babesiosis in the United States. A small number of cases of *B duncani* cases have been reported in California and the Pacific Northwest. *B divergens*–like human infections have been reported in Arkansas, Kentucky, Michigan, Missouri, and Washington State (**Fig. 1**A, B).[16,31]

Human babesiosis is most prevalent in the summer and in places where tick vectors, vertebrate reservoirs, and deer are in close proximity to humans. Cases may present throughout the year, and incubation periods may be prolonged if transfusion is acquired. Babesiosis is underreported to a greater extent than Lyme disease, given its nonspecific symptoms and higher proportion of subclinical asymptomatic cases.[29] Seroprevalence of antiantibody ranges from 2% to 10% in the general population and from less than 1% to 4.9% in blood donors, depending on endemicity of the infection in the studied population.[29,32–34]

PATHOGENESIS

The pathogenesis of babesiosis infection in humans has been associated with a diminished immune response, a dysfunctional immune response, and the effects of RBC lysis. Severe disease is prevalent in the immunocompromised, especially those with asplenia, HIV/AIDS, malignancy, immunosuppressive therapy, neonates, and those over the age of 50 years.[16] The spleen has a critical role in the initial clearance of

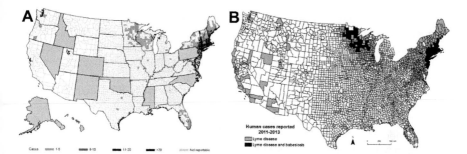

Fig. 1. (A) Geographic distribution of 2417 human cases of babesiosis in 40 states of the United States, 2019. The figure shows the incidence of babesiosis (number of cases per 100,000 persons) by county of residence in 2019. Human babesiosis caused by *Babesia microti* has been reported from the Northeast, from Maine to Maryland. *B microti* also causes disease in the upper Midwest, particularly in Wisconsin and Minnesota. *B duncani* has been the etiologic agent along the northwest Pacific Coast. Cases of *B divergens*–like infection have been reported from Arkansas, Kentucky, Missouri, and Washington State. Cases that occur outside of endemic regions may have been acquired in endemic regions and diagnosed in a nonendemic area or through transport of a contaminated blood unit for blood transfusion from an endemic region to a nonendemic region. (B) Human babesiosis and Lyme disease in the United States, by county 2011 to 2013. Human babesiosis and Lyme disease have been nationally notifiable conditions since 2011 and 1991, respectively. The names of counties that reported cases of Lyme disease and/or babesiosis from 2011 to 2013 were obtained from the Centers for Disease Control and Prevention. Counties with 3 or more cases of Lyme disease but fewer than 3 cases of babesiosis are depicted in green. Counties with 3 or more cases of Lyme disease and 3 or more cases of babesiosis are depicted in gray. No county reported 3 or more cases of babesiosis but fewer than 3 cases of Lyme disease. (*From* [A] CDC. Babesiosi Maps. Centers for Disease Control and Prevention. Available at https://www.cdc.gov/parasites/babesiosis/data-statistics/maps/maps.html; and [B] Diuk-Wasser MA, Vannier E, Krause PJ. Coinfection by the tick-borne pathogens Babesia microti and Borrelia burgdorferi: ecological, epidemiological and clinical consequences. Trends Parasitol. 2016;32(1):30-42; with permission.)

infected erythrocytes.[35,36] Both T- and B-cell–mediated immune responses are important in the control of *Babesia* infections.[16] B cells and the production of antibody are particularly important in eradication of infection, which may relapse in treated patients with severe B-cell dysfunction or B-cell–associated lymphoid malignancy and rituximab therapy. Multiple studies conducted in patients following acute *Babesia* infection or asymptomatically infected blood transfusion donors show that parasitemia can persist for months, or even years, in a subset of patients with impaired or absent antibody response.[17,20,37] RBC infection alters the cellular structure of the cell, resulting in lysis or enhanced clearance, but *Babesia* parasites have evolved responses to promote persistence. Persistent infection in animal hosts ensures transmission to the tick vector. Erythrocyte cytoadherence is a mechanism by which infected RBC express proteins on their surface, causing adherence to endothelial cells lining blood vessels. This allows *Babesia* to complete their life cycle without circulating through the spleen, where they may be destroyed.[35,38–40] Another mechanism that may contribute to persistence of *Babesia* infection in hosts is their ability to slow their rate of reproduction after a robust initial replication period. This allows extended time within the red cell and protection against host immune factors that circulate in the bloodstream. Alteration of replication speed has been demonstrated in studies of *B divergens*.[39] Proliferation accelerates once optimum extracellular conditions return.[39] These mechanisms have yet to be documented in humans.

Just as a diminished immune response can result in severe disease, an inappropriately intense immune response can do so as well. High parasitemia levels are thought to trigger an overproduction of host proinflammatory cytokines, such as interferon-gamma and interleukin-6. Cytokine storm may cause increased vascular permeability, leading to acute respiratory distress syndrome (ARDS) and shock.[35] Finally, hemolytic anemia results from the egress of *Babesia* from erythrocytes and occasional immune damage of infected red cells. The *Babesia* organism within the RBC matures to trophozoites, which undergo asexual budding and result in 2 or 4 daughters called merozoites. These are released in the bloodstream and invade other erythrocytes. In most cases, the degree of hemolysis is mild, possibly because babesia reproduction, unlike malaria, is asynchronous.[35,40] Lysis can be intense with high parasitemia, however, resulting in severe hemolytic anemia. In asplenic patients, an independent warm antibody autoimmune hemolysis has been described several weeks following apparently effective treatment of babesiosis.[41] Disseminated intravascular coagulation (DIC) may further complicate hematologic management.

CLINICAL MANIFESTATIONS

The incubation period for *B microti* infection is usually 1 to 4 weeks following a tick bite and 3 to 7 weeks (up to 6 months) after transfusion of contaminated blood products.[2,16,18] Concurrent infection with *B microti* may be seen with one or more tick-borne pathogens transmitted by *I scapularis* ticks. This may increase the number and duration of acute symptoms.[42,43] *B microti* infection may result in asymptomatic, mild to moderate disease, or severe disease. Symptoms in outpatient and inpatient disease are summarized in **Table 1**.

Asymptomatic

In a 10-year cohort study in a highly endemic location, the percentage of *B microti*–infected patients who experienced asymptomatic and symptomatic infection was determined. The ratio of symptomatic to asymptomatic *B microti* infection was found to be 80%/20% in adults and 60%/40% in children.[29] Parasitemia may persist

Table 1
Symptoms of babesiosis

Symptoms	Outpatients (%) (n = 41)	Inpatients (%) (n = 249)	All Patients (%) (n = 290)
Fever	88	89	89
Fatigue	85	82	82
Chills	63	68	67
Sweats	73	58	60
Anorexia	56	53	53
Headache	68	44	47
Myalgia	66	39	43
Nausea	32	44	42
Cough	34	27	28
Arthralgia	46	22	25

Outpatient cases are from Reubush et al,[45] Krause et al,[42] and Krause et al.[43] Inpatient cases are from White et al,[44] Krause et al,[79] Hatcher et al,[46] and Joseph et al.[58]

From Vannier EG, Diuk-Wasser MA, Ben Mamoun C, Krause PJ. Babesiosis. Infect Dis Clin North Am. 2015;29(2):357-370. https://doi.org/10.1016/j.idc.2015.02.008; with permission.

asymptomatically for months to years, but relapsing symptomatic disease is rare, except in immunocompromised patients.[29]

Mild to Moderate Disease

Most patients experience gradual onset of fatigue, fever, and malaise. On occasion, however, an abrupt onset of spiking fever may occur. Other common symptoms include chills, sweats, headache, and myalgia. Less common symptoms are anorexia, dry cough, nausea, abdominal pain, vomiting, shortness of breath, dark urine, and weight loss.[2,44–46] Other than fever, which can be high, the physical examination is often unremarkable. Splenomegaly and/or hepatomegaly may be present in a minority of patients. Scleral icterus and jaundice may develop secondary to hemolysis. There are rare reports of retinopathy with splinter hemorrhages.[2,44,46] Splenic infarct and rupture are rare but life-threatening complications that may occur in patients with otherwise mild infections.[47] Laboratory findings are nonspecific with the exception of abnormalities owing to hemolytic anemia. Thrombocytopenia is common, and leukopenia may occur. Other common findings are elevation in serum concentrations of liver enzymes, total and indirect bilirubin, blood urea nitrogen, and serum creatinine levels.[2,48,49] With the exception of hemolysis, there is frequent overlap in the clinical presentation of babesiosis, anaplasmosis, and *Babesia miyamotoi* infection.

Severe Disease

Severe babesiosis is mostly seen in older and/or immunocompromised patients. Severe babesiosis is frequently associated with systemic complications and, in immunocompromised patients, persistent or relapsing disease.[44,46,50,51] Clinical symptoms are similar to those seen in mild to moderate disease but are more severe. Nausea, vomiting, and diarrhea may be predictive of severe infection and hospitalization.[52] In endemic areas in late spring, summer, and early autumn, babesiosis should be considered in the differential diagnosis of persons with fever of unknown origin.

The abnormalities in laboratory tests associated with severe babesiosis are similar to those seen in mild to moderate infection, but are more pronounced and may last longer.[16] Complications described in severe babesiosis include ARDS, pulmonary edema, severe anemia, DIC, congestive heart failure, renal failure, splenic rupture, coma, and prolonged relapsing course of illness despite appropriate therapy.[44,46,53–55] The death rate in hospitalized patients has ranged from 0% to 9% but may be as high as 20% for the immunocompromised or patients who have contracted the disease by blood transfusion.[44,46,52,56–58]

Relapse and Reinfection

Babesiosis may relapse despite appropriate antimicrobial therapy in severely immunocompromised individuals, such as in patients with B-cell lymphoma and rituximab treatment, organ or stem cell transplantation, or HIV/AIDS with low CD4 counts.[56,59–61] Patients experiencing relapsing babesiosis often are asplenic; however, asplenia alone does not result in relapsing illness. Relapse usually occurs within days or a week after antibiotics are discontinued but may occur months later. Babesia parasitemia on thin blood smear confirms relapse. Babesiosis relapses are often less severe than the initial infection; however, with persistent infection, fatal outcome has occurred in about 20% of treated cases.[56,59]

Reinfection with babesiosis has recently been described in a single patient.[62]

DIAGNOSIS
Clinical Diagnosis

The diagnosis of babesiosis should be considered in febrile patients with fatigue, malaise, chills, sweats, headache, and/or myalgia in *Babesia* endemic areas, primarily in the late spring, summer, or early autumn. Babesiosis is a consideration in patients with typical symptoms and a history of blood transfusion in the preceding 6 months. Patients with Lyme disease experiencing a slow or incomplete response to effective treatment may have babesia coinfection.[57] A history of tick exposure may help but is often absent, as ticks are small and their bites are usually painless, so an attached tick may go unnoticed.[2]

Laboratory Diagnosis

The diagnosis of babesiosis is confirmed by microscopic identification of ringlike parasites inside erythrocytes on Giemsa or Wright-stained thin blood smears and/or by detection of amplified *Babesia* DNA using polymerase chain reaction (PCR).

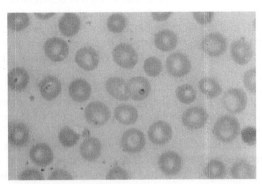

Fig. 2. Ring-staged *B microti* parasite in a sample of infected human blood (magnification of 1125X). (*From* CDC/ Dr. George R. Healy. Available at https://phil.cdc.gov/Details.aspx?pid=18984.)

On blood smear, *B microti* trophozoites appear as pleiomorphic ring forms (**Fig. 2**).[2,63] Parasitemia, reflecting parasite density seen on blood smear, is expressed in percentage and usually ranges from 0.1% to 10%, although can rarely be as high as 80%. Multiple blood smears may need to be examined in the early stage of the disease when parasitemia is often low. A parasitemia level less than 4% is usually seen in mild to moderate disease, whereas parasitemia ≥4% is associated with severe babesiosis.[2,16] Use of PCR for detection of *Babesia* DNA has replaced blood smear examination for initial diagnosis in some centers, but smear examination remains an important measure to follow for clearance of parasitemia. Real-time PCR assays, which target the *Babesia* 18S rRNA gene, have considerably lowered the limit of detection.[34,64–67] Use of quantitative PCR may be useful in following immunocompromised hosts at risk of relapse but is not needed in immunocompetent hosts. In addition, a transcription-mediated amplification test for tick-borne parasite is currently approved in the United States for screening the blood supply.[68]

Serology for *Babesia*-specific antibody can be used for diagnostic confirmation if acute and convalescent sera document a fourfold increase in antibody. Single-antibody positivity is not adequate for diagnostic confirmation.[69] Antibody tests should be interpreted with caution, as it is difficult to distinguish current from recent or past infection. The antigen used for serology should be that of the suspected *Babesia* species. The most common serologic test used is indirect fluorescent antibody testing (IFAT).[70,71] The complete *B microti* antigen-based IFAT has a sensitivity of 88% to 96% and a specificity of 90% to 100%.[70] The antibody titer that defines the threshold for a positive serologic test can differ between species and between laboratories. *B microti* immunoglobulin G (IgG) titers usually exceed 1:1024 during the acute phase of illness and may markedly decline over 6 months to a year or persists for several years.[37,72] A positive IgM titer, which can be detected 2 weeks after onset of symptoms, is suggestive of recent infection.[16,73]

B divergens, *B duncani*, and *B venatorum* antibodies are not detected in *B microti* antibody assays, although cross-reactivity has been reported between different *Babesia* species. There have been insufficient cases of *B duncani* infection to validate an IFAT.[8,74,75]

TREATMENT

Treatment of *Babesia* initially was largely based on case reports or small series and was extrapolated from rodent and animal model studies.[76–78] The combination of clindamycin and quinine, the first effective antimicrobial therapy for babesiosis, was not discovered until more than 20 years after the first case of human babesiosis was reported and about 10 years after it was first recognized to be endemic on Nantucket Island.[76] Twenty years later, the first and only randomized controlled therapeutic trial for babesiosis was carried out. Atovaquone and azithromycin were found to be as effective as clindamycin and quinine with fewer side effects and became the combination of choice except for life-threatening disease.[79] In the year 2020, the Infectious Diseases Society of America issued treatment guidelines for babesiosis (**Table 2**).[69,80]

Asymptomatic Babesia microti Infection

Although spontaneous resolution of infection is expected in immunocompetent individuals with asymptomatic *B microti* infection, antimicrobial treatment should be considered.[81] Asymptomatic patients with isolated positive serology should not be treated unless they develop symptoms and a positive smear or PCR.

Table 2
Treatment regimens for babesiosis[80]

Disease Severity	Treatment Regimen	
	Adult Doses	**Pediatric Doses**
Ambulatory patients: mild to moderate disease[a]	Preferred [a]Atovaquone 750 mg orally (with a fatty meal) Q12h plus azithromycin 500 mg orally on day 1, then 250 mg Q24h for 7 to 10 days Alternative [c]Clindamycin 600 mg orally Q8h plus quinine sulfate 650 mg orally Q8h for 7 to 10 days	[b]Atovaquone 20 mg/kg (up to 750 mg/dose) orally Q12h plus azithromycin 10 mg/kg (up to 500 mg/dose) orally on day 1, then 5 mg/kg (up to 250 mg/dose) orally Q24h for 7 to 10 days [c]Clindamycin 7–10 mg/kg (up to 600 mg/dose) orally Q6h-8h plus quinine sulfate 8 mg/kg (up to 650 mg/dose) orally Q8h for 7 to 10 days
Hospitalized patients: acute severe disease[d]	Preferred [e]Atovaquone 750 mg orally Q12h plus azithromycin 500 mg IV Q24h until symptoms abate, then convert to all oral therapy (see step-down therapy) Alternative [c]Clindamycin 600 mg IV Q6h plus quinine sulfate 650 mg orally Q8h until symptoms abate, then convert to all oral therapy (see step-down therapy)	[f]Atovaquone 20 mg/kg (up to 750 mg/dose) orally Q12h plus azithromycin 10 mg/kg (up to 500 mg/dose) IV Q24h until symptoms abate, then convert to all oral therapy (see step-down therapy) [c]Clindamycin 7–10 mg/kg (up to 600 mg/dose) IV Q6h-8h plus quinine sulfate 8 mg/kg (up to 650 mg/dose) orally Q8h until symptoms abate, then convert to all oral therapy (see step-down therapy)

Hospitalized patients: step-down therapy (transition to oral therapy)	**Preferred** Azithromycin 250 to 500 mg orally once daily plus Atovaquone 750 mg orally every 12 hours. Treatment of acute disease plus step-down therapy typically lasts 7–10 days in total. A high dose of azithromycin (500–1000 mg) orally should be considered for immunocompromised patients. **Alternative** [c]Clindamycin 600 mg orally Q8h plus quinine sulfate 650 mg orally Q8h. Treatment of acute disease plus step-down therapy typically lasts 7–10 days in total.	Atovaquone 20 mg/kg (up to 750 mg/dose) orally Q12h plus azithromycin 5–10 mg/kg (up to 500 mg/dose) orally Q24h. Treatment of acute disease and step-down therapy typically last 7–10 days in total [c]Clindamycin 7–10 mg/kg (up to 600 mg/dose) orally Q6h-8h plus quinine sulfate 8 mg/kg (up to 650 mg/dose) orally Q8h. Treatment of acute disease plus step-down therapy typically lasts 7–10 days in total
Immunocompromised patients	Start with one of the regimens recommended for hospitalized patients: acute severe disease and follow with one of the step-down therapies but treat for at least 6 consecutive weeks, including 2 final weeks during which parasites are no longer detected on peripheral blood smear. When oral azithromycin is used, a 500–1000 mg daily dose should be considered.	

[a] These patients usually are immunocompetent, experience mild to moderate symptoms, have a parasitemia <4%, and do not require hospital admission.

[b] Azithromycin modestly increases the risk of pyloric stenosis for infants less than 6 weeks old.

[c] Clindamycin plus quinine is preferred when parasitemia and symptoms have failed to abate following initiation of atovaquone plus azithromycin. Some physicians have used parenteral quinidine instead of ora quinine; however, quinidine is no longer available in the United States. All quinine doses listed are for the sulfate salt, which is the only quinine salt available in the United States; 650 mg quinine sulfate is equivalent to 542 mg quinine base and 8 mg quinine sulfate/kg is equivalent to 6 mg base/kg.

[d] Exchange transfusion should be considered for patients with high-grade parasitemia (>10%) or moderate to high-grade parasitemia and any one or more of the following: severe hemolytic anemia and/or severe pulmonary, renal, or hepatic compromise. Expert consultation with a transfusion services physician or hematologist in conjunction with an infectious disease specialist is strongly advised.

[e] Azithromycin 1000 mg given orally, in combination with other antibiotics, has been used successfully to clear Babesia microti infection in immunocompromised patients. A one-time dose of azithromycin 1000 mg ir travenously has been used for severe babesiosis but with very limited experience. While this dose has been shown to be safe, there are no published reports of the use this 1000 mg dose for severe babesiosis. If intravenous azithromycin 1000 mg is given to an immunocompromised patient, subsequent doses should be reduced to 500 mg daily.

[f] This regimen has not yet been reported for the treatment of children with severe babesiosis.

Adapted from Corrigendum to: Clinical Practice Guidelines by the Infectious Diseases Society of America (IDSA): 2020 Guideline on Diagnosis and Management of Babesiosis. Clin Infect Dis. 2021;73(1):172-173. https://doi.org/10.1093/cid/ciab275; with permission.

Mild to Moderate Babesia microti Disease

Patients with mild to moderate disease, typically seen in immunocompetent hosts, usually have a parasitemia less than 4% and do not require hospital admission. Following confirmation of the diagnosis, azithromycin plus atovaquone is the preferred regimen, prescribed for 7 to 10 days. The alternative option is a combination of quinine and clindamycin.[69,80] A randomized control trial conducted on 58 adults with non–life-threatening babesiosis compared a 7-day treatment with either azithromycin plus atovaquone with the combination of clindamycin plus quinine. Both treatment regimens resulted in clearance of parasitemia and symptoms at 3 months after completion of therapy. Atovaquone plus azithromycin was associated with fewer adverse effects (15%).[79] Most patients begin to experience resolution of symptoms within 48 hours after initiation of antimicrobial therapy. Fatigue may persist for weeks after an acute episode but will eventually resolve within 3 months in most cases.[2]

Severe Babesia microti Disease

Severe *B microti* infection is usually associated with high parasitemia greater than 4% and may lead to complications and relapsing infection. Patients are usually hospitalized and may require RBC exchange transfusion in addition to antimicrobial therapy. Risk factors for severe disease include age greater than 50 years, splenectomy, malignancy, HIV with low CD4 counts, or other immunosuppression.[44,46]

The preferred regimen is the combination of intravenous (IV) azithromycin plus oral atovaquone. Clindamycin (IV) plus oral quinine is the alternative option. A recent retrospective study of 46 patients with severe babesiosis, some of whom had life-threatening disease, resulted in only 2 treatment failures.[82] Transitioning to oral therapy is possible after reduction in parasitemia level and clinical improvement. The typical duration of treatment is 7 to 10 days but is usually prolonged in patients who are immunocompromised, especially when they experience persistent parasitemia and symptoms (**Table 1**).[69,80,82] Parasitemia level should be monitored with peripheral smear in the immunocompromised patient to ensure resolution of the infection.

In patients with relapsed or persistent parasitemia, development of resistance to azithromycin and/or atovaquone has been reported.[59,83] When a patient fails to respond to either the preferred or the alternative regimen, the optimal approach is difficult and based on a small amount of data. A combined therapy of azithromycin, atovaquone, and clindamycin may be used.[16,63,84] Other combinations have been tried.[85] There is a need for additional treatment options for severe or relapsing babesiosis. Recent studies conducted on immunocompromised mice demonstrated the potential efficacy of treatment of *B microti* infection with clofazimine, tafenoquine, or a combination of an endochin-like quinolone plus atovaquone.[86–89]

Exchange RBC transfusion is warranted in patients with parasitemia greater than 10%, severe hemolysis, or organ impairment (particularly cardiac, pulmonary, renal, or liver).[16,63,69,90] No prospective trials have been conducted to determine the benefit and optimal use of this approach. Exchange transfusion can lower parasitemia in blood and is thought to remove inflammatory mediators and toxic by-products of RBC lysis.[91,92] When parasitemia remains high or resurges after an initial exchange transfusion, a repeat exchange transfusion may be warranted.[84,93]

Prevention

Prevention of babesiosis is based on a combination of minimizing exposure to ticks and environmental management. Patients at high risk of severe babesiosis should avoid *Babesia* endemic areas particularly during tick transmission season (late spring, summer, and early fall).[16,63] Personal protection through vaccination or use of monoclonal antibodies may be possible in the future based on murine studies using particular merozoite antigens.[94] There is no current babesiosis vaccine available for humans, and no prophylactic antibiotic therapy is available.

SUMMARY

Babesiosis is an emerging tick-borne zoonosis caused by parasites of the genus *Babesia*. The primary mode of transmission is a tick bite. *B microti* is the most common cause of human babesiosis and is endemic in the Northeastern and upper Midwestern United States. *B divergens* is the main species causing human babesiosis in Europe, whereas *B crassa*-like agent, *B microti*, and *B venatorum* are endemic in China. Most *Babesia* infections are mild to moderate and clear with appropriate antibiotic, but some cases are asymptomatic, whereas others are fatal. Fever, fatigue, chills, sweats, and myalgia are the most common symptoms; however, disease can be associated with hematologic, cardiovascular, pulmonary, renal, and liver complications. Diagnosis should be suspected in a patient with typical symptoms and laboratory features with relevant epidemiologic exposure. Diagnostic confirmation of babesiosis relies on blood smear for microscopic identification of *Babesia* organisms and/or PCR for detection of *Babesia* DNA. Treatment is based on a combination of antimicrobials given for 7 to 10 days in immunocompetent hosts, but longer courses may be required in severely immunocompromised patients. Exchange RBC transfusion may be warranted in severe cases.

CLINICS CARE POINTS

- Human babesiosis is an emerging tick-borne zoonosis caused by a hemoprotozoan parasite that is transmitted by tick vectors or less frequently through blood transfusion, organ transplantation, or transplacental transfusion.

- Babesia infections are usually mild to moderate in severity but range from asymptomatic to fatal, and generally are severe in elderly and immunocompromised individuals.

- *Babesia microti*, the predominant cause for human babesiosis, is treated with a combination of atovaquone plus azithromycin, with clindamycin and quinine as an alternative.

- Red blood cell exchange transfusion remains an adjunct to antimicrobial therapy for treatment of severely ill patients, but clinical trials are needed to demonstrate its efficacy.

REFERENCES

1. Gray EB. Babesiosis surveillance — United States, 2011–2015. MMWR Surveill Summ 2019;68. https://doi.org/10.15585/mmwr.ss6806a1.
2. Vannier EG, Diuk-Wasser MA, Ben Mamoun C, et al. Babesiosis. Infect Dis Clin North Am 2015;29(2):357–70.
3. Shih CM, Liu LP, Chung WC, et al. Human babesiosis in Taiwan: asymptomatic infection with a Babesia microti-like organism in a Taiwanese woman. J Clin Microbiol 1997;35(2):450–4.
4. Gray J, Zintl A, Hildebrandt A, et al. Zoonotic babesiosis: overview of the disease and novel aspects of pathogen identity. Ticks Tick Borne Dis 2010;1(1):3–10.
5. Smith RP, Hunfeld KP, Krause PJ. Management strategies for human babesiosis. Expert Rev Anti Infect Ther 2020;18(7):625–36.

6. CDC. Recent Lyme disease surveillance data | CDC. Centers for Disease Control and Prevention. 2021. Available at: https://www.cdc.gov/lyme/datasurveillance/recent-surveillance-data.html. Accessed November 23, 2021.

7. Conrad PA, Kjemtrup AM, Carreno RA, et al. Description of Babesia duncani n.sp. (Apicomplexa: Babesiidae) from humans and its differentiation from other piroplasms. Int J Parasitol 2006;36(7):779–89.

8. Herwaldt BL, de Bruyn G, Pieniazek NJ, et al. Babesia divergens-like infection, Washington State. Emerg Infect Dis 2004;10(4):622–9.

9. Levine ND, Corliss JO, Cox FE, et al. A newly revised classification of the protozoa. J Protozool 1980;27(1):37–58.

10. Lemieux JE, Tran AD, Freimark L, et al. A global map of genetic diversity in Babesia microti reveals strong population structure and identifies variants associated with clinical relapse. Nat Microbiol 2016;1(7):16079.

11. Goethert HK, Molloy P, Berardi V, et al. Zoonotic Babesia microti in the northeastern U.S.: evidence for the expansion of a specific parasite lineage. PLoS One 2018;13(3):e0193837.

12. Spielman A, Wilson ML, Levine JF, et al. Ecology of Ixodes dammini-borne human babesiosis and Lyme disease. Annu Rev Entomol 1985;30:439–60.

13. Telford SR, Gorenflot A, Brasseur P, et al. CHAPTER 1 - Babesial infections in humans and wildlife. In: Kreier JP, editor. Parasitic Protozoa. 2nd edition. Academic Press; 1993. p. 1–47. https://doi.org/10.1016/B978-0-12-426015-3.50006-6. ISBN 9780124260153. Available at: https://www.sciencedirect.com/science/article/pii/B9780124260153500066.

14. Tufts DM, Diuk-Wasser MA. Vertical transmission: a vector-independent transmission pathway of Babesia microti in the natural reservoir host Peromyscus leucopus. J Infect Dis 2021;223(10):1787–95.

15. Armstrong PM, Katavolos P, Caporale DA, et al. Diversity of Babesia infecting deer ticks (Ixodes dammini). Am J Trop Med Hyg 1998;58(6):739–42.

16. Vannier E, Krause PJ. Human babesiosis. N Engl J Med 2012;366(25):2397–407.

17. Moritz ED, Winton CS, Tonnetti L, et al. Screening for Babesia microti in the U.S. blood supply. N Engl J Med 2016;375(23):2236–45.

18. Herwaldt BL, Linden JV, Bosserman E, et al. Transfusion-associated babesiosis in the United States: a description of cases. Ann Intern Med 2011;155(8):509–19.

19. Ngo V, Civen R. Babesiosis acquired through blood transfusion, California, USA. Emerg Infect Dis 2009;15(5):785–7.

20. Young C, Krause PJ. The problem of transfusion-transmitted babesiosis. Transfusion 2009;49(12):2548–50.

21. Brennan MB, Herwaldt BL, Kazmierczak JJ, et al. Transmission of babesia microti parasites by solid organ transplantation. Emerg Infect Dis 2016;22(11):1869–76.

22. Krause PJ, Vannier E. Transplacental transmission of human babesiosis. Infect Dis Clin Pract 2012;20(6):365–7.

23. Peniche-Lara G, Balmaceda L, Perez-Osorio C, et al. Human babesiosis, Yucatán State, Mexico, 2015. Emerg Infect Dis 2018;24(11):2061–2.

24. Paleau A, Candolfi E, Souply L, et al. Human babesiosis in Alsace. Med Mal Infect 2020;50(6):486–91.

25. Bloch EM, Kasubi M, Levin A, et al. Babesia microti and malaria infection in Africa: a pilot serosurvey in Kilosa District, Tanzania. Am J Trop Med Hyg 2018; 99(1):51–6.

26. Zhou X, Xia S, Huang JL, et al. Human babesiosis, an emerging tick-borne disease in the People's Republic of China. Parasit Vectors 2014;7(1):509.

27. Paparini A, Senanayake SN, Ryan UM, et al. Molecular confirmation of the first autochthonous case of human babesiosis in Australia using a novel primer set for the beta-tubulin gene. Exp Parasitol 2014;141:93–7.

28. Gray EB, Herwaldt BL. Babesiosis surveillance - United States, 2011-2015. MMWR Surveill Summ 2019;68(6):1–11.

29. Krause PJ, McKay K, Gadbaw J, et al. Increasing health burden of human babesiosis in endemic sites. Am J Trop Med Hyg 2003;68(4):431–6.

30. Dunn JM, Krause PJ, Davis S, et al. Borrelia burgdorferi promotes the establishment of Babesia microti in the northeastern United States. PLoS One 2014;9(12): e115494.

31. Diuk-Wasser MA, Vannier E, Krause PJ. Coinfection by the tick-borne pathogens Babesia microti and Borrelia burgdorferi: ecological, epidemiological and clinical consequences. Trends Parasitol 2016;32(1):30–42.

32. Leiby DA, Chung APS, Gill JE, et al. Demonstrable parasitemia among Connecticut blood donors with antibodies to Babesia microti. Transfusion 2005;45(11): 1804–10.

33. Tonnetti L, Thorp AM, Deisting B, et al. Babesia microti seroprevalence in Minnesota blood donors. Transfusion 2013;53(8):1698–705.

34. Moritz ED, Winton CS, Johnson ST, et al. Investigational screening for Babesia microti in a large repository of blood donor samples from nonendemic and endemic areas of the United States. Transfusion 2014;54(9):2226–36.

35. Krause PJ, Daily J, Telford SR, et al. Shared features in the pathobiology of babesiosis and malaria. Trends Parasitol 2007;23(12):605–10.

36. Reis SP, Maddineni S, Rozenblit G, et al. Spontaneous splenic rupture secondary to Babesia microti infection: treatment with splenic artery embolization. J Vasc Interv Radiol 2011;22(5):732–4.

37. Krause PJ, Spielman A, Telford SR, et al. Persistent parasitemia after acute babesiosis. N Engl J Med 1998;339(3):160–5.

38. Allred DR. Babesiosis: persistence in the face of adversity. Trends Parasitol 2003; 19(2):51–5.

39. Lobo CA, Cursino-Santos JR, Singh M, et al. Babesia divergens: a drive to survive. Pathogens 2019;8(3):E95.

40. Lobo CA, Rodriguez M, Cursino-Santos JR. Babesia and red cell invasion. Curr Opin Hematol 2012;19(3):170–5.

41. Woolley AE, Montgomery MW, Savage WJ, et al. Post-babesiosis warm autoimmune hemolytic anemia. N Engl J Med 2017;376(10):939–46.

42. Krause PJ, Telford SR, Spielman A, et al. Concurrent Lyme disease and babesiosis. Evidence for increased severity and duration of illness. JAMA 1996;275(21): 1657–60.

43. Krause PJ, McKay K, Thompson CA, et al. Disease-specific diagnosis of coinfecting tickborne zoonoses: babesiosis, human granulocytic ehrlichiosis, and Lyme disease. Clin Infect Dis 2002;34(9):1184–91.

44. White DJ, Talarico J, Chang HG, et al. Human babesiosis in New York State: review of 139 hospitalized cases and analysis of prognostic factors. Arch Intern Med 1998;158(19):2149–54.

45. Reubush TK, Cassaday PB, Marsh HJ, et al. Human babesiosis on Nantucket Island. Clinical features. Ann Intern Med 1977;86(1):6–9.

46. Hatcher JC, Greenberg PD, Antique J, et al. Severe babesiosis in Long Island: review of 34 cases and their complications. Clin Infect Dis 2001;32(8):1117–25.

47. Patel KM, Johnson JE, Reece R, et al. Babesiosis-associated splenic rupture: case series from a hyperendemic region. Clin Infect Dis 2019;69(7):1212–7.

48. Wormser GP, Villafuerte P, Nolan SM, et al. Neutropenia in congenital and adult babesiosis. Am J Clin Pathol 2015;144(1):94–6.

49. Kim N, Rosenbaum GS, Cunha BA. Relative bradycardia and lymphopenia in patients with babesiosis. Clin Infect Dis 1998;26(5):1218–9.

50. Cullen G, Sands BE, Yajnik V. Babesiosis in a patient on infliximab for Crohn's disease. Inflamm Bowel Dis 2010;16(8):1269–70.

51. Bogoch II, Davis BT, Hooper DC. Severe babesiosis in a patient treated with a tumor necrosis factor α antagonist. Clin Infect Dis 2012;54(8):1215–6.

52. Mareedu N, Schotthoefer AM, Tompkins J, et al. Risk factors for severe infection, hospitalization, and prolonged antimicrobial therapy in patients with babesiosis. Am J Trop Med Hyg 2017;97(4):1218–25.

53. Alvarez De Leon S, Srivastava P, Revelo AE, et al. Babesiosis as a cause of acute respiratory distress syndrome: a series of eight cases. Postgrad Med 2019; 131(2):138–43.

54. Dumic I, Patel J, Hart M, et al. Splenic rupture as the first manifestation of babesia microti infection: report of a case and review of literature. Am J Case Rep 2018; 19:335–41.

55. Li S, Goyal B, Cooper JD, et al. Splenic rupture from babesiosis, an emerging concern? A systematic review of current literature. Ticks Tick Borne Dis 2018; 9(6):1377–82.

56. Krause PJ, Gewurz BE, Hill D, et al. Persistent and relapsing babesiosis in immunocompromised patients. Clin Infect Dis 2008;46(3):370–6.

57. Fida M, Challener D, Hamdi A, et al. Babesiosis: a retrospective review of 38 cases in the upper midwest. Open Forum Infect Dis 2019;6(7):ofz311.

58. Joseph JT, Roy SS, Shams N, et al. Babesiosis in Lower Hudson Valley, New York, USA. Emerg Infect Dis 2011;17(5):843–7.

59. Wormser GP, Prasad A, Neuhaus E, et al. Emergence of resistance to azithromycin-atovaquone in immunocompromised patients with Babesia microti infection. Clin Infect Dis 2010;50(3):381–6.

60. Falagas ME, Klempner MS. Babesiosis in patients with AIDS: a chronic infection presenting as fever of unknown origin. Clin Infect Dis 1996;22(5):809–12.

61. Stowell CP, Gelfand JA, Shepard JAO, et al. Case records of the Massachusetts General Hospital. Case 17-2007. A 25-year-old woman with relapsing fevers and recent onset of dyspnea. N Engl J Med 2007;356(22):2313–9.

62. Ho J, Carey E, Carey DE, et al. Recurrence of human babesiosis caused by reinfection. Emerg Infect Dis 2021;27(10):2658–61.

63. Sanchez E, Vannier E, Wormser GP, et al. Diagnosis, treatment, and prevention of Lyme disease, human granulocytic anaplasmosis, and babesiosis: a review. JAMA 2016;315(16):1767–77.

64. Wang G, Villafuerte P, Zhuge J, et al. Comparison of a quantitative PCR assay with peripheral blood smear examination for detection and quantitation of Babesia microti infection in humans. Diagn Microbiol Infect Dis 2015;82(2): 109–13.

65. Teal AE, Habura A, Ennis J, et al. A new real-time PCR assay for improved detection of the parasite Babesia microti. J Clin Microbiol 2012;50(3):903–8.

66. Rollend L, Bent SJ, Krause PJ, et al. Quantitative PCR for detection of Babesia microti in Ixodes scapularis ticks and in human blood. Vector Borne Zoonotic Dis 2013;13(11):784–90.

67. Wilson M, Glaser KC, Adams-Fish D, et al. Development of droplet digital PCR for the detection of Babesia microti and Babesia duncani. Exp Parasitol 2015;149: 24–31.

68. Commissioner O of the. FDA approves first tests to screen for tickborne parasite in whole blood and plasma to protect the U.S. blood supply. FDA. 2020. Available at: https://www.fda.gov/news-events/press-announcements/fda-approves-first-tests-screen-tickborne-parasite-whole-blood-and-plasma-protect-us-blood-supply. Accessed January 3, 2022.

69. Krause PJ, Auwaerter PG, Bannuru RR, et al. Clinical practice guidelines by the Infectious Diseases Society of America (IDSA): 2020 guideline on diagnosis and management of babesiosis. Clin Infect Dis 2021;72(2):185–9.

70. Krause PJ, Telford SR, Ryan R, et al. Diagnosis of babesiosis: evaluation of a serologic test for the detection of Babesia microti antibody. J Infect Dis 1994; 169(4):923–6.

71. Levin AE, Williamson PC, Erwin JL, et al. Determination of Babesia microti sero-prevalence in blood donor populations using an investigational enzyme immuno-assay. Transfusion 2014;54(9):2237–44.

72. Ruebush TK, Chisholm ES, Sulzer AJ, et al. Development and persistence of anti-body in persons infected with Babesia microti. Am J Trop Med Hyg 1981;30(1): 291–2.

73. Krause PJ, Ryan R, Telford S, et al. Efficacy of immunoglobulin M serodiagnostic test for rapid diagnosis of acute babesiosis. J Clin Microbiol 1996;34(8):2014–6.

74. Herwaldt B, Persing DH, Précigout EA, et al. A fatal case of babesiosis in Mis-souri: identification of another piroplasm that infects humans. Ann Intern Med 1996;124(7):643–50.

75. Duh D, Jelovsek M, Avsic-Zupanc T. Evaluation of an indirect fluorescence immu-noassay for the detection of serum antibodies against Babesia divergens in hu-mans. Parasitology 2007;134(Pt 2):179–85.

76. Wittner M, Rowin KS, Tanowitz HB, et al. Successful chemotherapy of transfusion babesiosis. Ann Intern Med 1982;96(5):601–4.

77. Rowin KS, Tanowitz HB, Wittner M. Therapy of experimental babesiosis. Ann Intern Med 1982;97(4):556–8.

78. Bredt AB, Weinstein WM, Cohen S. Treatment of babesiosis in asplenic patients. JAMA 1981;245(19):1938–9.

79. Krause PJ, Lepore T, Sikand VK, et al. Atovaquone and azithromycin for the treat-ment of babesiosis. N Engl J Med 2000;343(20):1454–8.

80. Corrigendum to: Clinical Practice Guidelines by the Infectious Diseases Society of America (IDSA): 2020 guideline on diagnosis and management of babesiosis. Clin Infect Dis 2021;73(1):172–3.

81. Prevention CC for DC and. CDC - Babesiosis - resources for health professionals. 2019. Available at: https://www.cdc.gov/parasites/babesiosis/health_professionals/index.html. Accessed November 26, 2021.

82. Kletsova EA, Spitzer ED, Fries BC, et al. Babesiosis in Long Island: review of 62 cases focusing on treatment with azithromycin and atovaquone. Ann Clin Micro-biol Antimicrob 2017;16(1):26.

83. Simon MS, Westblade LF, Dziedziech A, et al. Clinical and molecular evidence of atovaquone and azithromycin resistance in relapsed Babesia microti infection associated with rituximab and chronic lymphocytic leukemia. Clin Infect Dis 2017;65(7):1222–5.

84. Li Y, Stanley S, Villalba JA, et al. Case report: overwhelming babesia parasitemia successfully treated promptly with RBC apheresis and triple therapy with clinda-mycin, azithromycin, and atovaquone. Open Forum Infect Dis 2020;7(10): ofaa448.

85. Vannier E, Gewurz BE, Krause PJ. Human babesiosis. Infect Dis Clin North Am 2008;22(3):469–88, viii-ix.
86. Lawres LA, Garg A, Kumar V, et al. Radical cure of experimental babesiosis in immunodeficient mice using a combination of an endochin-like quinolone and atovaquone. J Exp Med 2016;213(7):1307–18.
87. Mordue DG, Wormser GP. Could the drug tafenoquine revolutionize treatment of Babesia microti infection? J Infect Dis 2019;220(3):442–7.
88. Tuvshintulga B, Sivakumar T, Nugraha AB, et al. A combination of clofazimine–atovaquone as a potent therapeutic regimen for the radical cure of Babesia microti infection in immunocompromised hosts. J Infect Dis 2021;19:jiab537.
89. Vannier E, Gelfand JA. Clofazimine for babesiosis: preclinical data support a clinical trial. J Infect Dis 2021;19:jiab538.
90. Padmanabhan A, Connelly-Smith L, Aqui N, et al. Guidelines on the use of therapeutic apheresis in clinical practice - evidence-based approach from the writing committee of the American Society for Apheresis: the eighth special issue. J Clin Apher 2019;34(3):171–354.
91. Spaete J, Patrozou E, Rich JD, et al. Red cell exchange transfusion for babesiosis in Rhode Island. J Clin Apher 2009;24(3):97–105.
92. Saifee NH, Krause PJ, Wu Y. Apheresis for babesiosis: therapeutic parasite reduction or removal of harmful toxins or both? J Clin Apher 2016;31(5):454–8.
93. Radcliffe C, Krause PJ, Grant M. Repeat exchange transfusion for treatment of severe babesiosis. Transfus Apher Sci 2019;58(5):638–40.
94. Wang H, Wang Y, Huang J, et al. Babesia microti protein BmSP44 is a novel protective antigen in a mouse model of babesiosis. Front Immunol 2020;11:1437.

Powassan Virus Encephalitis

Anne Piantadosi, MD, PhD[a,b,*], Isaac H. Solomon, MD, PhD[c]

KEYWORDS

• Powassan virus • Deer tick virus • Encephalitis • Neuropathology

KEY POINTS

• Powassan virus is an *Ixodes*-borne flavivirus that can cause severe encephalitis.
• Prevalence studies in ticks and seroprevalence studies in wild mammals and humans suggest that human exposure to Powassan virus is more common than currently appreciated, and non-neuroinvasive disease is likely under-recognized.
• Diagnosis is typically established by serologic testing of blood or cerebrospinal fluid but also can be confirmed by reverse transcription– polymerase chain reaction or sequencing from cerebrospinal fluid or immunohistochemistry, in situ hybridization, or molecular testing of brain tissue.

INTRODUCTION

Powassan virus is a tick-borne flavivirus that is endemic to the United States, causes severe encephalitis, and is diagnosed with increasing frequency. Since its discovery in 1958, approximately 270 cases have been reported in the United States and Canada; however, multiple lines of epidemiologic evidence suggest that it may be more prevalent than is currently appreciated. This article briefly summarizes the virology, ecology, and epidemiology of Powassan virus and reviews clinical features of infection, with a focus on brain imaging, diagnostic testing, and neuropathology.

Powassan virus belongs to the *Flaviviridae* family and is a small enveloped virus, with an approximately 10.8-kb, positive-sense RNA genome that encodes a single open reading frame.[1] It is a member of the flavivirus genus, which is primarily composed of arthropod-borne viruses, and it is closely related to tick-borne encephalitis virus (TBEV). TBEV is a relatively well-studied cause of encephalitis in Europe and Asia, and several of its features are worth considering, because they may parallel Powassan virus. First, TBEV causes a substantial burden of disease, with more than 10,000 cases per year despite the availability of a vaccine.[2] Many TBEV infections

[a] Department of Pathology and Laboratory Medicine, Emory University School of Medicine, Atlanta, GA, USA; [b] Department of Medicine, Division of Infectious Diseases, Emory University School of Medicine, Atlanta, GA, USA; [c] Department of Pathology, Brigham and Women's Hospital, Harvard Medical School, 75 Francis Street, AL360U.2, Boston, MA 02115, USA
* Corresponding author. Woodruff Memorial Research Building 7207A, 101 Woodruff Circle, Atlanta, GA 30322.
E-mail address: anne.piantadosi@emory.edu

Infect Dis Clin N Am 36 (2022) 671–688
https://doi.org/10.1016/j.idc.2022.03.003
0891-5520/22/© 2022 Elsevier Inc. All rights reserved.
id.theclinics.com

are asymptomatic,[3] and its seroprevalence ranges from 2% to 5% or higher in high-risk populations.[4–6] Finally, within TBEV, there are three viral subtypes that differ by approximately 5% at the amino acid level, have different (but overlapping) geographic distributions, and cause different frequencies of neuroinvasive disease and fatality.[7]

Compared with TBEV, relatively less is known about Powassan virus. It was discovered in 1958 in Ontario, Canada,[8] and only approximately 25 cases were reported over the subsequent 40 years.[9] In part, this may have been due to under-recognition and limited testing. Infection may truly have been infrequent, however, because the canonical Powassan virus lineage I is transmitted by tick species rarely encountered by humans, Ixodes cookei and I marxi. In 1996, a second lineage of Powassan virus was discovered and termed deer tick virus (DTV), because it is transmitted by the common vector of human disease, I scapularis.[10] Unlike other Ixodes-borne infections, Powassan virus can be transmitted within a very short period of tick attachment.[11,12] To date, more than 240 cases have been reported. The two Powassan virus lineages differ by approximately 15% at the nucleotide level and 5% at the amino acid level[13] and thus can be distinguished by molecular testing, such as polymerase chain reaction (PCR) and sequencing. All recent human infections for which molecular characterization was performed have been due to lineage II/DTV.[14–21] However, because most Powassan virus infections are diagnosed by serology and lineages I and II are serologically indistinguishable, they are clinically diagnosed together as Powassan virus encephalitis.

ECOLOGY

Powassan virus is maintained in an enzootic cycle that is composed of small mammal reservoir hosts and tick vectors. Ticks can become infected by feeding on a viremic host or cofeeding with an infected tick, even on a nonviremic host. The virus persists through later stages of the tick life cycle, for example, an infected larval tick remains infected as a nymph and adult (through transstadial transmission), and ticks can pass the virus on to progeny (through transovarial transmission).[22] Large mammals, including humans, become infected as incidental, dead-end hosts. In addition to being transmitted by different vectors, Powassan virus lineages I and II are maintained by different small mammal reservoir species in different geographic regions. Lineage I has been detected primarily in woodchucks and squirrels in regions of Canada and the United States surrounding the Great Lakes. By contrast, Powassan virus lineage II/DTV is found in the northeast and north central United States. Shrews have recently been implicated as a primary reservoir,[23] and there is little evidence that it is maintained in white-footed mice, which are the primary reservoir for other I scapularis–borne pathogens.

Powassan virus has a prevalence of approximately 1% to 3% in I scapularis ticks in endemic regions of the northeast and north central United States and has higher prevalence in adult ticks.[24–29] By comparison with other tick-borne pathogens, a study of I scapularis from New York found a prevalence of 3.4% for Powassan virus, 3.2% for Babesia microti, 18% for Anaplasma phagocytophilum, and 55% for Borrelia burgdorferi.[29] Experimental work has demonstrated that other tick species, Amblyomma americanum and Dermacentor variabilis, are competent vectors for Powassan virus.[30] Relatively little is known, however, about how frequently these vectors carry Powassan virus in the wild[31] and to what extent Powassan virus is present in parts of the United States with lower prevalence of I scapularis. Interestingly, Powassan virus is found in Ixodes ticks and humans in Far Eastern Russia and is proposed to have been introduced from Canada through fur trade in the twentieth century.[32]

Multiple wild mammals have high seroprevalence for Powassan virus. A study in Ontario identified positive sera in 50% of coyotes, 47% of skunks, 26% of foxes, and 10% of raccoons,[33] although another study identified only 1 positive elk from 217 total cervid samples.[34] In the United States, Powassan virus seroprevalence increased in white-tailed deer between 1979 and 2009, reaching over 80% in Connecticut in 2005, 2006, and 2009.[35] In nearby Vermont and Maine, 11% and 13% of deer were seropositive, respectively, in 2010.[35] In New York, serologic evidence of Powassan virus infection was detected in woodchucks (4/6), an opossum (1/6), and birds (4/727).[28] The relatively widespread seropositivity in mammals, combined with the prevalence in ticks and the expansion of the tick vector itself,[36] suggest increasing risk of human exposure to Powassan virus, similar to what has been observed with other *Ixodes*-borne infections.

EPIDEMIOLOGY

The high prevalence of Powassan virus in ticks and wild mammals raises the question of whether human infection may be more common than is currently appreciated. Powassan virus neuroinvasive disease was formally added to the list of notifiable diseases in the United States in 2001, and non-neuroinvasive infection was added in 2004, whereas Canada has no national reporting requirements. Diagnosis of Powassan virus infection has increased from approximately 1 case/y between 1958 and 2005, to 7.7 cases/y from 2006 to 2015,[13] to 21 to 43 cases/y from 2016 to 2019.[37,38] The true incidence of Powassan virus infections in North America is unknown, however, and likely well above the number of reported cases. Because there is limited to no testing in patients without neuroinvasive symptoms, little is known about subclinical or mild infection.

The few recent human seroprevalence studies that have been conducted to date have yielded a range of results.[13] Positive serology was detected in 9/95 (9.5%) of patients with suspected tick exposure and 2/50 (4%; $P = .33$) of patients without suspected tick exposure in Wisconsin in 2015.[39] Similarly, seroprevalence was significantly higher in samples submitted for Lyme disease testing in Wisconsin (10/106; 9.4%) than in samples from patients in the northeastern United States without tick exposure or symptoms of tick-borne disease (2/100, 2%; $P = .034$).[40] A seroprevalence study identified Powassan virus neutralizing antibodies in 1% of individuals in a general population In Sussex County, New Jersey, where a cluster of recent encephalitis cases was described.[41] Only a single equivocal result was detected among 230 serum samples from individuals bitten by *I scapularis* or *I cookei* ticks in Maine from 2009 to 2013.[42] Among samples from 52 patients with confirmed Lyme disease in New York between 2011 and 2015, only one was positive for IgM, and this sample was negative by confirmatory testing for neutralizing antibodies.[43] Given the variability in reported seroprevalence rates, it would be of value to conduct larger studies across the broader geographic area from which Powassan virus has been reported.

With the important caveat that most available information is from patients with neuroinvasive disease, epidemiologic information can be derived from approximately 270 cases described in case reports and case series (**Table 1**) and reported by the Centers for Disease Control and Prevention (CDC) national arbovirus surveillance system (ArboNET). The geographic distribution of Powassan virus cases in North America centers around the Great Lakes region and the east coast (**Fig. 1**). The first case was identified in Ontario in 1958,[8] and a majority of subsequent cases from Canada have been from Ontario (approximately 8) and Quebec (approximately 5). Single cases also have been reported from Newfoundland and New Brunswick.[44,45] The first case in

Table 1
Published cases of Powassan virus infection

Case Number	Age/ Sex	Year/Location	Fatal (Yes/ No)	Immunocompromised (Yes/No)	PubMed Identifier(s)
1	5 M	1958 Canada (Ontario)	Y	N	13652010
2	57 F	1970 New Jersey	N	N	4684890
3	7 M	1971 New York	N	N	222159; 4856896
4	5 F	1972 New York	N	N	4856896
5	12 M	1972 New York	N	N	222159; 4856896
6	14m M	1972 New York	N	N	222159; 4856896
7	8 M	1972 Canada (Quebec)	N	N	4829843
8	6–15 M	1974 New York	N	N	222159; 1059007
9	3 M	1975 Canada (Quebec)	N	N	N/A: Can Dis Wkly Rep 1976;2:85–7
10	6–15 M	1975 New York	N	N	222159; 267829
11	6–15 M	1975 New York	N	N	222159; 267829
12	82 M	1975 New York	Y	N	222159; 267829
13	15 F	1976 Canada (Ontario)	N	N	N/A: Can Dis Wkly Rep 1976; 2:202–3
14	13m F	1977 Canada (Ontario)	N	N	223757
15	0–5 F	1977 New York	N	N	222159
16	8 M	1978 New York (Canada [Nova Scotia])	N	N	6297420
17	19 F	1979 Canada (Ontario)	N	N	N/A: Can Dis Wkly Rep 1979;5:129–30
18	7 M	1979 Canada (Ontario)	N	N	6254625
19	9 F	1980 Canada (Quebec)	N	N	N/A: Can Dis Wkly Rep 1982; 8:185–91
20	62 M	1987 Canada (Ontario)	N	N	2547526
21	76 M	1988 Canada (New Brunswick)	N	N	21233909
22	49 F	1994 Massachusetts	N	N	7643850
23	4 M?	1994–1995 Canada	N	N	9502462
24	64 M	1997 Canada (Ontario)	Y	N	10906899
25	66 M	1999 Vermont	N	N	18959500; 11693145
26	25 M	2000 Maine	N	N	18959500; 11693145

(continued on next page)

Table 1
(*continued*)

Case Number	Age/ Sex	Year/Location	Fatal (Yes/ No)	Immunocompromised (Yes/No)	PubMed Identifier(s)
27	53 F	2000 Maine	N	N	18959500; 12771287; 11693145
28	70 M	2001 Maine	N	N	18959500; 11693145
29	60 F	2002 Michigan	N	N	18959500
30	69 M	2003 Wisconsin	N	N	20443328; 18959500
31	74 F	2004 Maine	N	N	18959500
32	91 F	2004 New York	N	N	24274334; 18959500
33	83 M	2005 New York	N	N	24274334; 18959500
34	49 M	2006 Wisconsin	N	N	20443328
35	47 F	2007 Wisconsin	N	N	20443328
36	81 ?	2007 New York	Y	?	24274334
37	81 ?	2007 New York	N	?	24274334
38	77 ?	2007 New York	Y	?	24274334
39	62 M	2007 New York	Y	Y	24274334; 19439744
40	5 ?	2007 New York	N	?	24274334
41	70 ?	2007 New York	Y	?	24274334
42	61 M	2008 Canada (Quebec)	N	N	20929710
43	9 F	2008 New York	N	N	24274334; 20736878
44	22 M	2009 New York	N	N	23969017
45	73 ?	2009 New York	N	?	24274334
46	76 ?	2009 New York	N	?	24274334
47	4 ?	2009 New York	N	?	24274334
48	77 M	2010 New York	Y	N	24274334; 23166187
49	67 F	2011 Minnesota	Y	Y	23017222
50	69 M	2011 Minnesota; North Dakota	N	N	23111001
51	61 M	2011 Minnesota	N	Y	23111001
52	60 M	2011 Minnesota; North Dakota	N	N	23111001
53	18 M	2011 Minnesota	N	N	23111001
54	43 M	? Minnesota	N	N	22040725
55	32/34 M	2012 New York	N	N	24274334; 23969017

(continued on next page)

Table 1
(continued)

Case Number	Age/ Sex	Year/Location	Fatal (Yes/ No)	Immunocompromised (Yes/No)	PubMed Identifier(s)
56	44 M	2013 New Hampshire	N	N	26668338
57	35 F	2013 Wisconsin	N	N	29431163
58	49 M	2014 Massachusetts	Y	N	26668338
59	52 M	2014 Massachusetts	N	N	26668338
60	65 F	2014 Massachusetts	N	N	26668338
61	67M	2014 Massachusetts	N	N	26668338
62	21 M	2014 Massachusetts	N	N	26668338
63	74 M	2015 Massachusetts	N	Y	26668338
64	82 M	2015 Massachusetts	Y	N	26668338
65	81 F	2016 Rhode Island	N	N	29942757
66	61 M	2016 Massachusetts	N	Y	29020227
67	63 M	2016 Massachusetts	Y	Y	33094116; 29554185
68	5m M	2016 Connecticut	N	N	33111953, 28426641
69	72 F	? Maine	Y	N	28903511
70	55 M	2017 Massachusetts	N	N	31538917
71	56 M	2017 New York	N	N	32007325
72	8 F	2017 Wisconsin	N	N	32060042
73	51 M	2017 New Jersey	N	Y	34283672
74	70 M	? Pennsylvania	N	Y	30104234
75	68 F	? Canada (Quebec; Ontario)	N	N	30559280
76	79 M	2018 Massachusetts	Y	N	33094116
77	30 F	2018 Indiana	N	Y	32539111
78	62 M	? Canada (Newfoundland; Ontario)	N	N	31158072
79	88 M	2018 Wisconsin	Y	N	33020816
80	87 M	? New York	N	N	31712240
81	75 F	2019 Massachusetts	Y	N	33094116
82	2m M	2019 Connecticut	N	N	33111953
83	42 M	2019 Wisconsin	N	N	33227515
84	76 M	? Wisconsin	N	N	33758161
85	62 M	? Connecticut	N	Y	34430178
86	82 F	? New York	Y	Y	34596868

Abbreviations: F, female; M, male; m, month; N, no; N/A, not applicable; ?, unknown; Y, yes;

the United States was identified in New Jersey in 1970,[46] and an additional 10 cases were described in New York in the 1970s.[47–49] Subsequently, Powassan virus was not reported until 1994 in Massachusetts,[50] 1999 in Vermont,[51] and 2000 in Maine,[51,52] coinciding with the recognition of DTV (lineage II). The first cases reported in the Midwest include Michigan in 2002, Wisconsin in 2003, and Minnesota in 2008.[51,53]

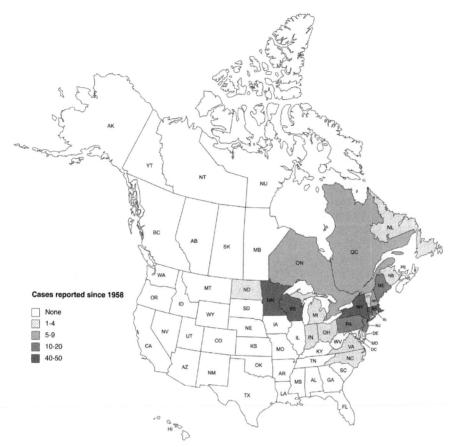

Fig. 1. Geographic distribution of 273 human Powassan virus infections reported between 1958 and 2021. (Created with mapchart.net.)

Altogether in the United States, more than 250 cases have been reported from 16 states. The greatest number of cases of have been reported from New York (n = 50), Wisconsin (n = 46), Minnesota (n = 45), and Massachusetts (n = 44). Fewer cases have been reported from Maine (n = 16), New Jersey (n = 14), Connecticut (n = 13), and Pennsylvania (n = 10), with a handful from Rhode Island (n = 5), New Hampshire (n = 5), and North Dakota (n = 2), and 1 case each in Indiana, Michigan, North Carolina, Ohio, Vermont, and Virginia.

Detailed clinical descriptions are available for 86 cases (see **Table 1**), and general information from annual or aggregated summaries is available for another 147 cases.[38,54–56] Of these 233 patients, a majority were male (n = 167, 72%) and over age 60 (n = 135, 58%), with 59 (25%) ages 18 to 59 and 39 (17%) under age 18. Illness onset most often occurred from April to June (n = 104, 45%), followed by July to September (n = 71, 30%) and October to December (n = 51, 22%), with only rare cases in January to March (n = 3, 1%). A vast majority of reported cases were from hospitalized patients (n = 217, 93%) and patients with neuroinvasive disease (n = 218, 94%), likely reflecting a bias in testing. The overall number of deaths was 28 (12%), including deaths from sequelae of hospitalization for Powassan virus disease.

TICK IDENTIFICATION AND SKIN PATHOLOGY

Patients may present at the time of, or soon after, a known tick bite, and ticks may be submitted for laboratory identification.[57] The female *I scapularis* is characterized by a red abdomen; a black, ovoid scutum covering up to half of the dorsum; black capitulum and legs; narrow and elongated, straight club-like palps; no eye spots or festoons; and an inverted U-shaped anal groove (**Fig. 2**A). *I scapularis* nymphs appear increasingly black during feeding, with an unchanged black ovoid scutum. The length of feeding can be estimated by the scutal index, the ratio of tick body length to scutum width,[58] although the relevance to Powassan virus disease is negligible due to the short time required to transmit infection.[11,12]

Skin at the site of a tick bite can appear normal to markedly erythematous while the tick is attached, and papular and nodular rashes may develop once removed.[59] Acute lesions may show histologic evidence of tick mouthparts attached to the epidermis, with an intradermal cavity containing red blood cells and a predominantly neutrophilic inflammatory infiltrate, which transitions to eosinophilic over time. Chronic lesions contain a dense inflammatory infiltrate of lymphocytes and eosinophils in a wedge shape, with overlying acanthotic and pseudoepitheliomatous epidermis, and associated with granulomata. Although the features of Powassan virus infection in skin have not been well described, mouse models do provide some insight into the distribution of virus and inflammatory response.[60,61]

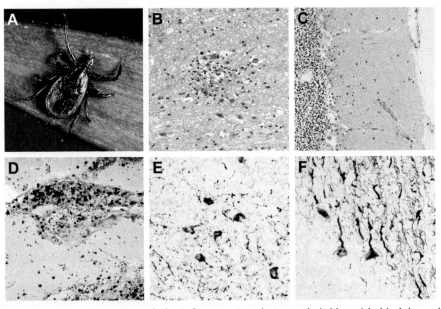

Fig. 2. Powassan virus neuropathologic features. Female *I scapularis* (deer tick; black-legged tick) can be grossly identified by characteristic U-shaped anal groove (*A*). Sections from fatal Powassan encephalitis cases show a microglial nodule with neuronophagia in the thalamus (*B*, *hematoxylin and eosin, image taken with 20x objective*), marked Purkinje cell loss and Bergmann gliosis in the cerebellum (*C, hematoxylin and eosin, image taken with 20x objective*), and CD3-positive T-cell infiltrate in the leptomeninges (*D, CD3 immunohistochemistry, image taken with 20x objective*). Powassan virus RNA in situ hybridization highlights infected neurons in the thalamus (*E, Powassan virus in situ hybridization, image taken with 20x objective*) and cerebellum (*F, Powassan virus in situ hybridization, image taken with 20x objective*). (*Image A Courtesy of* Michael L. Levin, PhD via the CDC Public Health Image Library.)

CLINICAL EVALUATION

Powassan virus has an incubation period of approximately 2 weeks, although this can range up to a month or longer.[31] Patients initially may experience nonspecific symptoms, such as fever and fatigue. Mild disease is identified occasionally (**Box 1**). However, neuroinvasive disease occurs in approximately 95% of recognized cases,[37,38] and patients often develop confusion and focal neurologic deficits requiring hospitalization.[19,62] Rarely, Powassan virus has been described to cause chororetinitis[63] (which also is seen in West Nile virus [WNV]), ophthalmoplegia,[64] and spinal cord (anterior horn) involvement leading to flaccid weakness.[44]

Although thrombocytopenia occasionally has been reported,[62,65] there are no peripheral laboratory abnormalities classically associated with Powassan virus. Cerebrospinal fluid (CSF) analysis generally demonstrates low to moderate elevation in protein, normal glucose, and pleocytosis in the range of hundreds of white blood cells (WBCs)/μL, which can be either lymphocyte or polymorphonuclear predominant.[62] It is worth considering that, like other tick-borne pathogens, Powassan virus may occur in coinfection,[66] so compatible clinical findings or laboratory abnormalities should prompt testing for Lyme disease, *Borrelia miyamotoi*, anaplasmosis, or babesiosis. Finally, although primarily associated with tick exposure, Powassan virus can be transmitted by blood transfusion[67] and is worth considering in the differential diagnosis for patients who receive transfusion in endemic areas.

IMAGING

Results of neuroradiological studies from head computed tomography or brain magnetic resonance imaging (MRI) have been reported for approximately 60 cases of Powassan virus encephalitis, and the wide range of findings is consistent with a similarly wide spectrum of clinical symptoms. Approximately 25% of published cases reported no acute abnormalities or nonspecific findings, including in two fatal cases.[9,68] The most common abnormalities reported were T2/fluid-attenuated inversion

---

Box 1
Case title: a 67-year-old woman with systemic illness

Case presentation: A 67-year-old woman presented to an outpatient clinic with a subacute systemic illness. She initially had a week of fever, headache, and profound fatigue. Following resolution of her fevers, she felt tremulous with dysregulated temperature, had difficulty concentrating, and noted decreased quality in handwriting; these symptoms were gradually improving. She had a persistently poor appetite and mild nausea without vomiting. Her gastrointestinal symptoms worsened with doxycycline. Over the past 2 days, she developed a pruritic rash on the extensor surface of her hands, elbows, and knees. Notable exposures include ticks, mosquitoes, and her baby grandchild. On physical examination, she had an erythematous papular rash most notable on her knees and extensor surfaces of her hands. Neurologic examination was unremarkable, including cranial nerves, motor strength, sensation, fine motor coordination, balance, and gait.

Clinical questions: What are potential causes of this patient's improving systemic illness? What additional testing could be ordered to confirm the diagnosis?

Discussion: Recommended tests included Lyme test with Western blot, *Anaplasma/Ehrlichia* PCR, Powassan virus antibody, WNV antibody, and cytomegalovirus IgM and IgG. This patient's serum Powassan virus IgM was positive with PRNT of 1:20, indicating recent infection.

Learning point: Powassan virus may present with mild symptoms and minimal neurologic involvement.

recovery (FLAIR) hyperintensities (suggestive of edema and inflammation) in basal ganglia (50%), cerebellum (40%), thalamus (30%), brainstem (30%), cerebral cortex (30%), and temporal lobes (10%). Occasional diffusion restriction, suggesting cytotoxic edema, and nonspecific white matter hyperintensities also have been noted. Leptomeningeal contrast enhancement was present in 15% of cases, and parenchymal enhancement was rare. Cerebellar involvement has previously been suggested to be a poor prognostic factor for Powassan virus disease,[62] which is supported here by cerebellar abnormalities in approximately 70% of fatal cases compared with less than 20% of nonfatal cases ($P = .0004$). Overall, imaging findings range from mild to diffuse meningoencephalitis/rhombencephalitis and do not have distinguishing features compared with other viruses infecting the central nervous system (CNS).

DIAGNOSTIC APPROACH

The nonspecific nature of the symptoms, laboratory, and imaging findings associated with Powassan virus makes it incumbent on physicians to consider it as a potential cause of encephalitis and pursue dedicated diagnostic testing. Diagnostic criteria have been outlined by the Centers for Disease Control and Prevention (CDC) for Powassan virus and other arboviruses[68] (**Fig. 3**). Diagnosis can be made by direct detection, and, although Powassan virus is rarely recovered in culture, molecular tests frequently detect its RNA, and this may be particularly useful in immunocompromised patients who do not mount sufficient antibody responses.[14,16] Several studies have demonstrated the use of sequencing-based assays to detect Powassan virus RNA in CSF and brain tissue.[14–18] It also can be identified by PCR,[20,21] and a multiplex

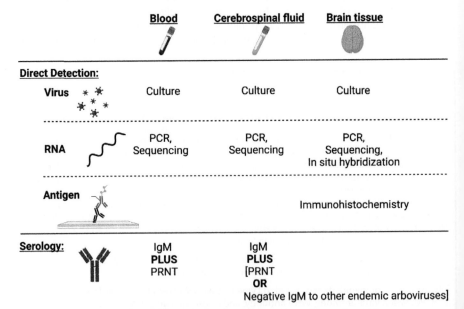

Fig. 3. Diagnostic approaches for Powassan virus. Testing modalities are listed for each specimen type (blood, CSF, and brain tissue) and target (virus, RNA, antigen, and antibody). (Created with BioRender.com.)

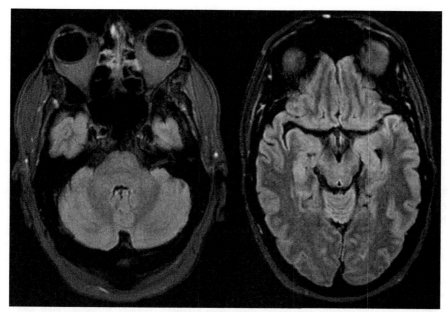

Fig. 4. Brain MRI from patient in **Box 2** at 4 days from initial symptom onset shows mild T2/FLAIR hyperintensity in the cerebellar vermis (left) and pons, midbrain, and medial temporal lobes (right). No significant contrast enhancement or diffusion restriction was identified.

Box 2
Case title: a 58-year-old immunocompromised man with subacute neurologic symptoms

Case presentation: A 58-year-old man with a history of hypertension, hyperlipidemia, hypothyroidism, nonalcoholic fatty liver disease, remote Hodgkin lymphoma treated with bone marrow transplant and rituximab, and hypogammaglobulinemia requiring IVIG infusions every 6 weeks, presented with 1 to 2 days of gradual-onset vertical diplopia, ataxia, dysarthria, and short-term memory loss. He reported a subjective fever. On examination, although alert and oriented, he had profoundly impaired short-term memory and an odd affect with mildly elevated mood and inappropriate laughter at times. MRI showed mild T2/FLAIR hyperintensity in the cerebellar vermis, pons, midbrain, and medial temporal lobes (left greater than right), with no significant contrast enhancement or diffusion restriction (**Fig. 4**). A lumbar puncture was performed at day 6 after symptom onset, with an opening pressure of 22 cm H_2O, and CSF analysis was notable for protein = 84.7 mg/dL (normal 10–44 mg/dL), glucose = 56 mg/dL (normal 40–70 mg/dL), and cell counts with 1 red blood cell/µL and 92 WBCs/µL (89% lymphocytes, 11% monocytes, and 0% neutrophils). Testing for specific pathogens was negative, including Powassan virus IgM from CSF.

Clinical questions: What are potential causes of this patient's illness? What additional testing could be ordered to confirm the diagnosis? What treatment should the patient receive?

Discussion: The patient was empirically treated with acyclovir, which was stopped when testing for herpes simplex virus was negative. All targeted viral studies were negative. The patient was treated empirically with 1g methylprednisolone daily for 3 days and received scheduled IVIG during admission. His symptoms improved during his hospital stay, with better speech and regained ability to walk. He was discharged to a subacute care facility on hospital day 7 (approximately 13 days after symptom onset) with mild residual ataxia and had no residual side effects at 1-year follow-up. Metagenomic next-generation sequencing performed on CSF was positive for Powassan virus.

Learning point: Powassan virus serology may be negative in patients with immunodeficiency, and molecular testing should be considered. In all patients with suspicion for Powassan virus infection and negative initial serology, convalescent serology testing should be pursued.

PCR for Powassan virus and other *Ixodes*-borne infections has been used in nonclinical applications.[69] Although these reports suggest that molecular diagnostics are generally higher yield for Powassan virus than other arboviral infections, such as WNV, they are rarely available outside of a research setting. Direct detection in brain tissue samples can also be useful, as discussed later.

Serology is the most common method used to diagnose Powassan virus infection. A diagnosis can be made by observing a four-fold rise in antibody titers between acute and convalescent sera (including seroconversion) or by detecting both virus-specific IgM and neutralizing antibodies in serum or CSF. Confirmation of neutralizing antibodies via a plaque reduction neutralization test (PRNT) is necessary due to the high overall antibody cross-reactivity between flaviviruses. According to CDC guidelines, neuroinvasive disease also can be diagnosed by detecting Powassan virus IgM in CSF and not detecting IgM to other endemic viruses, although in practice a positive IgM from CSF generally is followed-up with confirmation by PRNT.

NEUROPATHOLOGY

Information regarding the neuropathology of Powassan virus encephalitis has been derived from both biopsy and autopsy reports. Surgical brain biopsies may be collected for diagnostic purposes after less-invasive testing options have been exhausted or in conjunction with procedures to relieve intracranial pressure, whereas autopsies are performed to establish or confirm a suspected cause of death and to document the extent of the disease process. Neuropathologic findings have been published for 10 cases of Powassan virus encephalitis, including 2 nonfatal cases. Four cerebellar biopsies showed mild to severe T cell–predominant lymphocytic inflammation involving leptomeninges and cerebellar cortex, microgliosis with occasional microglial nodules, Purkinje cell loss with Bergmann gliosis, and thickened dura.[14–16,19,21] A thalamic biopsy showed hemorrhagic infarction with lymphoplasmacytic infiltrate.[70] These histologic features, including the lack of significant neutrophilic or granulomatous inflammation, are characteristic of arboviral encephalitis but require correlation with other laboratory and clinical findings to rule out other infectious and noninfectious causes of encephalitis.

Seven autopsies have been reported, with gross brain findings ranging from unremarkable,[8] to mild diffuse swelling of cerebral hemispheres,[9] and to marked edema resulting in herniation and Duret hemorrhages.[14,19,21] The degree of involvement of different brain regions varied between cases but included cerebellum, thalamus, basal ganglia, cerebral cortex, deep white matter, hippocampus, midbrain, medulla, pons, and spinal cord. Histologic findings at autopsy included leptomeningeal, perivascular, and parenchymal inflammation consistent with meningoencephalitis (**Fig. 2B–C**).[8,9,19,21,68] Mild to severe T lymphocyte–predominant inflammatory infiltrates were present in the meninges and Virchow-Robin spaces (**Fig. 2D**). Focal to dense perivascular T cell–predominant inflammation was observed surrounding parenchymal blood vessels without true vasculitis. Parenchymal inflammation (greater in gray matter than white matter) consisted of diffuse microgliosis with focal to dense microglial nodules, neuronophagia, and focal areas of tissue necrosis without true infarction. Severe loss of neurons was present, including cerebellar Purkinje cell and spinal cord anterior horn cells. These histologic findings likely reflect viral infection and death of neurons with associated host inflammatory responses. General autopsy findings have not suggested infection outside of the CNS, except in one patient who presented with orchitis and was found to have chronic inflammation and positive Powassan virus immunohistochemistry (IHC) in testicle sections.[14,16]

In contrast to many other causes of CNS viral infections, including herpesviruses, polyomaviruses, and rabies virus, no viral inclusions have been seen in biopsy or autopsy sections for any of the reported cases of Powassan virus, which is typical for arboviral encephalitis. Powassan virus IHC, available at reference laboratories, including the CDC Infectious Diseases Pathology Branch, has identified viral antigen in neurons and macrophages, likely representing the primary cellular targets in the CNS and subsequent clearance of infected cells.[14,16,19,21,68] Overall, the gross and histopathologic findings of Powassan virus infection are consistent with other causes of viral meningoencephalitis; thus, definitive diagnosis requires detection of viral antigen by IHC or viral RNA by in situ hybridization (**Fig. 2**E, F) or molecular studies.

THERAPEUTIC OPTIONS AND CLINICAL OUTCOMES

Treatment of Powassan virus is supportive, and no antiviral therapies have been tested to date. Because much of the disease is believed to be due to neuroinflammation, some patients have been treated with steroids, sometimes with apparent benefit[19,66] and other times without.[16,71] Given the small number of cases and the difficulty in assessing confounders, such as age and comorbidity, there are too few data to support or refute the use of steroids. Similarly, intravenous immunoglobulin (IVIG) has been used in some cases,[66] based on reports of success in WNV,[72] but its effectiveness is unclear.[62] The overall mortality for Powassan virus is approximately 10%, as discussed previously and in prior reviews.[73] Many patients have substantial long-term morbidity, including persistent neurologic symptoms in approximately a third of patients who survive.[31]

DISCUSSION

Given the substantial morbidity and mortality associated with known cases of Powassan virus encephalitis, as well as the likelihood that exposure and infection are more common than appreciated, there is substantial need to better understand the pathogenesis of this emerging virus and develop preventative and therapeutic strategies.

In vitro and animal studies of Powassan virus and the closely related TBEV suggest several salient features of pathogenesis. First, tick saliva enhances transmission and neuroinvasion,[74,75] likely by stimulation of an inflammatory response and recruitment of target cells. Thus, interventions targeting tick saliva represent an intriguing strategy to prevent this and other tick-borne infections.[36] Following transmission, dendritic cells and macrophages are thought to be among the first cells infected, allowing transport to lymph nodes, virus replication, and viremia.[76] Mechanisms of neuroinvasion are poorly understood, although a recent study suggests possible crossing of the blood-brain barrier through vascular endothelial cells.[77] Neuropathogenesis occurs through direct infection of neurons, and astrocytes restrict replication.[78] Although laboratory mice (BALB/c and C57BL/6) experience lethal infection with Powassan virus, the white-footed mouse *Peromyscus leucopus* is refractory to intraperitoneal infection and experiences only mild brain inflammation after intracranial infection.[79] This suggests the presence of one or more restriction factors,[10,79] which RNA sequencing analysis suggests may be an interferon-stimulated gene.[80] As an interesting parallel, TRIM79α was shown to restrict TBEV by degrading the NS5 polymerase.[81] Improved understanding of Powassan virus pathogenesis and host-virus interactions is needed to guide intervention strategies.

Currently, no antiviral medications are available to treat Powassan virus, although preclinical studies have identified several possibilities.[82,83] Vaccination is another compelling avenue of future research, especially given the successful implementation of vaccines against TBEV. Unfortunately, TBEV vaccines themselves do not provide cross-protection against Powassan virus, as they do for other tick-borne flaviviruses.[84] Recently, a lipid nanoparticle mRNA vaccine targeting the Powassan virus premembrane and envelope genes was shown to protect mice.[85] As further research into pathogenesis, treatment, and prevention continues, minimizing the effects of Powassan virus infection will rely on ecological approaches to decrease tick population as well as individual practices for tick avoidance and removal.[36]

CLINICS CARE POINTS

- Testing for Powassan virus infection should be considered in *Ixodes*-endemic regions in patients presenting in the spring, summer, and fall. A high index of suspicion is needed, because symptoms and clinical evaluation can be nonspecific.

- Diagnosis of Powassan virus infection generally is made by serology testing of blood or CSF. In immunocompromised patients who may not mount sufficient antibody response, molecular testing can be helpful.

- Treatment of Powassan virus is supportive. There is too little evidence to support or refute the use of high-dose steroids or IVIG.

DISCLOSURE

The authors have no financial or commercial conflicts of interest to report. A. Piantadosi is funded by the National Institute of Allergy and Infectious Diseases of the National Institutes of Health under award number K08AI139348. A. Piantadosi and I.H. Solomon are funded by the National Institute of Neurological Disorders and Stroke of the National Institutes of Health under award number R21NS119660.

REFERENCES

1. Mandl CW, Holzmann H, Kunz C, et al. Complete genomic sequence of Powassan virus: evaluation of genetic elements in tick-borne versus mosquito-borne flaviviruses. Virology 1993;194(1):173–84.
2. Lindquist L, Vapalahti O. Tick-borne encephalitis. Lancet 2008;371(9627): 1861–71.
3. Gritsun TS, Nuttall PA, Gould EA. Tick-borne flaviviruses. Adv Virus Res 2003;61: 317–71.
4. Rigaud E, Jaulhac B, Garcia-Bonnet N, et al. Seroprevalence of seven pathogens transmitted by the Ixodes ricinus tick in forestry workers in France. Clin Microbiol Infect 2016;22(8):735 e1-9.
5. Thortveit ET, Aase A, Petersen LB, et al. Human seroprevalence of antibodies to tick-borne microbes in southern Norway. Ticks Tick Borne Dis 2020;11(4): 101410.
6. Svensson J, Christiansen CB, Persson KEM. A serosurvey of tick-borne encephalitis virus in sweden: different populations and geographical locations. Vector Borne Zoonotic Dis 2021;21(8):614–9.
7. Ruzek D, Avsic Zupanc T, Borde J, et al. Tick-borne encephalitis in Europe and Russia: Review of pathogenesis, clinical features, therapy, and vaccines. Antivir Res 2019;164:23–51.
8. McLean DM, Donohue WL. Powassan virus: isolation of virus from a fatal case of encephalitis. Can Med Assoc J 1959;80(9):708–11.

9. Gholam BI, Puksa S, Provias JP. Powassan encephalitis: a case report with neuro-pathology and literature review. CMAJ 1999;161(11):1419–22.

10. Telford SR 3rd, Armstrong PM, Katavolos P, et al. A new tick-borne encephalitis-like virus infecting New England deer ticks, Ixodes Dammini. Emerg Infect Dis 1997;3(2):165–70.

11. Ebel GD, Kramer LD. Short report: duration of tick attachment required for trans-mission of powassan virus by deer ticks. Am J Trop Med Hyg 2004;71(3):268–71.

12. Feder HM, Telford S, Goethert HK, et al. Powassan virus encephalitis following brief attachment of connecticut deer ticks. Clin Infect Dis 2021;73(7):e2350–4.

13. Campbell O, Krause PJ. The emergence of human Powassan virus infection in North America. Ticks Tick Borne Dis 2020;11(6):101540.

14. Normandin E, Solomon IH, Zamirpour S, et al. Powassan virus neuropathology and genomic diversity in patients with fatal encephalitis. Open Forum Infect Dis 2020;7(10):ofaa392.

15. Piantadosi A, Kanjilal S, Ganesh V, et al. Rapid detection of powassan virus in a patient with encephalitis by metagenomic sequencing. Clin Infect Dis 2018;66(5): 789–92.

16. Solomon IH, Spera KM, Ryan SL, et al. Fatal powassan encephalitis (Deer Tick Virus, Lineage II) in a patient with fever and orchitis receiving rituximab. JAMA Neurol 2018;75(6):746–50.

17. Deng X, Achari A, Federman S, et al. Metagenomic sequencing with spiked primer enrichment for viral diagnostics and genomic surveillance. Nat Microbiol 2020;5(3):443–54.

18. Cavanaugh CE, Muscat PL, Telford SR 3rd, et al. Fatal Deer Tick Virus Infection in Maine. Clin Infect Dis 2017;65(6):1043–6.

19. El Khoury MY, Camargo JF, White JL, et al. Potential role of deer tick virus in Po-wassan encephalitis cases in Lyme disease-endemic areas of New York. U S A Emerg Infect Dis 2013;19(12):1926–33.

20. El Khoury MY, Hull RC, Bryant PW, et al. Diagnosis of acute deer tick virus en-cephalitis. Clin Infect Dis 2013;56(4):e40–7.

21. Tavakoli NP, Wang H, Dupuis M, et al. Fatal case of deer tick virus encephalitis. N Engl J Med 2009;360(20):2099–107.

22. Costero A, Grayson MA. Experimental transmission of Powassan virus (Flaviviri-dae) by Ixodes scapularis ticks (Acari:Ixodidae). Am J Trop Med Hyg 1996; 55(5):536–46.

23. Goethert HK, Mather TN, Johnson RW, et al. Incrimination of shrews as a reservoir for Powassan virus. Commun Biol 2021;4(1):1319.

24. Ebel GD, Campbell EN, Goethert HK, et al. Enzootic transmission of deer tick vi-rus in New England and Wisconsin sites. Am J Trop Med Hyg 2000;63(1–2): 36–42.

25. Brackney DE, Nofchissey RA, Fitzpatrick KA, et al. Stable prevalence of Powas-san virus in Ixodes scapularis in a northern Wisconsin focus. Am J Trop Med Hyg 2008;79(6):971–3.

26. Knox KK, Thomm AM, Harrington YA, et al. Powassan/Deer Tick Virus and Borre-lia Burgdorferi Infection in Wisconsin Tick Populations. Vector Borne Zoonotic Dis 2017;17(7):463–6.

27. Anderson JF, Armstrong PM. Prevalence and genetic characterization of Powas-san virus strains infecting Ixodes scapularis in Connecticut. Am J Trop Med Hyg 2012;87(4):754–9.

28. Dupuis AP 2nd, Peters RJ, Prusinski MA, et al. Isolation of deer tick virus (Powas-san virus, lineage II) from Ixodes scapularis and detection of antibody in

vertebrate hosts sampled in the Hudson Valley, New York State. Parasit Vectors 2013;6:185.

29. Aliota MT, Dupuis AP 2nd, Wilczek MP, et al. The prevalence of zoonotic tick-borne pathogens in Ixodes scapularis collected in the Hudson Valley, New York State. Vector Borne Zoonotic Dis 2014;14(4):245–50.

30. Sharma R, Cozens DW, Armstrong PM, et al. Vector competence of human-biting ticks Ixodes scapularis, Amblyomma americanum and Dermacentor variabilis for Powassan virus. Parasit Vectors 2021;14(1):466.

31. Corrin T, Greig J, Harding S, et al. Powassan virus, a scoping review of the global evidence. Zoonoses Public Health 2018;65(6):595–624.

32. Leonova GN, Kondratov IG, Ternovoi VA, et al. Characterization of Powassan viruses from Far Eastern Russia. Arch Virol 2009;154(5):811–20.

33. Artsob H, Spence L, Th'ng C, et al. Arbovirus infections in several Ontario mammals, 1975-1980. Can J Vet Res 1986;50(1):42–6.

34. Allen SE, Jardine CM, Hooper-McGrevy K, et al. Serologic evidence of arthropod-borne virus infections in wild and captive ruminants in Ontario, Canada. Am J Trop Med Hyg 2020;103(5):2100–7.

35. Nofchissey RA, Deardorff ER, Blevins TM, et al. Seroprevalence of Powassan virus in New England deer, 1979-2010. Am J Trop Med Hyg 2013;88(6):1159–62.

36. Eisen RJ, Eisen L. The blacklegged tick, ixodes scapularis: an increasing public health concern. Trends Parasitol 2018;34(4):295–309.

37. Piantadosi A, Kanjilal S. Diagnostic approach for arboviral infections in the United States. J Clin Microbiol 2020;58(12):e01926-19..

38. Vahey GM, Mathis S, Martin SW, et al. West nile virus and other domestic nationally notifiable arboviral diseases - United States, 2019. MMWR Morb Mortal Wkly Rep 2021;70(32):1069–74.

39. Frost HM, Schotthoefer AM, Thomm AM, et al. Serologic evidence of powassan virus infection in patients with suspected lyme disease(1). Emerg Infect Dis 2017;23(8):1384–8.

40. Thomm AM, Schotthoefer AM, Dupuis AP 2nd, et al. Development and validation of a serologic test panel for detection of powassan virus infection in u.s. patients residing in regions where lyme disease is endemic. mSphere 2018;3(1): e00467-17.

41. Vahey GM, Wilson N, McDonald E, et al. Seroprevalence of powassan virus infection in an area experiencing a cluster of disease cases: sussex county, New Jersey, 2019. Open Forum Infect Dis 2022;9(3):ofac023.

42. Smith RP Jr, Elias SP, Cavanaugh CE, et al. Seroprevalence of borrelia burgdorferi, b. miyamotoi, and powassan virus in residents bitten by ixodes ticks, maine, USA. Emerg Infect Dis 2019;25(4):804–7.

43. Wormser GP, McKenna D, Scavarda C, et al. Co-infections in Persons with Early Lyme Disease, New York, USA. Emerg Infect Dis 2019;25(4):748–52.

44. Picheca C, Yogendrakumar V, Brooks JI, et al. Polio-like manifestation of powassan virus infection with anterior horn cell involvement, Canada. Emerg Infect Dis 2019;25(8):1609–11.

45. Fitch WM, Artsob H. Powassan encephalitis in new brunswick. Can Fam Physician 1990;36:1289–90.

46. Goldfield M, Austin SM, Black HC, et al. A non-fatal human case of Powassan virus encephalitis. Am J Trop Med Hyg 1973;22(1):78–81.

47. Deibel R, Srihongse S, Woodall JP. Arboviruses in New York State: an attempt to determine the role of arboviruses in patients with viral encephalitis and meningitis. Am J Trop Med Hyg 1979;28(3):577–82.

48. Smith R, Woodall JP, Whitney E, et al. Powassan virus infection. A report of three human cases of encephalitis. Am J Dis Child 1974;127(5):691–3.
49. Embil JA, Camfield P, Artsob H, et al. Powassan virus encephalitis resembling herpes simplex encephalitis. Arch Intern Med 1983;143(2):341–3.
50. Centers for Disease Control and Prevention. Arboviral disease–United States, 1994. MMWR Morb Mortal Wkly Rep 1995;44(35):641–4.
51. Hinten SR, Beckett GA, Gensheimer KF, et al. Increased recognition of Powassan encephalitis in the United States, 1999-2005. Vector Borne Zoonotic Dis 2008; 8(6):733–40.
52. From the Centers for Disease Control and Prevention. Outbreak of powassan encephalitis–maine and vermont, 1999-2001. JAMA 2001;286(16):1962–3.
53. Johnson DK, Staples JE, Sotir MJ, et al. Tickborne Powassan virus infections among Wisconsin residents. WMJ 2010;109(2):91–7.
54. Krow-Lucal ER, Lindsey NP, Fischer M, et al. Powassan virus disease in the United States, 2006-2016. Vector Borne Zoonotic Dis 2018;18(6):286–90.
55. Curren EJ, Lehman J, Kolsin J, et al. West nile virus and other nationally notifiable arboviral diseases - United States, 2017. MMWR Morb Mortal Wkly Rep 2018; 67(41):1137–42.
56. McDonald E, Martin SW, Landry K, et al. West nile virus and other domestic nationally notifiable arboviral diseases - United States, 2018. MMWR Morb Mortal Wkly Rep 2019;68(31):673–8.
57. Laga AC, Mather TN, Duhaime RJ, et al. Identification of hard ticks in the united states: a practical guide for clinicians and pathologists. Am J Dermatopathol 2022;44(3):163–9.
58. Pritt BS. Scutal index and its role in guiding prophylaxis for lyme disease following tick bite. Clin Infect Dis 2018;67(4):617–8.
59. Castelli E, Caputo V, Morello V, et al. Local reactions to tick bites. Am J Dermatopathol 2008;30(3):241–8.
60. Hermance ME, Santos RI, Kelly BC, et al. Immune cell targets of infection at the tick-skin interface during powassan virus transmission. PLoS One 2016;11(5): e0155889.
61. Hermance ME, Thangamani S. Utilization of RNA in situ Hybridization to Understand the Cellular Localization of Powassan Virus RNA at the Tick-Virus-Host Interface. Front Cell Infect Microbiol 2020;10:172.
62. Piantadosl A, Rubin DB, McQuillen DP, et al. Emerging cases of powassan virus encephalitis in New England: clinical presentation, imaging, and review of the literature. Clin Infect Dis 2016;62(6):707–13.
63. Nord JM, Goldberg NR. Novel case of multifocal choroiditis following powassan virus infection. Ocul Immunol Inflamm 2021;1–3.
64. Lessell S, Collins TE. Ophthalmoplegia in Powassan encephalitis. Neurology 2003;60(10):1726–7.
65. Raval M, Singhal M, Guerrero D, et al. Powassan virus infection: case series and literature review from a single institution. BMC Res Notes 2012;5:594.
66. Dumic I, Glomski B, Patel J, et al. Double trouble": severe meningoencephalitis due to borrelia burgdorferi and powassan virus co-infection successfully treated with intravenous immunoglobulin. Am J Case Rep 2021;22:e929952.
67. Taylor L, Condon T, Destrampe EM, et al. Powassan virus infection likely acquired through blood transfusion presenting as encephalitis in a kidney transplant recipient. Clin Infect Dis 2021;72(6):1051–4.
68. Yu Q, Matkovic E, Reagan-Steiner S, et al. A fatal case of powassan virus encephalitis. J Neuropathol Exp Neurol 2020;79(11):1239–43.

69. Tokarz R, Tagliafierro T, Cucura DM, et al. Detection of Anaplasma phagocytophilum, Babesia microti, Borrelia burgdorferi, Borrelia miyamotoi, and Powassan Virus in Ticks by a Multiplex Real-Time Reverse Transcription-PCR Assay. mSphere 2017;2(2):e00151-17.

70. Choi EE, Taylor RA. A case of Powassan viral hemorrhagic encephalitis involving bilateral thalami. Clin Neurol Neurosurg 2012;114(2):172–5.

71. Kroopnick A, Jia DT, Rimmer K, et al. Clinical use of steroids in viral central nervous system (CNS) infections: three challenging cases. J Neurovirol 2021;27(5):727–34.

72. Haley M, Retter AS, Fowler D, et al. The role for intravenous immunoglobulin in the treatment of West Nile virus encephalitis. Clin Infect Dis 2003;37(6):e88–90.

73. Hermance ME, Thangamani S. Powassan virus: an emerging arbovirus of public health concern in North America. Vector Borne Zoonotic Dis 2017;17(7):453–62.

74. Hermance ME, Thangamani S. Tick saliva enhances powassan virus transmission to the host, influencing its dissemination and the course of disease. J Virol 2015;89(15):7852–60.

75. Santos RI, Hermance ME, Reynolds ES, et al. Salivary gland extract from the deer tick, Ixodes scapularis, facilitates neuroinvasion by Powassan virus in BALB/c mice. Sci Rep 2021;11(1):20873.

76. Kemenesi G, Banyai K. Tick-borne flaviviruses, with a focus on powassan virus. Clin Microbiol Rev 2019;32(1). https://doi.org/10.1128/CMR.00106-17.

77. Conde JN, Sanchez-Vicente S, Saladino N, et al. Powassan viruses spread cell to cell during direct isolation from ixodes ticks and persistently infect human brain endothelial cells and pericytes. J Virol 2022;96(1):e0168221.

78. Lindqvist R, Mundt F, Gilthorpe JD, et al. Fast type I interferon response protects astrocytes from flavivirus infection and virus-induced cytopathic effects. J Neuroinflammation 2016;13(1):277.

79. Mlera L, Meade-White K, Saturday G, et al. Modeling Powassan virus infection in Peromyscus leucopus, a natural host. PLoS Negl Trop Dis 2017;11(1):e0005346.

80. Mlera L, Meade-White K, Dahlstrom E, et al. Peromyscus leucopus mouse brain transcriptome response to Powassan virus infection. J Neurovirol 2018;24(1):75–87.

81. Taylor RT, Lubick KJ, Robertson SJ, et al. TRIM79alpha, an interferon-stimulated gene product, restricts tick-borne encephalitis virus replication by degrading the viral RNA polymerase. Cell Host Microbe 2011;10(3):185–96.

82. Eyer L, Svoboda P, Balvan J, et al. Broad-spectrum antiviral activity of 3'-deoxy-3'-fluoroadenosine against emerging flaviviruses. Antimicrob Agents Chemother 2021;65(2):e01522-20.

83. Flint M, McMullan LK, Dodd KA, et al. Inhibitors of the tick-borne, hemorrhagic fever-associated flaviviruses. Antimicrob Agents Chemother 2014;58(6):3206–16.

84. McAuley AJ, Sawatsky B, Ksiazek T, et al. Cross-neutralisation of viruses of the tick-borne encephalitis complex following tick-borne encephalitis vaccination and/or infection. NPJ Vaccin 2017;2:5.

85. VanBlargan LA, Himansu S, Foreman BM, et al. An mRNA vaccine protects mice against multiple tick-transmitted flavivirus infections. Cell Rep 2018;25(12):3382–92.e3.

When to Think About Other Borreliae:
Hard Tick Relapsing Fever (*Borrelia miyamotoi*), *Borrelia mayonii*, and Beyond

Kyle G. Rodino, PhD[a], Bobbi S. Pritt, MD, MSc[b],*

KEYWORDS

- Lyme disease • Relapsing fever • Tickborne

KEY POINTS

- Although *Borrelia burgdorferi* is the most common pathogenic *Borrelia* species in North America, other hard tick-transmitted *Borrelia* species such as *Borrelia miyamotoi* and *Borrelia mayonii* can cause human disease and are likely underrecognized.
- *B. miyamotoi* is a relapsing fever (RF) spirochete transmitted by *Ixodes* species ticks that causes a flu-like illness, and rarely, meningoencephalitis. Relapses are occasionally seen if infection is not treated.
- *Borrelia mayonii* is a less common cause of Lyme disease (LD) in North America found only in the upper Midwest that is characterized by diffuse rashes and high spirochetemia.
- Doxycycline is the most cited treatment of *Borrelia* infections and it has the added benefit of activity against other tickborne bacterial pathogens that may coexist.

INTRODUCTION

Several hard tick-transmitted *Borrelia* species cause human disease. While *Borrelia burgdorferi* sensu stricto (hereafter referred to as *B. burgdorferi*) is the most common cause of Lyme disease (LD) in North America and thus the most important tickborne pathogen on this continent, other important hard tick-transmitted *Borrelia* in North America include *B. miyamotoi*, the cause of *B. miyamotoi* disease (BMD), and *B. mayonii*, a second, less common cause of LD in the upper Midwestern United States.[1,2] *Borrelia bissettii* is an additional hard tick-transmitted species occasionally detected in individuals in North America, but its potential as a public health threat is

[a] Department of Pathology and Laboratory Medicine, Perelman School of Medicine, University of Pennsylvania, 3400 Spruce Street, Philadelphia, PA 19104, USA; [b] Department of Laboratory Medicine and Pathology, Division of Clinical Microbiology, Mayo Clinic, 200 1st Street Southwest, Rochester, MN 55905, USA
* Corresponding author.
E-mail address: Pritt.bobbi@mayo.edu

Infect Dis Clin N Am 36 (2022) 689–701
https://doi.org/10.1016/j.idc.2022.04.002
0891-5520/22/© 2022 Elsevier Inc. All rights reserved.

not well understood.[3] This article will discuss these other hard tick-transmitted *Borrelia* species and describe what is known about the clinical manifestations, laboratory diagnosis, and treatment of their associated infections. While the number of reported cases with these organisms is significantly lower than those of LD due to *B. burgdorferi*, the overlapping clinical syndromes and limitations of commonly used diagnostic options likely result in an under-appreciation of total infections.

ETIOLOGY, ECOLOGY, AND EPIDEMIOLOGY

Borrelia species are spirochetal bacteria within the family Spirochaetaceae. The genus contains many species including several known and potential human pathogens transmitted by hard (ixodid) ticks, soft (argasid) ticks, and body lice (*Pediculus humanus humanus*). The genus is traditionally partitioned into members of the *B burgdorferi* sensu lato (Bbsl) complex (housing the LD-causing species) and the non–LD-causing, relapsing fever (RF) species, based on genetic and biological differences between these groups.[4] Recently, some investigators suggested that sufficient genetic diversity exists between the two groups to warrant placing the Bbsl into a new genus, *Borreliella*[5]. However, *Borrelia* taxonomy has become increasingly complex, with many new proposed species and the discovery of a third *Borrelia* group that does not cluster with either the LD or RF clades.[4,6] Thus, this proposed taxonomic scheme has not been widely accepted by the bacteriology community, and this article will retain the *Borrelia* genus designation for both the RF and Bbsl members.

There are currently 22 named and several proposed Bbsl species,[6] all of which are transmitted by hard ticks. Ten Bbsl species are known to infect humans, including 3 species in North America: *B. burgdorferi*, *B. mayonii*, ad *B. bissettii*. The RF group is more diverse and contains species transmitted by soft ticks, hard ticks, and body lice. Of these, *B. miyamotoi* is the only known human pathogenic RF species that is transmitted by hard ticks. The following sections provide further details about *B. miyamotoi* and *B. mayonii*. Other *Borrelia* species found in North America are also briefly covered.

Borrelia miyamotoi

B. miyamotoi belongs to the RF clade of the genus *Borrelia* and is therefore more genetically similar to tickborne relapsing fever (TBRF) species transmitted by soft ticks than the LD-causing *Borrelia*.[7,8] Within the RF clade, *B. miyamotoi* is most closely related to *Borrelia lonestari* and *Borrelia theileri*. Genomic characterization of *B. miyamotoi* initially placed strains into 2 distinct groups: *B. miyamotoi* sensu stricto, the strains isolated from Japan, and the globally present *B. miyamotoi* sensu lato, encompassing strains detected in Russia, Europe, and North America.[9] However, further molecular characterization has revealed increased genetic diversity among the known isolates, with at least recognized 3 clades (Asian, European, and North American), and complex intermingling of genotypes within geographic regions and vectors.[7,10,11] In the United States, genetic diversity between *B. miyamotoi* found on the west coast and east coast has been described, resulting in at least 4 region-specific clades. Further studies are needed to determine the impact, if any, of this gene-level heterogeneity on human infection or disease.[11–13]

B. miyamotoi is found throughout the Northern hemisphere and transmitted primarily by species of hard ticks in the *Ixodes ricinus*-complex. *B. miyamotoi* was first discovered in 1994 by Fukunaga and colleagues, who isolated the bacterium from *Ixodes persulcatus* ticks in Japan.[14] The authors named this bacterium after Kenji Miyamoto, a renowned Japanese entomologist. Other *Ixodes* species, including *Ixodes pavlovski, Ixodes ovatus* and *I. ricinus*, in addition to *Hyalomma concinna*, have since been identified as vectors in Asia.[7] In Russia, whereby the bacterium was first linked to human infection, the previously mentioned *Ixodes* spp. in Asia, with the addition of *I persulcatus*, are the primary vectors. *I. ricinus* is also the dominant tick-vector of *B. miyamotoi* throughout Europe.[7,15] In North America, *Ixodes scapularis* is the major vector, primarily in the Northeast and upper Midwest regions.[7,16] However, on the west coast of the United States, *B. miyamotoi* is transmitted by *Ixodes pacificus*, whereby tick prevalence studies report higher rates of *B. miyamotoi* carriage than *B. burgdorferi*.[7] These *Ixodes* species also transmit *B. burgdorferi* and other pathogens in these regions.

Rodents, including mice, voles, squirrels, and chipmunks, are the main animal reservoirs for *B. miyamotoi*. In particular, the white-footed mouse (*Peromyscus leucopus*) is a common reservoir host for *B. miyamotoi* in North America, in addition to serving as a primary host for *B burgdorferi*.[13,17] Birds have also been shown to carry the pathogen.[18]

Unlike *B burgdorferi*, *B. miyamotoi* can be passed transovarially (ie, via infection of the developing egg in the gravid female tick), in addition to transradially (ie, from larva to nymph, and/or nymph to adult). Thus, the pathogen can be at least partially maintained through vertical transmission in the tick vector.[19,20]

Tick surveillance studies around the globe provide varied estimates of prevalence, but generally fall in the range of 1%-6%, with a few studies showing isolated tick populations highly enriched with *B. miyamotoi,* such as Napa county, northern California (15.4%).[7,10,15] A recent study in the United States assessing nearly 40,000 human-biting ticks detected *B. miyamotoi*-infected ticks in 19 states with a 1%-1.8% prevalence.[21] Prevalence in nymph and adult stage ticks is consistently higher than the larval stage, demonstrating that the acquisition of *B. miyamotoi* during blood meals is an important contributor to tick carriage, despite the potential for transovarial transmission.

Human seroprevalence studies conducted in endemic regions of the United States have found baseline rates of 0.12%-3.9% in otherwise healthy control populations.[9,22,23] As expected, the seroprevalence is higher in populations with a known history of tick-bites, compatible clinical syndromes, or activities or occupations potentially leading to more frequent exposure, with rates ranging from 3.2% to 21.0%.[8,9,22,23]

Borrelia mayonii

B. mayonii is a member of the Bbsl genospecies complex closely related to *B. burgdorferi,* with 94.7% to 94.9% similarity identified by multilocus sequence analysis (MLSA)[24] and 93.83% average nucleotide identity with all known species by whole chromosomal genome sequence analysis.[25] The organism was first reported in a series of 6 symptomatic patients from the upper Midwestern United States in 2016.[26] All 6 reported exposure to tick bites in Minnesota and Wisconsin and had blood (n = 5) or synovial fluid (n = 1) submitted for Bbsl species testing by real-time PCR targeting the *oppA2* gene during 2012 to 2014.[26] This assay uses melting temperature (Tm) to detect and differentiate *B. burgdorferi, Borrelia afzelii,* and *Borrelia garinii.* Infection with a novel *Borrelia* species was suspected based on the presence of an unexpected Tm peak (**Fig. 1**), which prompted confirmatory culture and molecular analyses. The unexpected Tm peak, later shown to be indicative of *B. mayonii,* was not detected among 24,786 clinical specimens tested during the same time frame (2012–2014) from 44 other states, suggesting a limited, regional distribution of this organism.[26] It was also not detected in the 66,562 clinical specimens from all 50 states

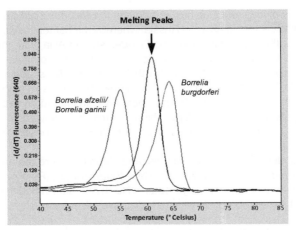

Fig. 1. Representative melting temperature (Tm) peaks for *B. afzelii/B. garinii, B. burgdorferi,* and *B. mayonii (arrow).* The Y-axis displays the negative derivative of the ratio of fluorescence resonance energy transfer (FRET) signal and background fluorescence.

that had been tested during 2003 to 2011 by the same method, suggesting that it was an emerging pathogen in the upper Midwest.[26]

The limited geographic distribution of *B. mayonii* was further supported by a subsequent analysis of 7292 additional clinical specimens submitted by health care providers throughout the United States for tickborne pathogen testing from 2014 to 2015.[27] Use of a *Borrelia* PCR and multilocus sequence typing (MLST) detected *B. mayonii* from 9 specimens, of which all were submitted by providers in Minnesota and Wisconsin. MLST revealed limited sequence diversity across the 8 housekeeping genes for these *B. mayonii* positive specimens.[27] Even when considering these 9 cases, the number of human cases remains less than 25 to date (unpublished Mayo Clinic data).

I. scapularis is the likely vector of *B. mayonii.* It is the most significant vector of human disease in the upper Midwestern United States, and its vector competence for *B. mayonii* has been experimentally demonstrated in mice, including *P. leucopus.*[28,29] *B. mayonii* has been detected in host-seeking ticks in Minnesota and Wisconsin, with combined nymph and adult prevalence rates of 0.3% to 2.9%.[30–33] The Michigan Department of Health and Human Services also reported the detection of *B. mayonii* in 2 of 38 (5.3%) host-seeking *I. scapularis* ticks from southeastern Michigan in 2019.[34] It is unknown if the prevalence rates of *B. mayonii* in host-seeking ticks vary over time, but a recent study examining the prevalence of *B. burgdorferi* and *Anaplasma phagocytophilum* in host-seeking *I. scapularis* at 28 longitudinal sampling sites in Minnesota, Wisconsin and Michigan found significant variation in prevalence across sites and among different years of sampling within sites.[35] There is currently no evidence for transovarial transmission of *B. mayonii* by infected *I. scapularis* females.[36] This also holds true for *B. burgdorferi,* the other cause of LD in the US.

Importantly, *B. mayonii* has not been detected from ticks collected in regions outside of the upper Midwestern US, providing further evidence for the limited geographic distribution of this organism. The largest tick surveillance study for *B. mayonii* to date tested greater than 11,000 host-seeking *I. scapularis* collected from 5 geographic US regions from 2013 to 2019, and only detected this bacterium in ticks from Minnesota and Wisconsin.[33] A smaller study of greater than 500 ticks by Tokarz and colleagues also failed to detect *B. mayonii* in *I. scapularis* collected in New York and Connecticut, despite these states having a high prevalence of other *I. scapularis* transmitted pathogens.[37] *B. mayonii* was also not detected in 3122 *I. ricinus* nymphs collected from an endemic region of LD in France.[38] Despite the lack of *B. mayonii* detection in *I. scapularis* from the northeastern United States, Eisen and colleagues demonstrated that *I. scapularis* from Connecticut have equal vector efficiency to those from Minnesota.[39] Thus, factors other than vector competence are likely responsible for the geographic restriction of *B. mayonii* to the upper Midwest.

B. mayonii has been detected by culture and PCR from naturally infected *P. leucopus* [4 (2.6%) of 151 *Peromyscus* spp. tested] and 2 American red squirrels [*Tamiasciurus hudsonicus*; 2 (40%) of 5] in Minnesota, implicating these animals as potential reservoir hosts.[40] *B. mayonii* has also been detected by PCR in *Peromyscus* spp. and *Tamias striatus* (eastern chipmunk) in Northern Wisconsin, with prevalence rates of 1.19% (5/420) and 23.5% (4/17), respectively.[41] The high prevalence of *B. mayonii* in *T. striatus* and *T. hudsonicus* suggests that they may be important natural hosts, although the number of sampled individuals in these studies was low, and further research is recommended to confirm these findings. Recently, the reservoir competence of *P. leucopus* for *B. mayonii* was confirmed by showing that these mice could acquire infection from infected feeding *I. scapularis* nymphs and subsequently transmit infection to uninfected feeding larval ticks.[29] While the length of infectivity is unknown in *P. leucopus*, an experimental mouse model showed that the CD-1 strain outbred white mouse can remain infected with *B. mayonii* for approximately 1 year.[42] *B. mayonii* were detected from ear biopsies, bladder, heart, and spinal cord of these infected mice by PCR and/or culture.

CLINICAL PRESENTATION
Borrelia miyamotoi

Clinical signs and symptoms of BMD generally manifest 2 weeks after exposure and are consistent with a flu-like illness, without unique findings to differentiate it from other tickborne diseases (TBDs). Fever, fatigue, and headache are the most common symptoms, followed by myalgias, arthralgias, chills, and nausea.[43,44] The classic LD rash, erythema migrans (EM), is rarely present with BMD.[9] It has been suggested that cases of BMD presenting with EM are actually manifestations of coinfection with LD-causing *Borrelia*, in which case the EM rash would be universally absent with *B. miyamotoi*.[45,46] Relapsing febrile episodes can occur with BMD, with an average interval of 9 days (range 2–14 days), but occur less frequently and with fewer cycles than other TBRF *Borrelia*.[15] Laboratory findings include leukopenia, thrombocytopenia, and increased AST and ALT, features shared with other TBDs, such as anaplasmosis, ehrlichiosis, and babesiosis.[8,47] Cases of meningoencephalitis have been reported, exclusively in immunocompromised populations.[46,48–50]

Borrelia mayonii

Only 7 cases of LD due to *B. mayonii* have been described to date.[26,30] These patients ranged in age from 10 to 67 years (median 42 years) and 5 were male. Patients presented with fever (6/7), headache (6/7), myalgias (5/7), nausea/vomiting (4/6), rash (4/5), arthralgias (2/7), lymphopenia (4/6), mild thrombocytopenia (2/5), and elevated hepatic transaminases (3/4). None had a known immunocompromising condition. All febrile patients tested PCR positive for *B. mayonii* from EDTA whole blood and made a full recovery with antibiotic therapy. The remaining patient had a positive PCR for *B. mayonii* from synovial fluid and reported residual joint pain 6 months after

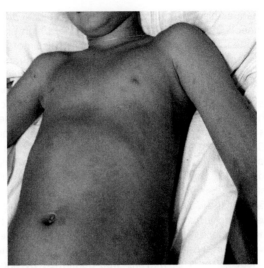

Fig. 2. Truncal rash from a young boy infected with *B. mayonii*. Note the diffuse nature of the rash, with the lack of the characteristic erythema migrans lesion.

treatment, despite antibiotic therapy. Two febrile patients were admitted to the hospital during acute illness (max 4 days). There were no deaths. While there is some overlap between the symptoms of *B. mayonii* and *B. burgdorferi* infection, the diffuse nature of rashes in 2 patients with *B. mayonii* (including the reported involvement of the palms and soles in one patient) are in stark contrast to the characteristic EM rash of LD due to *B. burgdorferi* [26] (**Fig. 2**). The lack of a classic EM rash may hinder the diagnosis, as it is used to make a clinical diagnosis of LD.[51] Four patients in the initial report also had nausea or vomiting, 2 had fever exceeding 39°C, and 3 had symptoms suggestive of neurologic involvement; these are not features typically associated with LD due to *B. burgdorferi*.[26]

EVALUATION
Borrelia miyamotoi

Laboratory diagnosis of *B. miyamotoi* centers around nucleic acid amplification testing (NAAT) and serology. *B. miyamotoi* NAATs are available at select reference laboratories in the United States from a variety of specimen types, including blood, CSF, and joint fluid. There are no FDA-approved or cleared assays at this time. Compared with the molecular detection of *B. burgdorferi*, *B. miyamotoi* NAATs show improved sensitivity in whole blood, derived from the higher spirochete burden in peripheral blood for BMD. Despite the increase in circulating *Borrelia*, peripheral blood smears have poor diagnostic sensitivity, with organisms unlikely to be seen on peripheral blood smear.[52] While there are reports of spirochetes detected from CSF Gram stain or Giemsa stain, direct visualization is not a recommended diagnostic modality.[48,49] *B. miyamotoi*-specific serology is available at the CDC and limited reference laboratories. After disease onset, antibodies to *B. miyamotoi* most reliably appear within 11 to 20 days for IgM class antibodies and 21 to 50 days for IgG class antibodies, leading to the low sensitivity of acute-phase testing. However, initial serology results can be helpful in establishing a baseline for comparison with convalescent testing, usually

2 to 4 weeks apart. Cross-reactivity has been reported with LD serologic assays, namely those that used *B. burgdorferi* whole-cell sonicate or C6 antigens due to shared epitopes with *B. miyamotoi*.[53] In such cases, *B. miyamotoi*-specific serology help differentiates BMD from LD. Finally, *B. miyamotoi* can be isolated in modified Barbour-Stoenner-Kelly (BSK) media, but culture is not used for routine diagnosis, due to the availability of faster and easier diagnostic methods.[54] Future TBD diagnostics may include broad pathogen detection using a single next-generation sequencing (NGS) assay, as 2 recent publications demonstrated the ability to detect *B. miyamotoi* and *B. mayonii*, in addition to other tickborne bacteria, from whole blood samples.[55,56]

Borrelia mayonii

As with *B. miyamotoi*, laboratory diagnosis of *B. miyamotoi* centers around NAATs and serology. Serology is the primary laboratory test for diagnosis of LD, and published cases of *B. mayonii* infection showed serologic reactivity patterns similar to those of patients with *B. burgdorferi* infection when using commercially available serology tests for *B. burgdorferi*. In the original report of 6 patients,[26] all 4 patients with blood collected 3 or more days after illness onset were positive by *B. burgdorferi* C6 enzyme immunoassay (EIA). Three of these 4 patients were also tested by whole-cell EIA and all were positive. The traditional 2-tiered LD testing algorithm requires confirmatory serologic testing of EIA positive specimens by IgM and/or IgG immunoblot,[57] and this was mostly achieved in this case series.[26] Two patients failed to produce a detectable IgG immunoblot response in specimens collected greater than 30 days from symptom onset, which may be due to a blunted immune response following antibiotic treatment (as previously observed with *B. burgdorferi* infection), or to decreased sensitivity of *B. burgdorferi* tests for detecting *B. mayonii* antibodies.

While it is reassuring that patients with *B. mayonii* infection would likely be detected using Lyme serology tests, commercially available tests are not capable of distinguishing infections with *B. mayonii* and *B. burgdorferi*. Treatment recommendations do not differ for infection with the 2 organisms, but specific identification is important for understanding the biology and epidemiology of emerging pathogens such as *B. mayonii*. For this reason, PCR performed on blood is the preferred test for specific diagnosis of acute *B. mayonii* infection. *B. mayonii* infections are associated with high spirochetemia levels, similar to those of RF borreliosis and in stark contrast to those of *B. burgdorferi* infection; these high spirochetemia levels facilitate the detection of *B. mayonii* in blood by PCR. *B. mayonii* has also been detected by PCR in synovial fluid. Multiplex laboratory-developed assays that detect and differentiate multiple *Borrelia* species have been described, but there are currently no FDA-approved/cleared assays.[26,58]

Spirochetes can be occasionally seen on peripheral blood thin films, but this is not a reliable means of diagnosis and does not allow for the differentiation of RF spirochetes (**Fig. 3**).[26,30] Finally, *B. mayonii* can be isolated in modified BSK media.[54] Culture is not used for routine diagnosis but is useful for research, and conclusive demonstration of active infection. Future routine diagnosis of *B. mayonii* and other tickborne pathogens may use broad range NGS testing as a means of simultaneously detecting multiple organisms with a single test.[55,56]

THERAPEUTIC OPTIONS

Official guidelines for the treatment of BMD and LD due to *B mayonii* have not been published, but doxycycline (100 mg twice per day for 14 days) is the most cited treatment of *Borrelia* infections, and it has the added benefit of activity against other

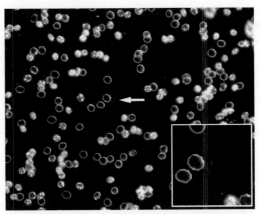

Fig. 3. Dark-field microscopic visualization of a single spirochete in diluted blood from a patient with *B. mayonii* infection (400 × magnification). (*Courtesy of* Adam Replogle, Centers for Disease Control and Prevention, Atlanta, GA)

tickborne bacterial pathogens that may coexist.[8,9] Secondary options in patients whereby doxycycline may be contraindicated include amoxicillin and cefuroxime.[9] Intravenous ceftriaxone followed by a switch to intravenous penicillin G has been used successfully in patients presenting with *B. miyamotoi* meningoencephalitis.[49]

OTHER *BORRELIA* SPECIES

In addition to the species mentioned above, a number of other *Borrelia* species have occasionally been detected in humans and proposed to cause human disease. Among members of the Bbsl complex detected in humans are *B. bissettii* (North America), *Borrelia lusitaniae* and *Borrelia spielmanii* (Europe), *Borrelia valaisiana* (Europe and Asia), and *Borrelia yangtzensis* (Asia).[59] *Borrelia americana* and *Borrelia andersonii* have also been detected in specimens from humans residing in Florida and Georgia, but further study is needed to understand the significance of these findings.[60] Similarly, a hard tick-transmitted RF species, *B. lonestari,* was initially suspected to be the causative agent of southern tick-associated rash illness (STARI) based on the detection of this bacterium by PCR in a patient with EM,[61] but this is now considered unlikely.[62]

Of these species, *B. bissettii* deserves additional mention as a possible cause of TBD in North America. *B. bissettii* is a member of the Bbsl complex found in North America and Europe. This organism was reported as a potential cause of human infection in 1996 based on DNA detection in CSF and skin specimens from patients in Slovenia.[63,64] Twelve years later, *B. bissettii* DNA was detected in a resected heart valve of a 59-year-old man from the Czech Republic with aortic valve stenosis and endocarditis.[65] The patient had been hospitalized 6 months before admission for aortic valve disease with a clinical and serologic diagnosis of LD and tickborne meningoencephalitis. Spirochetal culture was negative, but *B. bissettii* was detected from the valve by PCR targeting the Bbsl *flagellin* gene. No other *Borrelia* species were detected. Investigators from the same group also detected *B. bissettii* DNA in serum samples from 7 patients in the Czech Republic with suspected LD.[66] These patients had a wide range of symptoms, including fatigue, myalgia, arthralgia, headache, and flu-like symptoms. Of note, the authors detected *B. burgdorferi* in 4 of these patients, one of which also contained *B. garinii* DNA. The significance of these findings is unclear. In 2011, *Borrelia bissettii*-like DNA was detected in the serum from 3 to 114 (2.6%) north-coastal California residents at high risk for LD using PCR and sequence analysis of 5S-23S (*rrf-rrl*) rRNA intergenic spacer and *p66* gene loci.[67] Two of these patients had molecular evidence of *B. burgdorferi* coinfection. Clinical information was available for 2 of the 3 patients with *B. bissettii*-like sequences detected; the patient with only *B. bissettii*-like DNA in serum was asymptomatic, while the patient with *B. bissettii*-like and *B. burgdorferi* DNA in serum had a history of EM and joint pain.[67] This contrasts with reports of European patients, in which *B. bissettii* alone was associated with clinical symptoms.

In North America, *B. bissettii* has been detected from *Ixodes* species ticks, including *I. scapularis* and *I pacificus* ticks, as well as *Peromyscus* spp. mice and dusky-footed woodrats (*Neotoma fuscipes*).[67,68] Recently, investigators showed that *B. bissettii* induced disease in a mouse model, with the production of bladder, heart, and femorotibial join lesions.[69] Further research is indicated to understand the full spectrum and epidemiology of human disease due to *B. bissettii*.

PREVENTION

Avoidance of tick bites is paramount to the prevention of infections with *B. miyamotoi, B. mayonii,* and *B. bissettii*. Excellent guidelines exist for reducing the risk of tick exposure.[59,70] Commonly used methods include the use of chemical repellents on skin and clothing, avoidance of tick habitats, and frequent examination for ticks on humans and pets ("tick checks").

Attached ticks should be removed immediately to avoid transmission of TBPs. *B. miyamotoi* resides in tick salivary glands, as opposed to the midgut for *B. burgdorferi*, which potentially reduces the time for transmission to 24 hours.[71] In contrast, the time for *B. mayonii* transmission seems to be similar to rates observed for *B. burgdorferi*. Investigators used an outbred mouse model to determine the probability of *B. mayonii* transmission from a single *I. scapularis* nymph after feeding on uninfected mice for 24, 48, and 72 hours.[42] They did not detect evidence of transmission after 24 or 48 hours of feeding, but 31% (5/16) of mice were positive by ear biopsy culture at 72 hours, and 57% (8/14) were positive after a complete feed was acquired by the single nymph. The authors also inadvertently exposed some mice to 2 infected nymphs simultaneously, and 25% (1/4) of these animals were positive for *B. mayonii* at just 48 hours, while 71% (5/7) were positive at 72 hours, and 83% (5/6) were positive following a complete feed.[42] This suggests that exposure to more than one infected tick can shorten the time required for transmission of *B. mayonii* and increase the likelihood of infection. This has also been previously observed for *B. burgdorferi* [42].

DISCUSSION

Our understanding of TBDs continues to expand with the discovery of novel pathogens such as *B. miyamotoi, B. mayonii,* and *B. bissettii*. Infection with these *Borrelia* species causes overlapping clinical manifestations and thus molecular testing is indicated for definitive diagnosis. Fortunately, acute infection can be successfully treated using doxycycline and other antibiotics. Further studies are indicated to more fully characterize the biology, ecology, epidemiology, and pathogenicity of these emerging pathogens.

DISCLOSURES

The authors have nothing to disclose.

REFERENCES

1. Eisen RJ, Kugeler KJ, Eisen L, et al. Tick-borne zoonoses in the united states: Persistent and emerging threats to human health. ILAR J 2017;58(3):319–35.
2. Rosenberg R, Lindsey NP, Fischer M, et al. Vital signs: Trends in reported vector-borne disease cases - United States and territories, 2004-2016. MMWR Morb Mortal Wkly Rep 2018;67(17):496–501.
3. Golovchenko M, Vancova M, Clark K, et al. A divergent spirochete strain isolated from a resident of the Southeastern United States was identified by multilocus sequence typing as *Borrelia bissettii*. Parasit Vectors 2016;9:68.
4. Margos G, Gofton A, Wibberg D, et al. The genus *Borrelia* reloaded. PLoS One 2018;13(12):e0208432.
5. Adeolu M, Gupta RS. A phylogenomic and molecular marker based proposal for the division of the genus *Borrelia* into two genera: The emended genus *Borrelia* containing only the members of the relapsing fever *Borrelia*, and the genus *Borreliella* gen. Nov. Containing the members of the lyme disease *Borrelia* (*Borrelia burgdorferi* sensu lato complex). Antonie Van Leeuwenhoek 2014;105(6):1049–72.
6. Margos G, Fingerle V, Cutler S, et al. Controversies in bacterial taxonomy: The example of the genus *Borrelia*. Ticks Tick Borne Dis 2020;11(2):101335.
7. Cutler S, Vayssier-Taussat M, Estrada-Pena A, et al. A new borrelia on the block: *Borrelia miyamotoi* - a human health risk? Euro Surveill 2019;24(18).
8. Wagemakers A, Staarink PJ, Sprong H, et al. *Borrelia miyamotoi*: A widespread tick-borne relapsing fever spirochete. Trends Parasitol 2015;31(6):260–9.
9. Krause PJ, Fish D, Narasimhan S, et al. *Borrelia miyamotoi* infection in nature and in humans. Clin Microbiol Infect 2015;21(7):631–9.
10. Crowder CD, Carolan HE, Rounds MA, et al. Prevalence of *Borrelia miyamotoi* in *Ixodes* ticks in Europe and the United States. Emerg Infect Dis 2014;20(10):1678–82.
11. Hojgaard A, Osikowicz LM, Maes S, et al. Detection of genetic variability in *Borrelia miyamotoi* (spirochaetales: Spirochaetaceae) between and within the Eastern and Western United States. J Med Entomol 2021;58(6):2154–60.
12. Cook VJ, Fedorova N, Macdonald WP, et al. Unique strain of *Borrelia miyamotoi* in *Ixodes pacificus* ticks, California, USA. Emerg Infect Dis 2016;22(12):2205–7.
13. Salkeld DJ, Nieto NC, Bonilla DL, et al. *Borrelia miyamotoi* infections in small mammals, california, USA. Emerg Infect Dis 2018;24(12):2356–9.
14. Fukunaga M, Takahashi Y, Tsuruta Y, et al. Genetic and phenotypic analysis of *Borrelia miyamotoi* sp. Nov., isolated from the ixodid tick *Ixodes persulcatus*, the vector for lyme disease in Japan. Int J Syst Bacteriol 1995;45(4):804–10.
15. Platonov AE, Karan LS, Kolyasnikova NM, et al. Humans infected with relapsing fever spirochete *Borrelia miyamotoi*, Russia. Emerg Infect Dis 2011;17(10):1816–23.
16. Scoles GA, Papero M, Beati L, et al. A relapsing fever group spirochete transmitted by *Ixodes scapularis* ticks. Vector Borne Zoonotic Dis 2001;1(1):21–34.
17. Barbour AG, Bunikis J, Travinsky B, et al. Niche partitioning of *Borrelia burgdorferi* and *Borrelia miyamotoi* in the same tick vector and mammalian reservoir species. Am J Trop Med Hyg 2009;81(6):1120–31.
18. Hamer SA, Hickling GJ, Keith R, et al. Associations of passerine birds, rabbits, and ticks with *Borrelia miyamotoi* and *Borrelia andersonii* in Michigan. U.S.A Parasit Vectors 2012;5:231.

19. Rollend L, Fish D, Childs JE. Transovarial transmission of *Borrelia* spirochetes by *Ixodes scapularis*: A summary of the literature and recent observations. Ticks Tick Borne Dis 2013;4(1–2):46–51.

20. Han S, Lubelczyk C, Hickling GJ, et al. Vertical transmission rates of *Borrelia miyamotoi* in *Ixodes scapularis* collected from white-tailed deer. Ticks Tick Borne Dis 2019;10(3):682–9.

21. Xu G, Luo CY, Ribbe F, et al. *Borrelia miyamotoi* in human-biting ticks, United States, 2013-2019. Emerg Infect Dis 2021;27(12):3193–5.

22. Brummitt SI, Kjemtrup AM, Harvey DJ, et al. *Borrelia burgdorferi* and *Borrelia miyamotoi* seroprevalence in California blood donors. PLoS One 2020;15(12): e0243950.

23. Smith RP Jr, Elias SP, Cavanaugh CE, et al. Seroprevalence of *Borrelia burgdorferi, B. miyamotoi*, and Powassan virus in residents bitten by *Ixodes* ticks, Maine, USA. Emerg Infect Dis 2019;25(4):804–7.

24. Pritt BS, Respicio-Kingry LB, Sloan LM, et al. *Borrelia mayonii* sp. Nov., a member of the *Borrelia burgdorferi* sensu lato complex, detected in patients and ticks in the upper Midwestern United States. Int J Syst Evol Microbiol 2016;66(11): 4878–80.

25. Kingry LC, Batra D, Replogle A, et al. Whole genome sequence and comparative genomics of the novel Lyme borreliosis causing pathogen, *Borrelia mayonii*. PLoS One 2016;11(12):e0168994.

26. Pritt BS, Mead PS, Johnson DKH, et al. Identification of a novel pathogenic *Borrelia* species causing Lyme borreliosis with unusually high spirochaetaemia: A descriptive study. Lancet Infect Dis 2016;16(5):556–64.

27. Kingry LC, Anacker M, Pritt B, et al. Surveillance for and discovery of *Borrelia* species in US patients suspected of tickborne illness. Clin Infect Dis 2018; 66(12):1864–71.

28. Dolan MC, Hojgaard A, Hoxmeier JC, et al. Vector competence of the black-legged tick, *Ixodes scapularis*, for the recently recognized Lyme borreliosis spirochete candidatus *borrelia mayonii*. Ticks Tick Borne Dis 2016;7(5):665–9.

29. Parise CM, Breuner NE, Hojgaard A, et al. Experimental demonstration of reservoir competence of the white-footed mouse, *Peromyscus leucopus* (Rodentia: Cricetidae), for the Lyme disease spirochete, *Borrelia mayonii* (spirochaetales: Spirochaetaceae). J Med Entomol 2020;57(3):927–32.

30. Pritt BS, Fernholz EC, Replogle AJ, et al. *Borrelia mayonii* - a cause of Lyme borreliosis that can be visualized by microscopy of thin blood films. Clin Microbiol Infect 2021. https://doi.org/10.1016/j.cmi.2021.07.023. S1198-743X(21)00415-8.

31. Johnson TL, Graham CB, Maes SE, et al. Prevalence and distribution of seven human pathogens in host-seeking *Ixodes scapularis* (acari: Ixodidae) nymphs in Minnesota, USA. Ticks Tick Borne Dis 2018;9(6):1499–507.

32. Stauffer MT, Mandli J, Pritt BS, et al. Detection of zoonotic human pathogens from *Ixodes scapularis* in Wisconsin. J Vector Ecol 2020;45(1):147–9.

33. Lehane A, Maes SE, Graham CB, et al. Prevalence of single and coinfections of human pathogens in *Ixodes* ticks from five geographical regions in the United States, 2013-2019. Ticks Tick Borne Dis 2021;12(2):101637.

34. Michigan trends in tickborne disease 2016-2020. Available at: https://www.michigan.gov/documents/emergingdiseases/2021_Tickborne_Disease_Summary_Report_725827_7.pdf. Accessed March 17, 2022.

35. Foster E, Burtis J, Sidge JL, et al. Inter-annual variation in prevalence of *Borrelia burgdorferi* sensu stricto and *Anaplasma phagocytophilum* in host-seeking *Ixodes scapularis* (Acari: Ixodidae) at long-term surveillance sites in the upper

Midwestern United States: Implications for public health practice. Ticks Tick Borne Dis 2022;13(2):101886.

36. Breuner NE, Hojgaard A, Eisen L. Lack of evidence for transovarial transmission of the lyme disease spirochete *Borrelia mayonii* by infected female *Ixodes scapularis* (acari: Ixodidae) ticks. J Med Entomol 2018;55(3):739–41.

37. Tokarz R, Tagliafierro T, Sameroff S, et al. Microbiome analysis of *Ixodes scapularis* ticks from New York and Connecticut. Ticks Tick Borne Dis 2019;10(4): 894–900.

38. Boyer PH, De Martino SJ, Hansmann Y, et al. No evidence of *Borrelia mayonii* in an endemic area for Lyme borreliosis in France. Parasit Vectors 2017;10(1):282.

39. Eisen L, Breuner NE, Hojgaard A, et al. Comparison of vector efficiency of *Ixodes scapularis* (acari: Ixodidae) from the Northeast and upper Midwest of the United States for the Lyme disease spirochete *Borrelia mayonii*. J Med Entomol 2017; 54(1):239–42.

40. Johnson TL, Graham CB, Hojgaard A, et al. Isolation of the lyme disease spirochete *Borrelia mayonii* from naturally infected rodents in Minnesota. J Med Entomol 2017;54(4):1088–92.

41. Siy PN, Larson RT, Zembsch TE, et al. High prevalence of *Borrelia mayonii* (Spirochaetales: Spirochaetaceae) in field-caught *Tamias striatus* (Rodentia: Sciuridae) from northern Wisconsin. J Med Entomol 2021;58(6):2504–7.

42. Dolan MC, Breuner NE, Hojgaard A, et al. Duration of *Borrelia mayonii* infectivity in an experimental mouse model for feeding *Ixodes scapularis* larvae. Ticks Tick Borne Dis 2017;8(1):196–200.

43. Krause PJ, Barbour AG. *Borrelia miyamotoi*: The newest infection brought to us by deer ticks. Ann Intern Med 2015;163(2):141–2.

44. Molloy PJ, Telford SR 3rd, Chowdri HR, et al. *Borrelia miyamotoi* disease in the Northeastern United States: A case series. Ann Intern Med 2015;163(2):91–8.

45. Krause PJ, Narasimhan S, Wormser GP, et al. *Borrelia miyamotoi* sensu lato seroreactivity and seroprevalence in the Northeastern United States. Emerg Infect Dis 2014;20(7):1183–90.

46. Sato K, Takano A, Konnai S, et al. Human infections with *Borrelia miyamotoi*, Japan. Emerg Infect Dis 2014;20(8):1391–3.

47. Chowdri HR, Gugliotta JL, Berardi VP, et al. *Borrelia miyamotoi* infection presenting as human granulocytic anaplasmosis: A case report. Ann Intern Med 2013; 159(1):21–7.

48. Hovius JW, de Wever B, Sohne M, et al. A case of meningoencephalitis by the relapsing fever spirochaete *Borrelia miyamotoi* in europe. Lancet 2013; 382(9892):658.

49. Gugliotta JL, Goethert HK, Berardi VP, et al. Meningoencephalitis from *Borrelia miyamotoi* in an immunocompromised patient. N Engl J Med 2013;368(3):240–5.

50. Henningsson AJ, Asgeirsson H, Hammas B, et al. Two cases of *Borrelia miyamotoi* meningitis, sweden, 2018. Emerg Infect Dis 2019;25(10):1965–8.

51. Lantos PM, Rumbaugh J, Bockenstedt LK, et al. Clinical practice guidelines by the Infectious Diseases Society of America (IDSA), American Academy of Neurology (AAN), and American College of Rheumatology (ACR): 2020 guidelines for the prevention, diagnosis and treatment of Lyme disease. Clin Infect Dis 2021;72(1):1–8.

52. Telford SR, Goethert HK, Molloy PJ, et al. Blood smears have poor sensitivity for confirming *Borrelia miyamotoi* disease. J Clin Microbiol 2019;57(3).

53. Molloy PJ, Weeks KE, Todd B, et al. Seroreactivity to the C6 peptide in *Borrelia miyamotoi* infections occurring in the Northeastern United States. Clin Infect Dis 2018;66(9):1407–10.
54. Replogle AJ, Sexton C, Young J, et al. Isolation of *Borrelia miyamotoi* and other borreliae using a modified BSK medium. Sci Rep 2021;11(1):1926.
55. Kingry L, Sheldon S, Oatman S, et al. Targeted metagenomics for clinical detection and discovery of bacterial tick-borne pathogens. J Clin Microbiol 2020; 58(11).
56. Rodino KG, Wolf MJ, Sheldon S, et al. Detection of tick-borne bacteria from whole blood using 16s ribosomal RNA gene PCR followed by next-generation sequencing. J Clin Microbiol 2021;59(5).
57. Two-tiered testing decision tree. Available at: https://www.cdc.gov/lyme/healthcare/clinician_twotier.html. Accessed March 17, 2022.
58. Hojgaard A, Osikowicz LM, Eisen L, et al. Evaluation of a novel multiplex pcr amplicon sequencing assay for detection of human pathogens in *Ixodes* ticks. Ticks Tick Borne Dis 2020;11(6):101504.
59. Mead P. Epidemiology of lyme disease. Infect Dis Clin North Am 2022. In Press.
60. Clark KL, Leydet B, Hartman S. Lyme borreliosis in human patients in Florida and Georgia, USA. Int J Med Sci 2013;10(7):915–31.
61. James AM, Liveris D, Wormser GP, et al. *Borrelia lonestari* infection after a bite by an *Amblyomma americanum* tick. J Infect Dis 2001;183(12):1810–4.
62. Wormser GP, Masters E, Liveris D, et al. Microbiologic evaluation of patients from Missouri with erythema migrans. Clin Infect Dis 2005;40(3):423–8.
63. Picken RN, Cheng Y, Strle F, et al. Patient isolates of *Borrelia burgdorferi* sensu lato with genotypic and phenotypic similarities of strain 25015. J Infect Dis 1996;174(5):1112–5.
64. Strle F, Picken RN, Cheng Y, et al. Clinical findings for patients with Lyme borreliosis caused by *Borrelia burgdorferi* sensu lato with genotypic and phenotypic similarities to strain 25015. Clin Infect Dis 1997;25(2):273–80.
65. Rudenko N, Golovchenko M, Mokracek A, et al. Detection of *Borrelia bissettii* in cardiac valve tissue of a patient with endocarditis and aortic valve stenosis in the Czech republic. J Clin Microbiol 2008;46(10):3540–3.
66. Rudenko N, Golovchenko M, Ruzek D, et al. Molecular detection of *Borrelia bissettii* DNA in serum samples from patients in the Czech republic with suspected borreliosis. FEMS Microblol Lett 2009;292(2):274–81.
67. Girard YA, Fedorova N, Lane RS. Genetic diversity of *Borrelia burgdorferi* and detection of *B. bissettii*-like DNA in serum of north-coastal California residents. J Clin Microbiol 2011;49(3):945–54.
68. Margos G, Hojgaard A, Lane RS, et al. Multilocus sequence analysis of *Borrelia bissettii* strains from North America reveals a new *Borrelia* species, *Borrelia kurtenbachii*. Ticks Tick Borne Dis 2010;1(4):151–8.
69. Schneider BS, Schriefer ME, Dietrich G, et al. *Borrelia bissettii* isolates induce pathology in a murine model of disease. Vector Borne Zoonotic Dis 2008;8(5): 623–33.
70. Preventing tick bites. Available at: https://www.cdc.gov/ticks/avoid/on_people.html. Accessed March 17, 2022.
71. Breuner NE, Dolan MC, Replogle AJ, et al. Transmission of *Borrelia miyamotoi* sensu lato relapsing fever group spirochetes in relation to duration of attachment by *Ixodes scapularis* nymphs. Ticks Tick Borne Dis 2017;8(5):677–81.

The Role of the Infectious Disease Consultation in Lyme Disease

Jean Dejace, MD

KEYWORDS

- Consultation • Lyme • Borrelia • Chronic • PTLDS

KEY POINTS

- Clinical outcomes in Lyme disease are generally very good, contrary to commonly held public perceptions.
- Nonspecific somatic symptoms follow treatment of Lyme disease in a minority of patients, but the cause remains elusive.
- There is a multidisciplinary evidence-based international consensus on effective use of antibiotic therapy for Lyme disease treatment.
- Infectious disease consultation can aid in rectifying overdiagnosis and overtreatment of Lyme disease.

INTRODUCTION

The role of the infectious disease consultant in the assessment and management of a patient referred for persistent symptoms after treatment of Lyme disease is multidimensional. The first aspect is diagnostic and therapeutic, as in consultations provided for management of other infections. Optimal antibiotic selection and duration is explored in detail elsewhere in this volume, but assuring optimal treatment of a diagnosed infection is a primary goal. One may, however, be called on to redress an incorrect diagnosis—a not uncommon occurrence. Presuming a correct diagnosis of Lyme disease was made, patients may have questions that have not been answered regarding their recovery or symptoms that persist despite standard antibiotic treatment. In this case, the infectious disease consultant can provide important context for a diagnosis that may take on a life of its own. It behooves the consultant to enter these patient encounters prepared with an understanding of not only evidence-based diagnosis and treatment of Lyme disease and other black-legged tick transmitted infections but also the reasons that lead some patients and providers to pursue

Division of Infectious Disease, Department of Medicine, University of Vermont, The UVM Medical Center Campus, 111 Colchester Avenue, Smith 275, Burlington, VT 05401, USA
E-mail address: Jean.Dejace@uvmhealth.org

Infect Dis Clin N Am 36 (2022) 703–718
https://doi.org/10.1016/j.idc.2022.04.003
id.theclinics.com

unconventional and potentially dangerous treatment regimens. As in any discipline in medicine, a successful clinical encounter results in the patient feeling that they have gained an expert ally who cares about their welfare,[1] even if disagreement on the best path forward remains. This article attempts to provide a general overview from which you may derive an approach appropriate to your individual patient interactions and your practice.

BACKGROUND

Is there any basis for the apparent controversies surrounding Lyme disease? In broad terms, the salient issues contributing are (1) the disconnect between a public view or societal framing of Lyme disease and the general experience of Lyme disease encountered in most clinical practices and research studies; (2) acknowledged limitations of diagnostic testing; (3) unexplained long-lasting fatigue and other nonspecific symptoms following treatment in a small minority of patients; and (4) the potential for black-legged tick transmitted co-infection and a profusion of misinformation on this issue.

Lyme Disease and Social Construction of "Chronic Lyme Disease"

Controversies regarding the clinical spectrum, diagnosis, and treatment of Lyme disease are rooted in the early history of its description in North America, in the biology of untreated *B burgdorferi* infection with its tendency to relapse with different presentations, the limitations of laboratory diagnostics, and a social construction of the vaguely defined concept of "chronic Lyme disease" that encompasses a wide variety of commonly experienced symptoms of diverse origins. Although recognized by its cutaneous and neurologic manifestations in Europe in the late 1800s and early 1900s, Lyme disease was first described by Steere and colleagues in 1977 when investigating a cluster of cases of acute oligoarticular arthritis in Lyme, Connecticut. Thus, Lyme disease was first recognized by its later manifestations, both rheumatologic (North America) and neurologic (Europe). The bacterial cause was not identified for another 5 years after Steere's initial report.[2] In the interim, the characteristic rash of early Lyme disease was redescribed (having been first recognized in Europe in 1911), and the potential for disease relapse, if untreated, with extracutaneous manifestations was recognized.

The indolent course of untreated infection with cutaneous, neurologic, and cardiac complications led to initial parallels to another relapsing spirochetal infection, syphilis. Although studies of antibiotic treatment of both early and late Lyme disease reinforced the view of an effectively treatable bacterial disease (as with syphilis), the stage was set for ongoing concerns regarding the actual scope and natural history of Lyme disease, whether treated or not. Some persons had persistent fatiguing illness after treatment despite resolution of rashes, arthritis, or other inflammatory responses to infection. When these symptoms are disabling and persist for more than 6 months, the illness is often referred to as posttreatment Lyme disease syndrome (PTLDS). To add to concern regarding adequacy of treatment, 5% to 10% of patients with Lyme arthritis experience joint swelling and synovial inflammation that fails to resolve despite repeated courses of otherwise effective antibiotics, a condition now called postinfective Lyme arthritis (see Sheila L. Arvikar and Allen C. Steeres' article, "Lyme Arthritis," in this issue).

Within a few years of the celebration of the discovery of the bacterial cause of Lyme disease, a public debate was already underway regarding the nature of Lyme disease, its diagnosis, and treatment.[3] The concept that Lyme disease is essentially untreatable became established in the public view despite subsequent decades of clinical experience and research to the contrary. The unfortunate result of this view-point is a common belief in the value of prolonged courses of antibiotics for persons with persistent symptoms following initial treatment.[4] Controlled trials have repeatedly demonstrated harm but no reproducible benefit with this approach. Nevertheless, patient advocacy and at least one medical provider group contend that cure of Lyme disease may require months to years of antibiotic treatment. Confusion regarding Lyme disease was further promulgated by the extension of a diagnosis of Lyme disease to persons with medically unexplained illness in the absence of clinical or serologic evidence of B burgdorferi infection. The social construction of "chronic Lyme disease," although the entity remained not clearly defined, has been reinforced by anecdote, media narratives, and patient advocacy groups to the point that it is often the prevailing public view of Lyme disease.

Vagaries of Lyme Disease Diagnostic Testing

Lack of a means of direct detection of B burgdorferi during most phases of infection contributes to controversies regarding both diagnosis and treatment of Lyme disease. The history and current status of diagnostic testing for Lyme disease is reviewed in Takaaki Kobayashi and Paul G. Auwaerter article, "Diagnostic testing for Lyme disease", which outlines current approaches to serodiagnostic testing for B burgdorferi antibodies.

Antibody testing, of course, reveals only an immune fingerprint. A positive serology for antibodies to B burgdorferi may represent prior infection unrelated to a current illness or a false-positive test result. A negative serology might occur in a person with active Lyme infection who has yet to mount a sufficient immune response for detection. A negative antibody screen is to be expected in many cases of early localized Lyme disease using standard 2-tier testing of immunoassay followed by immunoblot[5]. Beyond lack of sensitivity in early disease, interpretation of immunoblot testing can add to confusion. Patients and providers may be presented with confirmatory immunoblot results listing the number of immunoglobulin M (IgM) or IgG "bands" detected as opposed to a confirmed "positive" or "negative" result. Interpretation of the immunoblot results should follow established guidelines, but reports vary in their clarity on this point. Even a reported "positive" result, if based on IgM alone in a patient with months of illness, would be misleading. Furthermore, immunoblots can be difficult to read in the laboratory, where weak bands may incorrectly be interpreted as positive.[6] Modified 2-tier testing with 2 immunoassays eliminates some of these complexities. Suffice it to say that these limitations and difficulties contribute to a milieu ripe for misunderstanding and controversy that is not present for many other common infections.

Some laboratories purporting to specialize in tick-borne diagnostics have arisen. Their diagnostic test offerings should be regarded with skepticism. These laboratories often provide alternative interpretive criteria and less specific testing methods. In one investigation by Fallon,[7] 40 healthy controls who had no history of Lyme disease and did not reside or recently travel to a Lyme endemic area had positive serology in 57% of samples sent to one specialty laboratory. None of these healthy controls were positive by standard 2-tier testing at reference laboratories. These specialty laboratories and their false-positive results are sometimes used by alternative practitioners to justify unconventional treatments.[8] It is important, therefore, for consultants to verify that reports of "positive Lyme tests" involved Food and Drug Administration–approved tests with appropriate laboratory and clinical interpretation.

Persistence of Unexplained Fatigue, Cognitive Symptoms Posttreatment

Postinfective symptoms such as fatigue may follow a variety of treated infections as well as Lyme disease. The causes vary but, as in Lyme disease, are often poorly understood. Therefore, any proposed treatment is directed at relieving patient symptoms, while avoiding use of unnecessary or possibly harmful therapies. Effective counseling of patients must include recognition of the multiple randomized, placebo controlled human studies (**Table 2**) that did address these symptoms and consistently found no overall benefit—but notable adverse reactions—from prolonged antibiotic therapy. The challenge for the infectious disease consultant is to recommend paths toward recovery for the patient with continued illness that ideally do not involve the potential adverse effects of unproven treatments. Because there is currently no evidence for effective pharmacologic approaches, the encouragement of interventions that have minimal adverse effects is preferable. From the perspective of the patient looking for a cure to what seems like a chronic infection, however, these generic approaches to chronic illness may seem inadequate.

Confusion Regarding Co-infection

Because new pathogens have been linked to black-legged tick infections and true co-infections with more than one pathogen described, the misconceptions surrounding persisting Lyme disease have been compounded by the concept that an array of other co-infections are contributing to long-lasting illness.

As a result, courses of multiple antibiotics may be prescribed to cover a variety of presumed co-infecting pathogens. Surprisingly, some patients receive treatment of putative co-infections that they would not have been exposed by the bite of a black-legged tick (ie, bartonellosis, *Babesia duncani*) or for which chronic infection has not been documented in humans (ie, anaplasmosis). Often the stated evidence for co-infection is based on serologic studies with low specificity or simply a patient symptom checklist. With very specific exceptions (in particular babesiosis), relapsed or chronic infection due to these agents following appropriate antibiotic therapy has not been documented.[9] That said, it is expected that infectious disease physicians will have a working knowledge of the potential array of pathogens in addition to *B burgdorferi* that might be transmitted by black-legged ticks to allay any patient concerns regarding co-infection.

COMPONENTS OF THE CONSULTATION

With that brief and necessarily compressed background, this article now addresses several factors that may be helpful to consider during interactions with patients referred for discussions of Lyme disease or other black-legged tick–associated infections. These issues include overall prognosis, validation of current symptoms, the frequency of misdiagnosis and misattribution, diagnostic uncertainty, and the role for instillation of hope for recovery. In addition, current scientific consensus regarding antibiotic use in Lyme disease as well as risks of fringe treatments are briefly addressed.

INITIAL PROGNOSIS

You may meet a patient early in their disease course. They want to know if the course of antibiotics they have been prescribed is adequate because they have read some concerning assertions on the Internet or heard from family and friends that longer courses of antibiotics are typically used.

Multiple studies have shown good outcomes in patients with early Lyme disease treated with shorter courses of antibiotic therapy (**Table 1**).

Long-term follow-up studies measuring health-related quality-of-life[13,14] years after Lyme infection have shown results similar to the general population.

If you are consulting on a patient at this point, certainly discuss any concerns regarding slow resolution of symptoms as well as contrary information they have gleaned from friends and media, but it is often reassuring to emphasize that the odds of a good outcome are overwhelmingly in their favor.

VALIDATION

Patients sometimes feel unheard or even dismissed by providers when they discuss feeling persistently unwell after treatment of Lyme disease. It is well established that a small but significant minority of patients with Lyme disease experience prolonged nonspecific symptoms such as fatigue, cognitive symptoms, or joint pains despite adequate treatment[15]. They are not making their symptoms up, and this consultation is an opportunity to impress on them that you are aware of this possible outcome and tell them that they are not alone. In a study following patients with erythema migrans,[16] 53%, 80%, and 92% were asymptomatic at 7 to 10 days, 21 to 28 days, and 6 months after initiation of antibiotics, respectively.

Some patients have categorized providers into those who do not believe them and will not give them antibiotics versus those who do believe them and will give them antibiotics; this creates a false dichotomy. Validation of symptoms does not, of course, indicate similar assessment of their likely cause or dictate particular medical interventions. It is important to convey that although you empathize with their experience of illness, your professional role necessitates judicious advice to guide patients away from unproven and harmful interventions, particularly as resolution of these symptoms with time is common. Although the causes of posttreatment Lyme disease have

Table 1			
Studies with patients with early Lyme disease treated with shorter courses of antibiotic therapy			
Study	**Population**	**Treatment**	**Outcome**
Luger et al,[10] 1995	232 patients with erythema migrans. Prospective.	2 groups: • 20 d cefuroxime • 20 d doxycycline	Success or improvement 1 mo posttreatment. • Doxycycline 95% • Cefuroxime 90%
Wormser et al,[11] 2003	180 patients with erythema migrans. Prospective.	3 groups: • 10 d doxycycline • Single-dose ceftriaxone + 10 d doxycycline • 20 d doxycycline	Complete response rate at 30 mo. Similar in all 3 groups 84%–90%. Highest in 10-d doxy group. A single treatment failure.
Kowalski et al,[12] 2010	607 patients with early localized or disseminated Lyme. Retrospective.	93% treated with doxycycline, 3% amoxicillin, 4% other. Grouped by antibiotic duration • </ = 10 d • 10–15 d • >16 d	Treatment failure free at 2 y. No significant difference in outcome, all ~99%.

eluded current science, there is substantial evidence that additional antibiotics cause more harm than benefit.

MISDIAGNOSIS AND MISATTRIBUTION

Although some patients manifest a clear temporal correlation between a convincingly diagnosed episode of Lyme disease and the onset of symptoms such as fatigue, joint pain, difficulties with concentration , and their concerns regarding long term effects of Lyme disease should be validated, these symptoms are quite common in the general population. In a recent prospective study that followed-up patients with erythema migrans and matched controls for 12 months and surveyed them for nonspecific symptoms often associated with PTLDS, no difference was found between patients and controls at 6 and 12 months.[17] In another study, however, 14% patients experienced PTLDS and only 4% of controls did.[18] Whatever the rate of PTLDS might be, misattribution of ongoing symptoms to Lyme disease is a factor in some patients, particularly when onset of infection was not recent.

Misdiagnosis of Lyme disease is not uncommon, particularly in patients experiencing long-term symptoms without response to treatment.[19,20] In some instances, the misdiagnosis is supported by use of unvetted or misleading diagnostic tests. Incorrect attribution of nonspecific symptoms to presumed Lyme disease is common, often in the absence of a compelling clinical history of Lyme disease or supportive serologic studies. The danger here is 2-fold: adverse effects of unwarranted antibiotic therapy and delaying the correct diagnosis that may be treatable.

One recent investigation of more than a thousand patients referred to an academic center for infectious disease consultation regarding Lyme disease found that an overwhelming majority had neither evidence of current Lyme disease nor a convincing history of prior *B burgdorferi* infection.[18] In another recent study of 301 patients with symptoms lasting more than 4 weeks evaluated for presumed Lyme disease by infectious disease consultants, less than 15% had confirmed or possible Lyme disease and most of the patients were diagnosed with other treatable disorders spanning a spectrum from depression to sleep apnea to multiple sclerosis.[21] Delayed diagnoses of cancer have also been reported.[22] Infectious disease consultants may uncover missed cases of other infections (ie, bacterial endocarditis, human immunodeficiency virus [HIV] disease and its opportunistic infections, mycobacterial infections) in patients treated for weeks to months for putative Lyme disease (personal experience). In addition, a careful evaluation of symptoms in patients on polypharmacy regimens for presumed Lyme disease may lead to prevention of progressive harm due to injudicious medication prescriptions.[23]

Providing a thorough evaluation for alternative etiologies, including other tick-borne diseases or infections, in patients with a dubious Lyme diagnosis is one of the most important roles that infectious disease providers can play.

EXPECTATIONS

"Polly Murray writes in The Widening Circle that she'd always revered the power of medicine; to come up against its limits was devastating. Acknowledging these limits is difficult—for doctors, for patients, for everybody. We've invested near-spiritual fervor in the medical realm: It holds our births and our deaths; it sees inside us and tell us what's wrong."[24]

When a patient presents to you feeling poorly, take a step back and think of what their expectations might be from both modern medicine and in terms of infections specifically.

We are presented with medical miracles on a regular basis. Myoelectric upper extremity prostheses to rival Luke Skywalker's have been available since the 1980s, and we have even transplanted cadaveric hands.[25] We have taken HIV from a death sentence to a relatively easily managed chronic disease.[26] Medicine is capable of amazing feats, but what is less obvious is how we often struggle with seemingly simple problems such as pain, persisting fatigue, and nausea.

Patients generally have different baseline expectations when it comes to infections than with a diagnosis of diabetes, systemic lupus erythematosus, or even a traumatic injury. If someone suffered multiple fractures in a car accident, they probably would not be shocked if they were unable to return to marathon running 6 months later. Infections are viewed as brief, and a return to baseline functional status is expected following the acute illness: a patient might typically think of something common such as an uncomplicated bacterial sinusitis. This brevity is unfortunately not true of all infections and by no means limited to Lyme disease. A person with *Staphylococcus aureus* vertebral osteomyelitis and epidural abscess might suffer from chronic back pain due to bone destruction or from chronic neurologic symptoms due to cord compromise despite bacterial eradication.[27] Fatigue often persists for months following Epstein-Barr virus mononucleosis,[28] and we are slowly familiarizing ourselves with post-COVID conditions.

Recognize these apparent inconsistencies and acknowledge to your patients that sometimes our relative lack of capabilities is counterintuitive. Doctors are frustrated too. We want our patients to regain their health as rapidly as possible.

Patients may react differently to being told no further antibiotic therapy is indicated. Some might be relieved because the antibiotics themselves have been making them feel unwell. Others will be less enthused, especially if they came into the visit expecting otherwise.

CONSENSUS

It can be helpful to discuss the strengths—and limitations—of clinical evidence-based consensus. Exploring the far reaches of the Internet with no guidance, one might come away with the impression that there is an ongoing debate about a multitude of topics ranging from whether humans contribute to global warming (they do[29]) to whether there is a link between childhood vaccines and autism (there is not[30]). That is what the weight of the current scientific evidence suggests; the rest consists of unsubstantiated or refuted hypotheses. If your patient has been vaccinated against COVID-19, there is a good chance they have an appreciation for scientific consensus in the face of a vocal fringe. Build on that.

Treatment of Lyme disease is discussed in detail elsewhere. There is a strong evidence basis for the recommended treatment of Lyme disease, specifically regarding the selection and duration of antibiotic therapy; this includes more than 12 randomized controlled trials of antibiotic treatment of early Lyme disease in North America and Europe. To address the question of persistent symptoms such as fatigue and arthralgias following recommended treatment, 4 randomized, placebo-controlled trials found no sustained benefit from long-term antibiotics (see The Fringe and **Table 2**).

Of course, experienced physicians are appropriately skeptical of the application of consensus guidance to every individual clinical scenario. Astute clinicians appreciate

Table 2
Four randomized, placebo-controlled trials on the benefits of long-term antibiotics

Study	Patients	Treatment	Outcome
Klempner et al,[48] 2001	129 patients previously treated for acute Lyme with persistent complaints (fatigue, body aches) for at least 6 mo	2 groups: • IV ceftriaxone x30 d then doxycycline x60 d • IV placebo x30 d then PO placebo x60 d	Health-Related Quality of Life SF36 at 180 d. No significant difference found between the 2 groups.
Krupp et al,[49] 2003	55 patients with history of Lyme disease and persistent fatigue at least 6 mo after antibiotic therapy	2 groups: • 28 d IV ceftriaxone • 28 d placebo	3 outcomes at 6 mo. • Reported fatigue. Improvement in antibiotic group although mean score still met study criteria for severe fatigue. • Measured cognitive processing speed. No significant difference. • Clearance of CSF antigen. No significant difference.
Fallon et al,[50] 2008	37 patients with history of treated Lyme disease and memory impairment.	2 groups: • 10 wk IV ceftriaxone • 10 wk IV placebo	Neuropsychological testing at 12 wk and 24 wk. Initial improvement in antibiotic group not sustained at 24 wk.
Berende et al,[43] 2016	280 patients with persistent symptoms attributed to Lyme	3 groups: • 14 d IV ceftriaxone followed by 12 wk doxycycline • 14 d IV ceftriaxone followed by 12 wk clarithromycin + hydroxychloroquine • 14 d IV ceftriaxone followed by 12 wk placebo	Health-Related Quality of Life SF-36. No significant difference between groups.

Abbreviations: CSF, cerebrospinal fluid; IV, intravenous.

that there are often shades of gray and unsettled questions in clinical medicine and are averse to pigeonholing their patient into arbitrary categories. Infectious disease physicians are well aware of the pitfalls of practicing "cookbook medicine" based on what has been characterized as "'because we said so" level of evidence from experts.[31] No clinical trial is perfect, and no clinical trial group can be extrapolated to every individual patient. Patients referred for an infectious disease consultation have sometimes seen multiple specialists, received multiple courses of antibiotics, and yet remain ill. There is a need for an "interpersonal medicine" approach in all chronically ill patients,[32] which may most naturally reside under the direction of the person's primary care provider, but may also involve a multidisciplinary team devoted to increasing well-being and improving function. With all that said, in the case of long-term antibiotics for Lyme disease, there is simply no clinical evidence of comparable quality to the 4 randomized controlled trials (see **Table 2**) to suggest sustained benefit from this practice, and the harm that is caused by this practice is repeatedly under-scored in these and other studies.[33,34]

The latest 2020 US guidelines for treatment of Lyme disease are endorsed by the Infectious Disease Society of America (IDSA), the American Academy of Neurology, and the American College of Rheumatology.[35] Multiple North American and European scientific bodies have reviewed the evidence and come to similar conclusions.[36–40] International recommendations on diagnostic strategies are similarly homogeneous.[41]

Acknowledging that science can be fluid and that past accepted medical practices have been retrospectively found to be harmful, barring compelling clinical evidence contrary to that compiled over the past several decades, this particular consensus is unlikely to change in the near future. Compared with the previous 2006 IDSA guidelines,[42] the trend based on ongoing review of the evidence is toward even shorter antibiotic courses and fewer indications for intravenous therapy. To date there has been no credible evidence to bring current practice into question. That does not diminish any individual patient's experience or suffering or completely dismiss the possibility that we might learn something revolutionary in the future, but the current body of evidence provides no justification for prescribing protracted courses of antibiotics. It is hoped, and indeed likely, that ongoing research into PTLDS and other postinfective syndromes will lead to novel avenues for more effective treatment.

DIAGNOSTIC UNCERTAINTY AND MANAGEMENT

Given diagnostic limitations discussed previously, at times you will be unable to confidently tell a patient whether or not their recent clinical syndrome was due to Lyme disease. Diagnostic uncertainty is often inadequately acknowledged in all medical practice and, given the vagaries of diagnostic testing, is a reality in some cases of putative Lyme disease.[43,44] Acknowledgment of areas of diagnostic uncertainty is a necessary aspect of physician-patient communication. Infectious disease physicians are experienced in weighing probabilities when a diagnosis is not certain, but patients often expect an absolute answer. The infectious disease consultant can provide a "diagnostic safety net" in the setting of uncertainty. The consultation for unresolved symptoms due to presumed Lyme disease is an opportunity to step back and consider the possibility of missed infectious disease diagnoses, including of course those that might be transmitted by the patient's regional tick exposures.[17] In almost all consultations your patient will already have received an appropriate antibiotic course for Lyme disease, so at the very least, it is also an opportunity to provide reassurance on adequate treatment while opening up consideration of others causes.

HOPE

Persistent fatigue and other nonspecific symptoms following *B burgdorferi* infection tend to improve with time. In the largest randomized, placebo-controlled clinical trial[45] of antibiotic treatment of these long-term symptoms, health-related quality-of-life scores in the placebo group improved over the study period, and there was no significant difference in scores between the placebo and treatment groups. Given what your patient may have gleaned from highly atypical or misleading anecdotal patient testimonials and media narratives—that persistent and even progressive decline is to be expected barring ongoing aggressive interventions—this may surprise them. If you have developed a degree of rapport during the consultation, there may be an opportunity here to reset expectations in the direction of recovery.

THE FRINGE

Although it is important for patients to understand that your counsel is in keeping with the evidence-based consensus, it is worthwhile to acknowledge alternative opinions they might find (or have already found) by word of mouth or on the Internet.

The spectrum of alternative therapies offered to patients with symptoms attributed to Lyme is vast and includes nutritional supplements, metal/chelation therapy, ultraviolet light, hyperbaric oxygen, urotherapy, enemas, and even stem cell transplantation.[46] There is no evidence to support these interventions, which are often costly and sometimes dangerous.

Overwhelmingly however, nonevidence-based management is manifested in prolonged courses of antibiotics.[47] Four significant randomized, placebo-controlled human clinical trials (**Table 2**) have shown no basis for this practice. Having a good command of the data and discussing it with patients can be helpful.

In the United States, the most prominent dissenting voice on Lyme management is the International Lyme and Associated Diseases Society who publish their own guidelines.[51] It is beyond the scope of this article to further critique their approach, but patients may choose to explore alternative medical approaches such as this. When a patient who strikes me as an independent learner brings up a website offering unorthodox strategies or an alternative provider, I suggest they perform a brief search on the following:

- What are the author's or provider's medical or scientific qualifications?
- If they have medical or scientific training, is it in a relevant area (eg, Infectious Disease, Neurology, Rheumatology)?
- Do they want you to pay for testing that is not covered by your insurance?

Are they selling you something? A book? An exclusive herbal remedy?

It is beneficial for patients if the consultant makes an effort to remain open to discussion of other sources of information and why they would or would not follow those recommendations. Remember, you are their expert ally.

CASE—"CHRONIC LYME DISEASE?"

A woman living in a Lyme-endemic area is referred to the infectious disease clinic by her primary care physician who is concerned about her chronic antibiotic use.

On review she has not traveled outside of New England and has no animal exposures, unusual hobbies, or dietary habits. She reported onset of postpartum fatigue several years before presentation and her fatigue has not relented since that time. She also experienced episodic arthralgias. These arthralgias are now constant, and although they go through periods of amelioration that can vary day to day, the pain never fully resolves. She had an episode of what was thought to be lower extremity cellulitis 2 years before presentation, which was treated with doxycycline. Throughout, she has had no fevers, no other neurologic findings, and her joints have not become swollen. She had extensive evaluation including neurology consultation and MRI of the brain and spine. She had normal complete blood count, comprehensive metabolic panel, C-reactive protein, and erythrocyte sedimentation rate.

Within this context, she was tested for Lyme disease at an academic medical center's laboratory before presentation, and this was negative. She then saw an

Integrative Medicine specialist who recommended she see a local solo private practitioner who purported to specialize in diagnosing and treating tick-borne illness. She was told she needed "advanced testing" for which she paid hundreds of dollars out of pocket. Her blood samples were sent to a private laboratory with self-proclaimed expertise in the diagnosis of Lyme disease. This testing was also negative. Nevertheless, she was started on doxycycline. She briefly followed with the initial prescriber, but that office closed. She found another "expert" via a family friend's recommendation. This person had an extensive website with protocols for long-term antibiotic use and elimination diets that he stated would treat the possibility of chronic Lyme disease and an array of proposed co-infections. At the time of infectious disease consultation, she has been on doxycycline for 2 years with the exception of summers when she switches to amoxicillin due to photosensitivity, and she stopped antibiotics briefly due to yeast infection. Repeated Lyme disease antibody testing was negative, but the patient was counseled by her Lyme specialist that her symptoms indicated ongoing Lyme disease and that testing was unreliable.

On specific questioning, by her own telling, none of the chronic, nonspecific symptoms she complained of for years have improved since starting antibiotic therapy, but she was fearful that her condition would worsen if she stopped.

CASE DISCUSSION

This narrative is a composite typical of cases I see in my clinic. Their ultimate outcomes are as varied as those in the studies and reports discussed previously (see Misdiagnosis) but rather than highlight memorable missed alternative diagnoses here we illustrate approaches to the initial encounter, which, while comparatively mundane, can be difficult to navigate.

We started by discussing her clinical symptoms and agreed that they could be caused by several medical disorders. We then moved on to what led to a presumed diagnosis of Lyme disease. We discussed her clinical presentation and that she did not have a history of typical signs and symptoms associated with early *B burgdorferi* infection. We did review the history of her "cellulitis" episode. We reviewed laboratory results, which were all negative, including recently repeated 2-tier testing for antibodies to *B burgdorferi* and testing for exposure to other tick-borne pathogens. I acknowledged that Lyme disease diagnostic testing is imperfect and that indeed a minority of patients with unquestioned Lyme diagnoses do develop long-term fatigue and joint pains as hers. We were left to reflect on the remote chance that she could have had atypical Lyme infection at onset and was in the small minority who developed persistent symptoms despite antibiotic treatment. I also emphasized the unlikelihood that, despite months of illness, her serologic testing would remain negative. I expressed that it is important to make sure an alternative, more likely, perhaps treatable diagnosis is not missed. She, similar to most patients, appreciated a thorough evaluation.

It is important to ascertain the patient's impression of the effect of antibiotic therapy as part of the discussion to minimize unnecessary antibiotic use and side effects thereof. This patient offered that the antibiotics made no difference in her symptoms. This is the middle ground and not uncommon. After all, if Lyme disease is an unlikely cause of the symptoms, then antibiotic therapy would not be expected to have an effect. In this context, the data on effectiveness of appropriate antibiotics in preventing recognized complications of untreated Lyme disease may reassure the patient that discontinuation of antibiotics is not only safe but preferable to taking medications with the potential for adverse effects.

In my experience, patients often report that antibiotics make them feel worse. This is unsurprising; infectious disease physicians are familiar with the side effects of antibiotics. Some patients are misled to believe that feeling worse on antibiotics is evidence of Lyme infection and that they are "herxing," a colloquialism based on the well-recognized but temporally limited Jarisch Herxheimer reaction. This reaction is a well-described phenomenon that may occur after initiation of syphilis treatment and has been reported with initiation of treatment in early Lyme disease. It is an acute febrile reaction in the first 24 to 48 hours of treatment that may be accompanied by flulike symptoms. It is self-limited, lasting hours or perhaps up to a couple of days. It is not tenable that persistent worsening or new symptoms on antibiotics are due to this reaction. In this situation I often review a pharmacy reference with the patient, listing the potential side effects of their therapy to see if they recognize any. Gastrointestinal side effects are well known; however, some side effects might be surprising. For instance, even doxycycline, although potentially antiinflammatory, has been associated with an increased rate of joint pain compared with placebo in treatment of other diseases.[52]

This patient and I discussed that, by her account, 2 years of antibiotic therapy had not made her better and that she had suffered some side effects (yeast infection, photosensitivity). I discussed with her other potential complications of antibiotic therapy such as *Clostridioides difficile* colitis. I told this patient that even if she had been infected with *B burgdorferi*, clinical trials and her own experience indicated that further antibiotic therapy was more likely to harm than benefit her. She was receptive to this. I encouraged her to explore other causes of her symptoms with her PCP. I offered her my email in case she wanted to run something she read on the Internet by me (remember, you hope to become an expert ally). If nothing else, it is important for patients to be exposed to the current mainstream scientific understanding of Lyme disease. Because of the availability of alternative providers, many are only aware of the fringe.

ROLE AS AN EDUCATOR

Because of the relative difficulty in diagnostic testing selection and interpretation as well as the challenge of dealing with patients who have been assaulted by misinformation, most medical providers welcome pragmatic teaching on Lyme disease management; this can be during the course of a routine consultation either verbally or in written form as part of your recommendations, a slightly more formal lunchtime lecture at your group practice's monthly meeting, or for a larger impact more innovative methods could be pursued.

One potential avenue is Project ECHO (Extension for Community Healthcare Outcomes), initially used for hepatitis C, which leverages video-conferencing to train and advise primary care providers regarding specialty treatment in rural and underserved areas. You can look for an ECHO hub or learn about starting your own ECHO program here: https://hsc.unm.edu/echo/embedded-content/locations-us.html.

FINAL THOUGHTS

Many pragmatic considerations may influence who you see in consultation. In an area with limited subspecialty care it is sometimes not feasible to see every consult that is requested. One may feel compelled to decline consultation on a patient who has already been treated appropriately for Lyme disease because you have no further treatment to offer and instead prioritize patients who may potentially benefit from antibiotics. With that said, patients are not best served if these consultations are systematically declined by infectious disease physicians.

Consultations regarding Lyme disease can be especially time consuming, and extensive counseling may be required. Depending on what the patient has read or been told before the visit, you may have an unsatisfying interaction. Poor outcomes despite application of our best efforts to treat infections are a reality of practice. We all accept that unfortunately not all infective endocarditis or prosthetic joint infections can be cured, but seeing a patient choose a path leading to adverse outcomes from misguided and dangerous polypharmacy,[21] avoidable intravenous line infections[32,53] or *C difficile colitis* can be particularly demoralizing. A failure rate does not make the work unworthy. Having done many of these consultations, I am not metaphorically batting a thousand or anywhere close but I have had very few interactions that became frankly disrespectful despite sometimes unbridgeable gaps in beliefs. If you are the archetypal infectious disease physician you will have more thoroughly reviewed the patient's history and spent more time with them than any other provider they have seen for this issue and that is lost on very few people. Many will thank you and heed your counsel.

As reports of the consequences of unsubstantiated Lyme therapies accumulate,[7,31,32] it would be unfortunate if for a disease with such a robust treatment consensus it becomes easier for patients to access alternative providers than to have a chance at receiving the current standard of care. The infectious disease physician can play an important role in rectifying this imbalance.

DISCLOSURES

None.

REFERENCES

1. Schattner A. The clinical encounter revisited. Am J Med 2014;127(4):268–74.
2. Burgdorfer W, Barbour AG, Hayes SF, et al. Lyme disease-a tick-borne spirochetosis? Science 1982;216(4552):1317–9.
3. Aronowitz RA. Lyme disease: the social construction of a new disease and its social consequences. Milbank Q 1991;69(1):79–112.
4. Macauda MM, Erickson P, Miller J, et al. Long-term Lyme disease antibiotic therapy beliefs among New England residents. Vector Borne Zoonotic Dis 2011; 11(7):857–62.
5. Moore A, Nelson C, Molins C, et al. Current Guidelines, Common Clinical Pitfalls, and Future Directions for Laboratory Diagnosis of Lyme Disease, United States. Emerg Infect Dis 2016;22(7):1169–77.
6. Seriburi V, Ndukwe N, Chang Z, et al. High frequency of false positive IgM immunoblots for Borrelia burgdorferi in clinical practice. Clin Microbiol Infect 2012; 18(12):1236–40.
7. Fallon BA, Pavlicova M, Coffino SW, et al. A comparison of lyme disease serologic test results from 4 laboratories in patients with persistent symptoms after antibiotic treatment. Clin Infect Dis 2014;59(12):1705–10. Feder HM et al. A critical appraisal of "chronic Lyme disease". NEJM 2007; 357: 1422- 1430.
8. Auwaerter PG, Bakken JS, Dattwyler RJ, et al. Antiscience and ethical concerns associated with advocacy of Lyme disease. Lancet Infect Dis 2011;11(9):713–9.
9. Lantos PM, Wormser GP. Chronic coinfections in patients diagnosed with chronic lyme disease: a systematic review. Am J Med 2014;127(11):1105–10.

10. Luger SW, Paparone P, Wormser GP, et al. Comparison of cefuroxime axetil and doxycycline in treatment of patients with early Lyme disease associated with erythema migrans. Antimicrob Agents Chemother 1995;39(3):661–7.

11. Wormser GP, Ramanathan R, Nowakowski J, et al. Duration of antibiotic therapy for early Lyme disease. A randomized, double-blind, placebo-controlled trial. Ann Intern Med 2003;138(9):697–704.

12. Kowalski TJ, Tata S, Berth W, et al. Antibiotic treatment duration and long-term outcomes of patients with early lyme disease from a lyme disease-hyperendemic area. Clin Infect Dis 2010;50(4):512–20.

13. Wormser GP, Weitzner E, McKenna D, et al. Long-term assessment of health-related quality of life in patients with culture-confirmed early Lyme disease. Clin Infect Dis 2015;61(2):244–7.

14. Wills AB, Spaulding AB, Adjemian J, et al. Long-term Follow-up of Patients With Lyme Disease: Longitudinal Analysis of Clinical and Quality-of-life Measures. Clin Infect Dis 2016;62(12):1546–51.

15. Rebman AW, Aucott JN. Post-treatment Lyme Disease as a Model for Persistent Symptoms in Lyme Disease. Front Med (Lausanne) 2020;7:57. https://doi.org/10.3389/fmed.2020.00057.

16. Nowakowski J, Nadelman RB, Sell R, et al. Long-term follow-up of patients with culture-confirmed Lyme disease. Am J Med 2003;115(2):91–6.

17. Wormser GP, McKenna D, Karmen CL, et al. Prospective Evaluation of the Frequency and Severity of Symptoms in Lyme Disease Patients With Erythema Migrans Compared With Matched Controls at Baseline, 6 Months, and 12 Months. Clin Infect Dis 2020;71(12):3118–24.

18. Aucott JN, Yang T, Yoon I, et al. Risk of post-treatment Lyme disease in patients with ideally-treated early Lyme disease: A prospective cohort study. Int J Infect Dis 2022;116:230–7.

19. Kortela E, Kanerva M, Kurkela S, et al. Suspicion of Lyme borreliosis in patients referred to an infectious diseases clinic: what did the patients really have? Clin Microbiol Infect 2021;27(7):1022–8.

20. Kobayashi T, Higgins Y, Samuels R, et al. Misdiagnosis of Lyme Disease With Unnecessary Antimicrobial Treatment Characterizes Patients Referred to an Academic Infectious Diseases Clinic. Open Forum Infect Dis 2019;6(7):ofz299.

21. Haddad E, Chabane K, Jaureguiberry S, et al. Holistic Approach in Patients With Presumed Lyme Borreliosis Leads to Less Than 10% of Confirmation and More Than 80% of Antibiotic Failures. Clin Infect Dis 2019;68(12):2060–6.

22. Nelson C, Elmendorf S, Mead P. Neoplasms misdiagnosed as "chronic lyme disease. JAMA Intern Med 2015;175(1):132–3.

23. Frankl S, Hadar PN, Yakhkind A, et al. Devastating Neurological Injury as a Result of Treatment of "Chronic Lyme Disease. Mayo Clin Proc 2021;96(7):2005–7.

24. Fischer M. Maybe It's Lyme. The Cut. 2019. Available at: https://www.thecut.com/2019/07/what-happens-when-lyme-disease-becomes-an-identity.html.

25. Zuo KJ, Olson JL. The evolution of functional hand replacement: From iron prostheses to hand transplantation. Plast Surg (Oakv) 2014;22(1):44–51.

26. Deeks SG, Lewin SR, Havlir DV. The end of AIDS: HIV infection as a chronic disease. Lancet 2013;382(9903):1525–33.

27. McHenry MC, Easley KA, Locker GA. Vertebral osteomyelitis: long-term outcome for 253 patients from 7 Cleveland-area hospitals. Clin Infect Dis 2002;34(10):1342–50.

28. Buchwald DS, Rea TD, Katon WJ, et al. Acute infectious mononucleosis: characteristics of patients who report failure to recover. Am J Med 2000;109(7):531–7.

29. Fahey DW, Doherty SJ, Hibbard KA, et al. Physical drivers of climate change. In: Wuebbles DJ, Fahey DW, Hibbard KA, et al, editors. Climate science special report: Fourth National Climate assessment, volume I. Washington, DC, USA: U.S. Global Change Research Program; 2017. p. 73–113.

30. Institute of Medicine. Adverse effects of vaccines: evidence and Causality. Washington, DC: The National Academies Press; 2012. https://doi.org/10.17226/13164.

31. Spellberg B, Shorr AF. Opinion-Based Recommendations: Beware the Tyranny of Experts. Open Forum Infect Dis 2021;8(11):ofab490.

32. Chang S, Lee TH. Beyond Evidence-Based Medicine. N Engl J Med 2018; 379(21):1983–5.

33. Marzec NS, Nelson C, Waldron PR, et al. Serious Bacterial Infections Acquired During Treatment of Patients Given a Diagnosis of Chronic Lyme Disease - United States. MMWR Morb Mortal Wkly Rep 2017;66(23):607–9.

34. Goodlet KJ, et al. Adverse events associated with antibiotics and intravenous therapies for post-Lyme disease syndrome in a commercially insured sample. CID 2018;67:1568.

35. Lantos PM, Rumbaugh J, Bockenstedt LK, et al. Clinical Practice Guidelines by the Infectious Diseases Society of America (IDSA), American Academy of Neurology (AAN), and American College of Rheumatology (ACR): 2020 Guidelines for the Prevention, Diagnosis and Treatment of Lyme Disease. Clin Infect Dis 2021;72(1):1–8.

36. Overview | Lyme disease | Guidance | NICE. The National Institute for Health and Care Excellence; 2018. Available at: https://www.nice.org.uk/guidance/ng95/.

37. Public Health Agency of Canada. For health professionals: Lyme disease - Canada.ca. 2021. Available at: https://Www.Canada.ca/En/Services/Health.Html; https://Www.Canada.ca/En/Services/Health.Html https://www.canada.ca/en/public-health/services/diseases/lyme-disease/health-professionals-lyme-disease.html.

38. Gocko X, Lenormand C, Lemogne C, et al. endorsed by the following scientific societies. Lyme borreliosis and other tick-borne diseases. Guidelines from the French scientific societies. Med Mal Infect 2019;49(5):296–317. Erratum in: Med Mal Infect. 2019 Oct;49(7):558-559. PMID: 31257066.

39. Hofmann H, Fingerle V, Hunfeld KP, et al, Consensus group. Cutaneous Lyme borreliosis: Guideline of the German Dermatology Society. Ger Med Sci 2017; 15:Doc14.

40. Rauer S, Kastenbauer S, Hofmann H, et al, Consensus group. Guidelines for diagnosis and treatment in neurology - Lyme neuroborreliosis. Ger Med Sci 2020;18:Doc03.

41. Eldin C, Raffetin A, Bouiller K, et al. Review of European and American guidelines for the diagnosis of Lyme borreliosis. Med Mal Infect 2019;49(2):121–32.

42. Wormser GP, Dattwyler RJ, Shapiro ED, et al. The clinical assessment, treatment, and prevention of lyme disease, human granulocytic anaplasmosis, and babesiosis: clinical practice guidelines by the Infectious Diseases Society of America. Clin Infect Dis 2006;43(9):1089–134.

43. Han PKJ, Strout TD, Gutheil C, et al. How Physicians Manage Medical Uncertainty: A Qualitative Study and Conceptual Taxonomy. Med Decis Making 2021; 41(3):275–91.

44. Meyer AND, Giardina TD, Khawaja L, et al. Patient and clinician experiences of uncertainty in the diagnostic process: Current understanding and future directions. Patient Educ Couns 2021;104(11):2606–15.

45. Berende A, ter Hofstede HJ, Vos FJ, et al. Randomized Trial of Longer-Term Therapy for Symptoms Attributed to Lyme Disease. N Engl J Med 2016;374(13): 1209–20.

46. Lantos PM, Shapiro ED, Auwaerter PG, et al. Unorthodox alternative therapies marketed to treat Lyme disease. Clin Infect Dis 2015;60(12):1776–82.

47. Tseng YJ, Cami A, Goldmann DA, et al. Incidence and Patterns of Extended-Course Antibiotic Therapy in Patients Evaluated for Lyme Disease. Clin Infect Dis 2015;61(10):1536–42.

48. Klempner MS, Hu LT, Evans J, et al. Two controlled trials of antibiotic treatment in patients with persistent symptoms and a history of Lyme disease. N Engl J Med 2001;345(2):85–92.

49. Krupp LB, Hyman LG, Grimson R, et al. Study and treatment of post Lyme disease (STOP-LD): a randomized double masked clinical trial. Neurology 2003; 60(12):1923–30.

50. Fallon BA, Keilp JG, Corbera KM, et al. A randomized, placebo-controlled trial of repeated IV antibiotic therapy for Lyme encephalopathy. Neurology 2008;70(13): 992–1003.

51. Cameron DJ, Johnson LB, Maloney EL. Evidence assessments and guideline recommendations in Lyme disease: the clinical management of known tick bites, erythema migrans rashes and persistent disease. Expert Rev Anti Infect Ther 2014;12(9):1103–35.

52. Periostat (doxycycline hyclate) [package insert]. Newton, PA: Collagenex Pharmaceuticals; 2001.

53. Shelton A, Giurgea L, Moshgriz M, et al. A case of Mycobacterium goodii infection related to an indwelling catheter placed for the treatment of chronic symptoms attributed to Lyme disease. Infect Dis Rep 2019;11(2):8108.

Printed and bound by CPI Group (UK) Ltd, Croydon, CR0 4YY

08/05/2025

01864722-0001